Clinical Outcomes Improvement and Perioperative Management of Surgical Patients

Clinical Outcomes Improvement and Perioperative Management of Surgical Patients

Editors

Dimitrios E. Magouliotis
Dimitris Zacharoulis

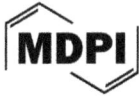

Basel • Beijing • Wuhan • Barcelona • Belgrade • Novi Sad • Cluj • Manchester

Editors

Dimitrios E. Magouliotis
Department of
Cardiothoracic Surgery
University of Thessaly
Larissa
Greece

Dimitris Zacharoulis
Department of Surgery
University of Thessaly
Larissa
Greece

Editorial Office
MDPI
St. Alban-Anlage 66
4052 Basel, Switzerland

This is a reprint of articles from the Special Issue published online in the open access journal *Journal of Clinical Medicine* (ISSN 2077-0383) (available at: https://www.mdpi.com/journal/jcm/special_issues/0IO98MY01D).

For citation purposes, cite each article independently as indicated on the article page online and as indicated below:

Lastname, A.A.; Lastname, B.B. Article Title. *Journal Name* **Year**, *Volume Number*, Page Range.

ISBN 978-3-7258-0471-9 (Hbk)
ISBN 978-3-7258-0472-6 (PDF)
doi.org/10.3390/books978-3-7258-0472-6

© 2024 by the authors. Articles in this book are Open Access and distributed under the Creative Commons Attribution (CC BY) license. The book as a whole is distributed by MDPI under the terms and conditions of the Creative Commons Attribution-NonCommercial-NoDerivs (CC BY-NC-ND) license.

Contents

About the Editors vii

Preface ix

Dimitrios E. Magouliotis, Thanos Athanasiou and Dimitrios Zacharoulis
Surgery and Reason: The End of History and the Last Surgeon
Reprinted from: *J. Clin. Med.* **2023**, *12*, 5708, doi:10.3390/jcm12175708 1

**Harm H. J. van Noort, Femke L. Becking-Verhaar, Wilmieke Bahlman-van Ooijen,
Maarten Pel, Harry van Goor and Getty Huisman-de Waal**
Three Years of Continuous Vital Signs Monitoring on the General Surgical Ward: Is It
Sustainable? A Qualitative Study
Reprinted from: *J. Clin. Med.* **2024**, *13*, 439, doi:10.3390/jcm13020439 5

**Jae-Hwan Kim, Kyoung-Sun Kim, Hye-Mee Kwon, Sung-Hoon Kim, In-Gu Jun,
Jun-Gol Song and Gyu-Sam Hwang**
Comparison of Fibrinogen Concentrate and Cryoprecipitate on Major Thromboembolic Events
after Living Donor Liver Transplantation
Reprinted from: *J. Clin. Med.* **2023**, *12*, 7496, doi:10.3390/jcm12237496 17

**Anna Caterina Milanetto, Claudia Armellin, Gloria Brigiari, Giulia Lorenzoni and
Claudio Pasquali**
Younger Age and Parenchyma-Sparing Surgery Positively Affected Long-Term Health-Related
Quality of Life after Surgery for Pancreatic Neuroendocrine Neoplasms
Reprinted from: *J. Clin. Med.* **2023**, *12*, 6529, doi:10.3390/jcm12206529 27

**Marica Giardini, Marco Guenzi, Ilaria Arcolin, Marco Godi, Massimo Pistono and
Marco Caligari**
Comparison of Two Techniques Performing the Supine-to-Sitting Postural Change in Patients
with Sternotomy
Reprinted from: *J. Clin. Med.* **2023**, *12*, 4665, doi:10.3390/jcm12144665 39

**Radu Petru Soroceanu, Daniel Vasile Timofte, Radu Danila, Sergiu Timofeiov,
Roxana Livadariu, Ancuta Andreea Miler, et al.**
The Impact of Bariatric Surgery on Quality of Life in Patients with Obesity
Reprinted from: *J. Clin. Med.* **2023**, *12*, 4225, doi:10.3390/jcm12134225 50

**Andrew Xanthopoulos, Angeliki Bourazana, Yuya Matsue, Yudai Fujimoto, Shogo Oishi,
Eiichi Akiyama, et al.**
Larissa Heart Failure Risk Score and Mode of Death in Acute Heart Failure: Insights from
REALITY-AHF
Reprinted from: *J. Clin. Med.* **2023**, *12*, 3722, doi:10.3390/jcm12113722 62

**Anna P. Karamolegkou, Maria P. Fergadi, Dimitrios E. Magouliotis, Athina A. Samara,
Evangelos Tatsios, Andrew Xanthopoulos, et al.**
Validation of the Surgical Outcome Risk Tool (SORT) and SORT v2 for Predicting Postoperative
Mortality in Patients with Pancreatic Cancer Undergoing Surgery
Reprinted from: *J. Clin. Med.* **2023**, *12*, 2327, doi:10.3390/jcm12062327 72

**Philip Deslarzes, Jonas Jurt, David W. Larson, Catherine Blanc, Martin Hübner and
Fabian Grass**
Perioperative Fluid Management in Colorectal Surgery: Institutional Approach to Standardized
Practice
Reprinted from: *J. Clin. Med.* **2024**, *13*, 801, doi:10.3390/jcm13030801 84

Nikolaos Manetas-Stavrakakis, Ioanna Myrto Sotiropoulou, Themistoklis Paraskevas, Stefania Maneta Stavrakaki, Dimitrios Bampatsias, Andrew Xanthopoulos, et al.
Accuracy of Artificial Intelligence-Based Technologies for the Diagnosis of Atrial Fibrillation: A Systematic Review and Meta-Analysis
Reprinted from: *J. Clin. Med.* **2023**, *12*, 6576, doi:10.3390/jcm12206576 . . . . **95**

Angelos Frisiras, Emmanuel Giannas, Stergios Bobotis, Ilektra Kanella, Arian Arjomandi Rad, Alessandro Viviano, et al.
Comparative Analysis of Morbidity and Mortality Outcomes in Elderly and Nonelderly Patients Undergoing Elective TEVAR: A Systematic Review and Meta-Analysis
Reprinted from: *J. Clin. Med.* **2023**, *12*, 5001, doi:10.3390/jcm12155001 . . . . **119**

Sascha Vaghiri, Dimitrios Prassas, Sarah Krieg, Wolfram Trudo Knoefel and Andreas Krieg
The Postoperative Effect of Sugammadex versus Acetylcholinesterase Inhibitors in Colorectal Surgery: An Updated Meta-Analysis
Reprinted from: *J. Clin. Med.* **2023**, *12*, 3235, doi:10.3390/jcm12093235 . . . . **137**

Dörte Wichmann, Olena Orlova, Alfred Königsrainer and Markus Quante
Is There a High Risk for GI Bleeding Complications in Patients Undergoing Abdominal Surgery?
Reprinted from: *J. Clin. Med.* **2023**, *12*, 1374, doi:10.3390/jcm12041374 . . . . **151**

About the Editors

Dimitrios E. Magouliotis

Dr. Dimitrios Magouliotis is a resident and post-doc researcher at the Department of Cardiothoracic Surgery, University of Thessaly. He has studied medicine at the University of Thessaly, and has completed two MSc degrees, one at the University of Thessaly and one at University College London. Dr. Magouliotis has also completed a PhD degree at the University of Thessaly. In addition, he has been an EACTS/FFF Fellow at the University of Michigan and MSTCVS Quality Collaborative. His research interests include cardiothoracic surgery, quality improvement, risk stratification tools, and surgical oncology.

Dimitris Zacharoulis

Dimitrios Zacharoulis is a Professor of Surgery and Chair at the Department of Surgery, University of Thessaly. Prof. Zacharoulis is a Fellow of the Royal College of Surgeons and the American College of Surgeons. His research interests include pancreatic surgery, liver surgery, surgical oncology, quality improvement, and translational research.

Preface

In recent years, the science of clinical outcome analysis, quality improvement initiatives, the perioperative management of surgical patients, and patient safety have continued to evolve at an increasingly rapid pace. In this context, over the years, novel concepts have arisen (risk stratification, shared decision-making—SDM, phase of care mortality analysis—POCMA, interdisciplinary meetings, prehabilitation, etc.), new initiatives have taken shape (e.g., state/nation-wide or international clinical databases), and new technologies and methods have been implemented across all surgical specialties (e.g., minimally invasive or robotic approaches). In order to care for our patients, raise the standards of healthcare services, and be successful in today's and tomorrow's rapidly changing healthcare environment, understanding and evolving these topics represents an essential duty of all surgeons, physicians, and professionals in relation to the care of surgical patients.

The present Special Issue covers a wide spectrum of topics on the perioperative management of surgical patients. We hope that you will enjoy reading the included articles while receiving the best currently available evidence on several aspects and core concepts of perioperative quality improvement. Finally, we would like to thank MDPI and Mrs. Monya Li for providing us with the opportunity to produce this Special Issue and for the support we received during the entire process.

Dimitrios E. Magouliotis and Dimitris Zacharoulis
Editors

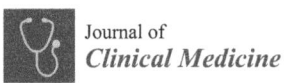

Editorial

Surgery and Reason: The End of History and the Last Surgeon

Dimitrios E. Magouliotis [1,*], Thanos Athanasiou [2] and Dimitrios Zacharoulis [3]

1. Unit of Quality Improvement, Department of Cardiothoracic Surgery, University of Thessaly, Biopolis, 41110 Larissa, Greece
2. Department of Surgery and Cancer, Imperial College London, St Mary's Hospital, London W2 1NY, UK; t.athanasiou@imperial.ac.uk
3. Department of Surgery, University of Thessaly, Biopolis, 41110 Larissa, Greece; zacharoulis@uth.gr
* Correspondence: dimitrios.magouliotis.18@ucl.ac.uk

Arguably, Georg Wilhelm Friedrich Hegel has been one of the most influential philosophers of the 19th century. In his Lectures on the Philosophy of World History [1], given at the University of Berlin between 1822 and 1830, he described world history not just as a sequence of random events but as rational progress toward a specific purpose. This purpose was identified as reaching the ultimate level of knowledge and freedom. In fact, in the introduction to these lectures, Hegel declared that there is reason in history and, vice versa, that world history is the progress of reason. However, reason also represents the moving force behind every progress and advance in the fields of medicine and surgery. Dating back to Hippocrates and the well-known phrase "Primum non nocere" or "First do no harm" reason in medicine and surgery mandates us not only to provide our best services to patients but, primarily, to provide them in a safe manner by creating and establishing a culture of safety. In other words, the reason that surgery passes through quality improvement (QI) in science.

QI and patient safety (PS) have become increasingly important in all surgical disciplines over the last two decades [2,3]. QI represents a continuous process whereby tools or methods are employed to promote measurable changes within a system which, in this case, is surgery [2,3]. QI interventions are at the core of this process, which is not a straight line but follows a spiral path of concentric circles dictated by reason (Figure 1). When a QI intervention is initiated, an established dogma is challenged. Through this clash of different theories, the practices associated with the best evidence-based outcomes prevail. A circle closes, and a new one opens with new clinical questions under examination. This process represents an analog to the progress of history proposed by Hegel, and we could admit that this is a process dictated by reason in surgery (Figure 1).

Given the pivotal role of reason in surgery and QI, we should further stress this point. One of the primary vehicles of advancement in QI science is the Plan-Do-Study-Act (PDSA) scheme [4]. Passing through each one of the four steps of the PDSA cycle leads to the establishment of a new clinical practice pattern. The PDSA cycle represents the assessment of a clinical practice that is opposed or subsidiary to the previously established model. The outcomes of these two alternative practices are compared, and through this clash of ideas and theories, only the system providing the best outcomes for patients prevails. Probably a great example of this clash of ideas has been the use of multiple arterial grafts (MAG) instead of single arterial grafting (SAG) in coronary artery bypass grafting (CABG). Over the past few years, there has been growing evidence favoring the utilization of multiple arterial conduits in appropriate patients undergoing CABG [5–7]. However, the adoption of multiple arterial conduits utilization has been relatively slow [8]. In this context, QI interventions were designed and implemented by courageous surgical societies, such as the Michigan Society of Thoracic and Cardiovascular Surgeons Quality Collaborative (MSTCVS-QC) [9]. These initiatives paved the way for a significant increase in MAG adoption [10], thus enhancing outcomes and providing more data on long-term outcomes.

Citation: Magouliotis, D.E.; Athanasiou, T.; Zacharoulis, D. Surgery and Reason: The End of History and the Last Surgeon. *J. Clin. Med.* **2023**, *12*, 5708. https://doi.org/10.3390/jcm12175708

Received: 8 August 2023
Accepted: 13 August 2023
Published: 1 September 2023

Copyright: © 2023 by the authors. Licensee MDPI, Basel, Switzerland. This article is an open access article distributed under the terms and conditions of the Creative Commons Attribution (CC BY) license (https://creativecommons.org/licenses/by/4.0/).

Based on increasing evidence favoring the use of multiple arterial conduits in patients undergoing CABG [11], a "Hegelian" circle, based on the superiority of the MAG approach, is about to close, and a new one is about to open, which will examine different strategies in conduits harvesting, treatment protocols on the extent of target vessel stenosis for radial artery conduits, along with post-discharge treatment protocols.

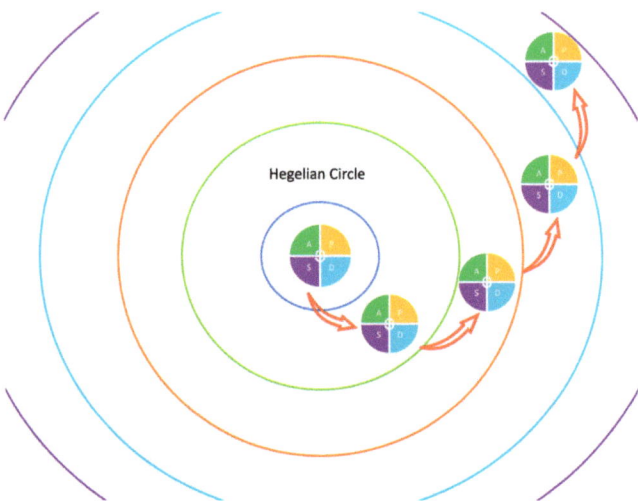

Figure 1. Representation of the merge between the Hegelian concentric circles of reason in history and the Plan-Do-Study-Act (PDSA) cycles of Quality Improvement in Surgery. This merge demonstrates the historical progress of reason in surgery.

The present Special Issue includes several articles that aim to answer important debates on different perioperative treatment pathways [12–18]. Two of them [14,15] validate risk-stratification tools, thus providing a necessary insight into preoperative planning and patient counseling while enhancing the shared decision-making process. In addition, Giardini et al. [12] compare two techniques in performing the supine-to-sitting postural change in patients with sternotomy, while Frisiras et al. [16] compare morbidity and mortality outcomes in elderly and nonelderly patients undergoing elective thoracic endovascular aortic repair (TEVAR). Such articles provide evidence that can enable the design and progression of different PDSA cycles, thus serving the unfolding of reason in surgical history.

Another core concept of the Hegelian dialectic is the provision of "world-historical individuals", the so-called "great men" of history, such as Socrates or Julius Caesar. In this context, world-historical individuals are able to influence, guide the tides of history and drive it forward through their actions and initiatives, thus leading to higher levels of knowledge and freedom. In surgery, there are many examples of world-historical individuals. Dr. Denton Cooley and Dr. Michael DeBakey in cardiac surgery, along with Dr. David Sugarbaker in thoracic surgery (mesothelioma surgery), perhaps represent such figures. These great surgeons have opened new paths in surgery through their actions and initiatives. In the QI context, the existence of such world-historical individuals is even more important, given the complexity of the tasks they undertake. Dr. Richard Prager is a characteristic world-historical individual in the field of QI in cardiothoracic surgery. From the very beginning of his efforts to establish a QI program in the State of Michigan, Dr. Prager faced certain great challenges, such as a) gathering all cardiothoracic surgeons of the State around a common table to discuss their outcomes and designing QI initiatives, b) unblinding performance data at the independent-institution level, and c) partnering the MSTCVS-QC with a payer which, in that case, was the Blue Cross Blue Shield of Michigan (BCBSM): the state's primary insurance payer [19]. Such disruptive individual actions are totally necessary for the progress of QI in surgery. In 1806, Hegel wrote a letter to his friend Friedrich Niethammer where he described Napoleon as "a world-soul [Weltseele] on horseback", indicating Napoleon to be a world-historical individual that drove forward reason's history. The well-known painting "Napoleon at the Saint-Bernard Pass" by Jacques-Louis David is the representation of Hegel's idea of Napoleon. Perhaps we can declare that disruptive surgeons like Dr. DeBakey, Dr. Cooley, or Dr. Prager are real-life representations of "a world-soul with scrubs".

A final crucial question is whether there is an end to the progress of history, and what is that end? As previously commented, Hegel is using the word "history" as the unfolding of reason in the progress of the consciousness of freedom. This has led some intellectuals like Francis Fukuyama to declare that the goal of self-consciousness and human freedom has been achieved in recent times, and the world has reached "the end of history" [20]. In this context, what Hegel means by an end of history is that the goal of history has been achieved, and the world is now conscious of freedom instead of lacking any further developments. In the context of surgery, the end of history could be reached through the awareness and adoption of QI methodology by the surgical community in their practice as a veil of safety for patients. The "last surgeon", the surgeon at the "end of history", would implement these principles in his practice and actively take part in QI initiatives. Perhaps, we are not far from such an end to history, and possibly many among us, there tends to be a resemblance to the "last surgeon". Nonetheless, the prevalence of such a heroic surgical idealism and culture in our time is totally necessary in order to protect and promote the best interests of patients, surgeons, and society as a whole.

Author Contributions: Conceptualization, D.E.M., T.A. and D.Z.; methodology, D.E.M., T.A. and D.Z.; software, D.E.M., T.A. and D.Z.; validation, D.E.M., T.A. and D.Z.; formal analysis, D.E.M., T.A. and D.Z.; investigation, D.E.M., T.A. and D.Z.; resources, D.E.M., T.A. and D.Z.; data curation, D.E.M., T.A. and D.Z.; writing—original draft preparation, D.E.M., T.A. and D.Z.; writing—review and editing, D.E.M., T.A. and D.Z.; visualization, D.E.M., T.A. and D.Z.; supervision, D.E.M., T.A. and D.Z.; project administration, D.E.M., T.A. and D.Z.; funding acquisition, D.E.M., T.A. and D.Z. All authors have read and agreed to the published version of the manuscript.

Conflicts of Interest: The authors declare no conflict of interest.

References

1. Hegel, G.W.F.; Nisbet, H.B. (Eds.) *Lectures on the Philosophy of World History: Introduction*; Cambridge University Press: Cambridge, UK, 1975.
2. Agency for Healthcare Quality and Research. Failure to Rescue. Available online: https://psnet.ahrq.gov/primer/failure-rescue (accessed on 12 April 2023).
3. National Quality Forum. Patient Safety 2017. Available online: http://www.qualityforum.org (accessed on 12 April 2023).
4. Taylor, M.J.; McNicholas, C.; Nicolay, C.; Darzi, A.; Bell, D.; Reed, J.E. Systematic review of the application of the plan-do-study-act method to improve quality in healthcare. *BMJ Qual. Saf.* **2014**, *23*, 290–298. [CrossRef] [PubMed]
5. Gaudino, M.; Benedetto, U.; Fremes, S.; Biondi-Zoccai, G.; Sedrakyan, A.; Puskas, J.D.; Angelini, G.D.; Buxton, B.; Frati, G.; Hare, D.L.; et al. Radial-artery or saphenous-vein grafts in coronary-artery bypass surgery. *N. Engl. J. Med.* **2018**, *378*, 2069–2077. [CrossRef] [PubMed]
6. Yi, G.; Shine, B.; Rehman, S.M.; Altman, D.G.; Taggart, D.P. Effect of bilateral internal mammary artery grafts on long-term survival: A meta-analysis approach. *Circulation* **2014**, *130*, 539–545. [CrossRef] [PubMed]
7. Taggart, D.P.; Altman, D.G.; Gray, A.M.; Lees, B.; Gerry, S.; Benedetto, U.; Flather, M. Randomized trial of bilateral versus single internal-thoracic-artery grafts. *N. Engl. J. Med.* **2016**, *375*, 2540–2549. [CrossRef] [PubMed]
8. Milojevic, M.; Head, S.J.; Mack, M.J.; Mohr, F.W.; Morice, M.-C.; Dawkins, K.D.; Holmes, D.R.; Serruys, P.W.; Kappetein, A.P. Influence of practice patterns on outcome among countries enrolled in the SYNTAX trial: 5-year results between percutaneous coronary intervention and coronary artery bypass grafting. *Eur. J. Cardio-Thorac. Surg.* **2017**, *52*, 445–453. [CrossRef] [PubMed]
9. Johnson, S.H.; Theurer, P.F.; Bell, G.F.; Maresca, L.; Leyden, T.; Prager, R.L. A statewide quality collaborative for process improvement: Internal mammary artery utilization. *Ann. Thorac. Surg.* **2010**, *90*, 1158–1164. [CrossRef] [PubMed]
10. Bond, C.J.; Milojevic, M.; He, C.; Theurer, P.F.; Clark, M.; Pruitt, A.L.; Gandhi, D.; DeLucia, A.; Jones, R.N.; Dabir, R.; et al. Quality Improvement: Arterial Grafting Redux, 2010:2019. *Ann. Thorac. Surg.* **2021**, *112*, 22–30. [CrossRef] [PubMed]

11. Magouliotis, D.E.; Fergadi, M.P.; Zotos, P.-A.; Rad, A.A.; Xanthopoulos, A.; Bareka, M.; Spiliopoulos, K.; Athanasiou, T. Differences in long-term survival outcomes after coronary artery bypass grafting using single vs multiple arterial grafts: A meta-analysis with reconstructed time-to-event data and subgroup analyses. *Gen. Thorac. Cardiovasc. Surg.* **2023**, *71*, 77–89. [CrossRef] [PubMed]
12. Giardini, M.; Guenzi, M.; Arcolin, I.; Godi, M.; Pistono, M.; Caligari, M. Comparison of Two Techniques Performing the Supine-to-Sitting Postural Change in Patients with Sternotomy. *J. Clin. Med.* **2023**, *12*, 4665. [CrossRef] [PubMed]
13. Soroceanu, R.P.; Timofte, D.V.; Danila, R.; Timofeiov, S.; Livadariu, R.; Miler, A.A.; Ciuntu, B.M.; Drugus, D.; Checherita, L.E.; Drochioi, I.C.; et al. The Impact of Bariatric Surgery on Quality of Life in Patients with Obesity. *J. Clin. Med.* **2023**, *12*, 4225. [CrossRef] [PubMed]
14. Xanthopoulos, A.; Bourazana, A.; Matsue, Y.; Fujimoto, Y.; Oishi, S.; Akiyama, E.; Suzuki, S.; Yamamoto, M.; Kida, K.; Okumura, T.; et al. Larissa Heart Failure Risk Score and Mode of Death in Acute Heart Failure: Insights from REALITY-AHF. *J. Clin. Med.* **2023**, *12*, 3722. [CrossRef] [PubMed]
15. Karamolegkou, A.P.; Fergadi, M.P.; Magouliotis, D.E.; Samara, A.A.; Tatsios, E.; Xanthopoulos, A.; Pourzitaki, C.; Walker, D.; Zacharoulis, D. Validation of the Surgical Outcome Risk Tool (SORT) and SORT v2 for Predicting Postoperative Mortality in Patients with Pancreatic Cancer Undergoing Surgery. *J. Clin. Med.* **2023**, *12*, 2327. [CrossRef] [PubMed]
16. Frisiras, A.; Giannas, E.; Bobotis, S.; Kanella, I.; Arjomandi Rad, A.; Viviano, A.; Spiliopoulos, K.; Magouliotis, D.E.; Athanasiou, T. Comparative Analysis of Morbidity and Mortality Outcomes in Elderly and Nonelderly Patients Undergoing Elective TEVAR: A Systematic Review and Meta-Analysis. *J. Clin. Med.* **2023**, *12*, 5001. [CrossRef] [PubMed]
17. Vaghiri, S.; Prassas, D.; Krieg, S.; Knoefel, W.T.; Krieg, A. The Postoperative Effect of Sugammadex versus Acetylcholinesterase Inhibitors in Colorectal Surgery: An Updated Meta-Analysis. *J. Clin. Med.* **2023**, *12*, 3235. [CrossRef] [PubMed]
18. Wichmann, D.; Orlova, O.; Königsrainer, A.; Quante, M. Is There a High Risk for GI Bleeding Complications in Patients Undergoing Abdominal Surgery? *J. Clin. Med.* **2023**, *12*, 1374. [CrossRef] [PubMed]
19. Milojevic, M.; Bond, C.; Theurer, P.F.; Jones, R.N.; Dabir, R.; Likosky, D.S.; Leyden, T.; Clark, M.; Prager, R.L. The Role of Regional Collaboratives in Quality Improvement: Time to Organize, and How? *Semin. Thorac. Cardiovasc. Surg.* **2020**, *32*, 8–13. [CrossRef] [PubMed]
20. Fukuyama, F. *The End of History and the Last Man*; Free Press: New York, NY, USA, 1992; ISBN 978-0-02-910975-5.

Disclaimer/Publisher's Note: The statements, opinions and data contained in all publications are solely those of the individual author(s) and contributor(s) and not of MDPI and/or the editor(s). MDPI and/or the editor(s) disclaim responsibility for any injury to people or property resulting from any ideas, methods, instructions or products referred to in the content.

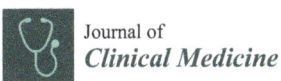

Article

Three Years of Continuous Vital Signs Monitoring on the General Surgical Ward: Is It Sustainable? A Qualitative Study

Harm H. J. van Noort *, Femke L. Becking-Verhaar, Wilmieke Bahlman-van Ooijen, Maarten Pel, Harry van Goor * and Getty Huisman-de Waal

Department of Surgery, Radboud University Medical Centre, 6500 HB Nijmegen, The Netherlands; femke.becking-verhaar@radboudumc.nl (F.L.B.-V.); wilmieke.vanooijen@radboudumc.nl (W.B.-v.O.); maarten.pel@radboudumc.nl (M.P.); getty.huisman-dewaal@radboudumc.nl (G.H.-d.W.)
* Correspondence: harm.vannoort@radboudumc.nl (H.H.J.v.N.); harry.vangoor@radboudumc.nl (H.v.G.); Tel.: +31-(0)24-36-134-38 (H.H.J.v.N.)

Citation: van Noort, H.H.J.; Becking-Verhaar, F.L.; Bahlman-van Ooijen, W.; Pel, M.; van Goor, H.; Huisman-de Waal, G. Three Years of Continuous Vital Signs Monitoring on the General Surgical Ward: Is It Sustainable? A Qualitative Study. *J. Clin. Med.* **2024**, *13*, 439. https://doi.org/10.3390/jcm13020439

Academic Editors: Dimitrios E. Magouliotis and Dimitris Zacharoulis

Received: 25 October 2023
Revised: 8 January 2024
Accepted: 10 January 2024
Published: 13 January 2024

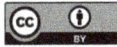

Copyright: © 2024 by the authors. Licensee MDPI, Basel, Switzerland. This article is an open access article distributed under the terms and conditions of the Creative Commons Attribution (CC BY) license (https://creativecommons.org/licenses/by/4.0/).

Abstract: Continuous monitoring of vital signs using a wireless wearable device was implemented in 2018 at a surgical care unit of an academic hospital. This study aimed at gaining insight into nurses' and patients' perspectives regarding the use and innovation of a continuous vital signs monitoring system, three years after its introduction. This qualitative study was performed in a surgical, non-intensive care unit of an academic hospital in 2021. Key-user nurses (nurses with additional training and expertise with the device) and patients were selected for semi-structured interviews, and nurses from the ward were selected for a focus group interview using a topic list. Transcripts of the audio tapes were deductively analysed using four dimensions for adoptions of information and communication technologies (ICT) devices in healthcare. The device provided feelings of safety for nurses and patients. Nurses and patients had a few issues with the device, including the size and the battery life. Nurses gained knowledge and skills in using the system for measurement and interpretations. They perceived the system as a tool to improve the recognition of clinical decline. The use of the system could be further developed regarding the technical device's characteristics, nurses' interpretation of the data and the of type of alarms, the information needs of patients, and clarification of the definition and standardization of continuous monitoring. Three years after the introduction, wireless continuous vital signs monitoring is the new standard of care according to the end-users at the general surgical ward.

Keywords: vital signs; clinical deterioration; monitoring; wearable electronic devices; continuous vital sign monitoring

1. Introduction

Measuring vital signs is crucial to evaluate the clinical condition of surgical patients. Subtle changes in vital signs such as respiratory rate, blood pressure, or heart rate can be the first signals of clinical deterioration. Nurses have crucial roles in the recognition of patients' clinical deterioration [1,2]. Nurses estimate modified Early Warning Scores (MEWSs) [3] indicating the clinical risk for clinical deterioration, admission to intensive care units (ICU), or severe events such as cardiac arrest or even death [4–10]. MEWSs are based on values of the vital signs: respiratory rate, blood oxygen saturation, blood pressure, heart rate, temperature, and level of consciousness. These parameters give the actual state of the physiological wellbeing of patients and indicate the need for medical treatment. Nurses also recognize subtle signs of deterioration by observing the patients and using their clinical judgement [2,10,11]. Nurses develop a sense of worry regarding the situation of their patients in cases of clinical deterioration [12]. While the nurses' sense of worry is sensitive to adverse events, deviations in vital signs are crucial factors that should be assessed and interpreted accordingly.

Compliance with MEWS protocols can be low, including subsequent follow ups according to the vital sign safety protocol [13–15]. Failures to timely escalate treatment still happen because of the insufficient measurement of vital signs [16,17]. Remote devices are introduced for the continuous monitoring of vital signs [18,19]. With the Visi Mobile as a wireless monitoring system, nurses mentioned an earlier identification of clinical decline, enhanced responses to clinical decline, and increased feelings of safety because of the higher frequency of vital signs measurements [20–22]. In our hospital, the introduction of the Visi Mobile in 2018 moved practice from the intermittent or periodic measurement of vital signs to continuous wireless monitoring. The Visi Mobile facilitates bedside and from-a-distance monitoring of vital signs by nurses. Since then, a decline in unplanned ICU admissions has been observed [23].

The CeHRes roadmap, a framework to achieve optimal uptake of eHealth technologies, suggests formatively evaluating the actual uptake or usage of technology to improve the technology and its use and to ensure sustainable use of the technology [24]. A post-implementation survey demonstrated that nurses were positive towards the use of the continuous vital signs monitoring system in daily practice [25]. However, understanding the nurses' and patients' perspectives for further development of the use of this system is lacking. Therefore, to proceed on the findings of Becking-Verhaar et al. [25], this study undertook a qualitative interview approach to provide in-depth insight into nurses' and patients' perspectives regarding the use of a continuous vital signs monitoring system, and how it can be further innovated to ensure the sustainable and effective use of this technology.

2. Materials and Methods

2.1. Design

This study was framed within the evaluation phase of the CeHRes Roadmap [24]. This study followed a qualitative approach by conducting individual interviews and a focus group interview with relevant stakeholders. This study was conducted between February and April 2021, which was three years after the introduction of the Visi Mobile. The Standards for Reporting Qualitative Research [26] were used to ensure transparent reporting. Furthermore, this study was performed according to the ethical guidelines of the declaration of Helsinki [27]. All participants provided informed consent a priori and data were treated anonymously. Under Dutch law there is no need for a formal ethical review for this type of study.

2.2. Setting

This study took place at a gastrointestinal surgical oncology unit of a Dutch academic hospital. In the 18-bed surgical ward, patients mainly recover from major abdominal surgical procedures, such as oesophageal resection, liver resection, pancreatic resection, colorectal surgery, and cytoreductive surgery with hyperthermic intraperitoneal chemotherapy.

System for Continuous Monitoring: Visi Mobile

The Visi Mobile (Sotera Wireless) was implemented on the surgical ward in May 2018 after a pilot phase (see Supplementary S1) [20]. The Visi Mobile is a wireless, wearable device with sensors at the thumb and chest for continuous measurement of oxygen saturation, heart frequency, body temperature, respiratory rate, heart rhythm, and blood pressure. These parameters are displayed on screens of the battery worn on the patients' wrist and on monitors at the nurse stations and lunchrooms [23]. The monitors provide nurses with continuous real-time vital sign data trends of the preceding 96 h and display single channel alarms when a single vital sign falls outside the pre-set safety limits. Vital signs data are automatically sent to electronic health records for automated MEWS calculation with on-demand monitoring by nurses. Nurses use the patients' data if they deem it to be necessary. Vital signs and the corresponding MEWSs are determined at least three times a day using the Visi Mobile device at the bedside. Nurses intervene depending on the MEWS or alarms given by the devices on the patient's wrist or on the dashboards. Alarms noted from a distance require evaluation by the nurse. Where alarms are accurate measurements of abnormal values, nurses validate the MEWSs at the bedside. Interventions are based on the hospital's MEWS protocol and the clinical judgement of the nurse. Key-user nurses were established for the Visi Mobile, having experience and providing supervising roles for other nurses at the unit regarding remote continuous monitoring for coaching and problem solving. They were involved during the initial implementation and were more experienced in the use of continuous monitoring.

2.3. Participant Selection

The main stakeholders were end-users of vital signs monitoring using the Visi Mobile at the gastrointestinal surgical oncology unit. The actual users of the system were nurses, key-user nurses, and patients admitted to the surgical unit.

Nurses were selected because they were continuously responsible for the safety of patients. From the nursing staff (n = 35), nurses were recruited for a focus group interview by using email and announcements during regular team meetings. A focus group was the preferred method due to its ability to facilitate optimal interaction between the nurses. Nurses were selected if they had worked for at least six months at the ward, to ensure sufficient experience with the remote continuous monitoring, and were not a key user.

Key-user nurses (n = 4) were recruited for individual interviews to collect in-depth insight into their perspectives on the uptake of the technology. Respondents were contacted face-to-face or by email for participation.

Also, patients were individually interviewed because they wore the device and experienced how nurses used it in daily practice. They were consecutively approached for participation if they were able to provide informed consent, were monitored by the Visi Mobile, understood and spoke the Dutch language, and were in a condition to talk about this topic based on the nurses' judgement. If they were open to an interview, an appointment was made to hold the interview.

2.4. Data Collection

All interviews were held face-to-face in calm and private rooms during the hospital stay of the patient in the afternoon at the patient's preferred time. Patients wore the particular device during data collection. The interviews with nurses lasted between 45 and 55 min and were conducted by one researcher (MP). The focus group interview took 75 min and was conducted by two researchers, of whom one was the interviewer (HN), and the other the observer (MP). The interviews with patients lasted for approximately 20 min and were undertaken by one of the researchers (MP, HN). MP was a Bachelor of Nursing student during this study and received supervision from HN and FBV. HN is a clinical academic nurse with experience in education, surgical nursing, and qualitative research. FBV is also a clinical academic nurse with experience in surgical nursing and pedagogy. All researchers had experience in individual interviewing, HN was also experienced in focus groups. The researchers discussed, before the first interviews and after each interview, their skills, the topic list, and the responses, to ensure quality of the data collection. All interviews were audio recorded and transcribed verbatim. For each group of respondents, a tailored topic guide was developed by MP, FB-V and HN, focusing on the aim of this study. The topic lists are shown in Supplementary S2.

2.4.1. Individual Interviews with Key-User Nurses

The themes during the interviews were: (a) experiences with continuous monitoring, (b) experiences regarding barriers, (c) possible improvements, and (d) preconditions (see Supplementary S3). The experiences with continuous monitoring were discussed by illustrating the facilitators and barriers to working with the system found in previous studies [20,25]. This enabled the comparison of similarities and differences between the previous and current perspectives, as was suggested by the CeHRes Roadmap [24].

Hence, the device was used for several years in which periodic improvements could have eliminated some barriers. The topic list continued to explore perspectives on possible improvements that could innovate the nurses' use of the continuous monitoring of vital signs. Therefore, the respondents were probed to suggest directions for solutions and subsequent requirements, and how these solutions could be integrated into daily nursing routines. In this phase, it was emphasized that a new role for a central nurse could focus on all kinds of tasks and activities that are related to the continuous monitoring of vital signs. Each interview ended by asking the respondent to prioritize a main current problem and direction for the solution.

2.4.2. Focus Group Interview with Nurses

The focus group started with attention as to how participants could discuss and interact with each other during the interview about the topics (see Supplementary S2). Then, the same topics as used in the individual interviews with nurses were introduced.

2.4.3. Individual Interviews with Patients

The topic list for patients included: (a) experiences with continuous monitoring, and (b) possible improvements (see Supplementary S2).

2.5. Data Analysis

A deductive content analysis approach was applied [28,29], guided by the list of factors that are related to the success or failure of information and communication technologies (ICT) adoption made by Gagnon et al. [30]. These factors are structured within four dimensions with (sub)indicators (see Table 1 and more detailed information in Supplementary S2). These dimensions were previously used to determine the feasibility of the Visi Mobile device [20] and were therefore used to explore what can be further innovated within each dimension. Two of three researchers (MP, HN, and FB-V) independently attributed the data of the transcripts to the dimensions and to the (sub)indicators of each dimension. Consensus was reached about the attribution of each citate afterwards. Then, data were summarized per indicator of the dimensions.

Table 1. Factors related to the adoption of ICT application based on the findings of Gagnon et al. (2012).

Dimension	Indicator
Factors related to ICT	Design and technical concerns
	Characteristics of the innovation
	System reliability
	Interoperability
	Legal issues
	Validity of the resources
	Cost issues
Individual factors of healthcare professionals	Knowledge
	Attitude
	Socio-demographic characteristics
Human environment	Factors associated with patients
	Factors associated with peers
Organizational aspects	Internal environment
	External environment

3. Results

Individual interviews were held with four key-user nurses and five patients. One of the four key-user nurses was male, all other respondents were female. Of the five patients, three were male. Six female nurses participated in the focus group interview. For the dimension 'Factors related to the ICT', citations were only attributed to the indicators 'design and technical concerns and characteristics of the innovation'. For the dimension 'Individual factors of healthcare professionals', citations were attributed to the indicator's 'knowledge' and 'attitude'. For the dimension of 'Human environment' and 'Organizational aspects', citations were attributed to both indicators. No data were attributed to the remaining indicators of the dimensions. The results of the analysis are demonstrated per attributed indicator. Citations are displayed in Table 2.

Table 2. Citations of the respondents per indicator.

Indicator	Respondent	Citation
Design and technical concerns	P4	"The device of the Visi Mobile is unfriendly for patients because the battery is too rude, and heavy. It never fits well, turns around my wrist and slides back and forth. It is not comfortable."
	R2	"In the future, there may be a possibility to apply artificial intelligence to handle and cluster the data overload."
Characteristics of the innovation	R1	"From a distance, you can estimate how your patient is doing, to some extent. Also, if your patient does not feel well, and you really want to be in the room all the time, which is not possible in a nursing ward, you feel you can better monitor your patient. So yes, it provides me a safe feeling."
	R3	"Recently, we had transferred a patient from the ICU to our unit, having a MEWS 6 and respiratory unstable. In that case, it would be great if there is someone who keep an extra eye on that patient, because I cannot constantly look to the display, and do not get an alarm on my pager."
	P3	"Tonight, a nurse entered my room because my oxygen level was too low. I understand the use of continuous monitoring and I think that the need differs for each ward. For me, this was not a minor operation, so I think this is perfect, for me, but also for them [nurses]."
Knowledge	R1	"Nine out of ten times you do not have to respond to a false alarm, but you just wait a few seconds before breathing frequency or saturation will improve. I have the idea we are on the right track in recognizing false alarms."
Attitude	FGR	"How skeptical we were about continuous monitoring... And now, three years later we cannot work without it."
	R1	"Some patients will be discharged soon, for example today or tomorrow. Why should you still monitor all vital signs and check trends?"
	FGR	"Sometimes, a saturation drops during the night as it also does at home. We check on the patient because of this saturation drop and then the patient seems to be okay."
Factors associated with patients	P2	"I like the idea of knowing my own vital signs, so that I know what I can expect. Firstly, I looked very often, but that became gradually less often."
Internal aspects	R2	"I think, for example, during evening and nightshifts we are much of our time present in the nursing office. During that shift, we do not need a dedicated nurse. During day shifts, when everyone is at the patient' rooms, I think a dedicated nurse is necessary. The question rises if you can deploy the dedicated nurse in patient care, and that he also receives all alarms, so that he can respond to the alarms."
	FGR	"I would like to maintain continuous monitoring, but I would also like to retain total care for my patients, without shifting tasks. That is very important to me".
	R3	"If the dedicated nurse signals a certain trend, and the nurse is not yet at the patient, then he [dedicated nurse] must inform me, so that I can visit the patient. If I [as nurse] do not get out, I can call the dedicated nurse to monitor trends."
Factors associated with peers	R4	"We can say that connecting the device can be a task for nurse assistants. It will give a nice touch to their job profile. It seemed that some nurse assistants do really like that, and they see it as a challenge."
External aspects	R3	"The difference between a high care ward and our general ward is getting smaller using this system. Subsequently, it is difficult to set boundaries, and to frame, between what you should do and not do."

P = Patient; FGR: Focus group Respondent R: Respondent.

3.1. Factors Related to ICT

3.1.1. Design and Technical Concerns

The nurses recognized several barriers that still affected the use of the continuous monitoring system. In particular, technical disturbing aspects were mentioned that required improvements. Disturbing aspects were clustered into four main aspects: (1) the connectivity between the device and the WIFI, (2) usability of the battery and cables, (3) reliability of the estimations, and (4) the amount of data that the system provides. Regarding the first aspect, the WIFI sometimes did not connect, which made it impossible to load the data from the electronic patient file. Secondly, patients mentioned that the battery was too big and heavy, and turned around on their wrist, which hampered the patient in daily activities. The battery had to be charged twice a day, which sometimes led to an empty battery and unavailable vital signs. Thirdly, nurses also mentioned that incorrectly placed cables (i.e., the ECG-leads, the thumb sensor, and the electro lead) led to measurement errors and false alarms. Moreover, some nurses described that patients' blood pressure measured by the Visi Mobile was not always a reliable estimation of the parameter. The blood pressure seemed to be less accurate the further away from calibration. Therefore, the reliability of estimations of the vital signs had to be improved, according to some nurses. Fourthly, the amount of data that continuously monitoring provides for nurses could be seen as an overload of data. The amount of data enables nurses to make trend analyses of vital signs such as falling blood pressure or a rising heart rate. Nurses indicated that they used trends to consult a physician. Some nurses explained that they learned how to handle the data overload over time by prioritizing and being aware of the clinical condition of the patient. Some of them also mentioned that the trend analysis was still far from optimal and may be improved using artificial intelligence. This could be helpful to deal with the overload of patient data and the use of trends for the recognition of clinical decline.

3.1.2. Characteristics of the Innovation

Nurses perceived continuous monitoring as an extra set of eyes of the nurse, enabling them to provide better care. Nurses did not have to be at the bedside the whole time in case of a sense of worry. The extra set of eyes provided feelings of trust. However, if a nurse was busy with a particular patient, she was not warned in case of abnormal vital signs of another patient. Some nurses mentioned this as a feeling of uncertainty. Moreover, some nurses stated they did not dare to let patients sleep without monitoring their vital signs continuously. Before the introduction of continuous monitoring, vital signs were measured three times a day (or more often, depending on the MEWS). Nurses described that deterioration of patients during night shifts was only noticed during the morning rounds. With the use of continuous monitoring, deterioration during nightshifts is recognized earlier, and interventions can be applied, which improves patient outcomes, according to nurses.

Patients also described that they felt safe due to the idea of their vital signs being monitored continuously. Some of them experienced a nurse coming to the bedside in case of abnormalities. They now knew that their vital signs were being monitored and that subsequent action would be taken.

3.2. Individual Factors of Healthcare Professionals

3.2.1. Knowledge

The nurses described that they gained knowledge about working with continuous monitoring. One of the nurses reported that during the introduction of this device (in 2018, red.) nurses immediately responded to an alarm by seeing the patient, also in the case of clear false alarms. One of the nurses mentioned an example of patients sleeping on their right or left side, whereby the Visi Mobile displayed no respiratory rate. Currently (in 2021, red.), nurses first look for the type of alarm and consider all measurements at that moment before acting on an alarm. In the case of alarm for breathing absence, nurses first look at saturation, heart rate, and whether the patient slept on a side (patients' attitude was measured with VM, red.), before they go to check on the patient. Three years after implementation, the nurses felt they understood all types of and reasons for alarms and that they handled the continuous data availability of vital signs efficiently. To work adequately and efficiently with continuous monitoring, knowledge regarding alarms must be integrated into training for nurses.

3.2.2. Attitude

The nurses felt mainly positive about the use of continuous monitoring, whereby their attitudes had changed over time from a more sceptical attitude to an enthusiastic attitude. Nurses described that CM became an essential part of their care, which facilitated them in anticipating patients' clinical deterioration. In addition, having patients' vital signs provided feelings of safety among the nurses. For example, nurses had experienced cases where resuscitation was initiated because of abnormal values of vital signs that came to nurses due to continuous monitoring. Nurses mentioned that the system guarantees more patient safety and better clinical conditions.

The nurses' attitude was also critical towards the use of trends. Due to the continuously available vital signs, a bored feeling among nurses could arise, which would affect their alertness to changes. When measuring the MEWS three times a day, changes in MEWS were always noted. However, these changes are less explicitly noticed now because vital signs are present all the time. Therefore, some nurses mentioned a critical note towards the possibility of only analysing trends, because small changes may be overlooked. Nurses explained the advantage of observing trends in vital signs, for example, regarding suspected false alarms such as breathing frequency. Thereby, although some nurses really examined the patients' situation, others only looked at the numbers instead of attending patients for physical examination. One of the nurses described a wish to actively discuss trends during the physicians' round, because this was currently no part of it. Another factor that affected the nurses' attitude towards monitoring was over-monitoring. It appeared that continuous monitoring was still used even if vital signs were stable for a long time, for instance, in the case of a patient who was to be discharged. This over-monitoring, measuring vital signs when the clinical added value was not clear, did provoke a tired feeling towards continuous monitoring.

3.3. Human Environment

3.3.1. Factors Associated with Patients

Patients had generally positive feelings about the use of continuous monitoring. Patients described that it was good for their health that someone was able to watch over them continuously and that, in case of abnormalities, nurses could respond immediately. Patients were soon used to the device and only noticed it during calibration by the nurse or changing batteries. Patients described increased comfort because blood pressure was measured all the time, while the burden of the blood pressure cuff happened only once in 24 h during calibration. Also, patients mentioned looking frequently at their own vital signs and health status, especially during the first postoperative days. Some patients noticed that they should not look at their screen that often because they interpreted the vital signs according to how they felt. Patients could feel worried when vital signs were going out of normal ranges, and confident after seeing good vital signs. Furthermore, patients indicated the value of interaction with a nurse who knew them, who applied the device, and who interacted with them about the vital signs. Some patients mentioned that the involvement of many different nurses in their care could be difficult because they wanted to be known personally. To further innovate the use of continuous monitoring, this value must be recognized.

Nurses also mentioned that patients might look frequently at their device, indicating that the patients might need some further information or support as to how they can interpret their own vital signs. They expressed the need to investigate how patients use the continuous monitoring system, to be able to supervise them better.

3.3.2. Factors Associated with Peers

The system for continuous monitoring was used by nurses and not by nurse assistants. Nurses stated that nurse-assistants could make an assisting contribution to the measurement of vital signs monitoring. They could change batteries, apply the system, and calibrate the blood pressure. They should be trained in these activities. Also, the nursing team should be properly aware of the expectations concerning continuous monitoring, such as changing responsibilities, policies on how to act on alarms, and whether high-risk medication could be administered while the patient is being monitored. The function of a dedicated nurse could be embedded into daily patient care by having a pager for incoming alarms. Nurses described the dedicated nurse as a partner for dialogue who addresses the practical implications of continuous monitoring, such as changing batteries or pasting stickers. Some nurses felt that such a position would remove their responsibilities and position in handling and responding to clinical decline. The majority described it as an appropriate task for nurse assistants. Therefore, the nurses concluded there was room for improvement through monitoring as a team with nurses and nurse-assistants.

3.4. Organizational Aspects
3.4.1. Internal Aspects

Regarding the organization of the use of the continuous monitoring system, nurses mentioned that they were not able to continuously watch the vital signs, as they were not all the time in one of the rooms where the dashboards were available. Therefore, the nurses notified each other in case of abnormal vital signs. In this matter, task-specific nursing in terms of a dedicated nurse was discussed as part of the topic guide. This possible new nursing function could be a supportive role for ward nurses by making them aware of abnormalities in patients' vital signs. The dedicated nurse first assesses the amount of data and possible false alarms before warning the ward nurses. However, such a role was not perceived as supportive by all nurses. Most nurses indicated that they wanted to have the final responsibility for patients' vital signs and the total care of patients. They expressed the wish to make a careful assessment themselves with a physical examination of patients and their clinical view before intervening. For newly graduated nurses, the help of a dedicated nurse can be supportive in facilitating a back-up for the nurse when she is unexperienced.

3.4.2. External Aspects

As the general ward is not organized according to intensive care standards, nurses mentioned that there is a difference between continuous monitoring and guarding vital signs. One of the participating nurses described that continuous monitoring provides more of an "own assessment" and "own feeling of concern". Nurses assess the vital signs of patients and use the system and their clinical judgement to intervene on a deviation. In intensive care facilities, every change is noticed and subsequently handled. Although nurses mentioned that a dedicated nurse for this task could facilitate responses to each alarm, they perceived that this was more guarding vital signs than monitoring vital signs. A clear definition of what continuous monitoring of vital signs at general wards is, and what kind of boundaries are determined, would enhance clarity as to the expectations towards nurses.

4. Discussion

This study assessed perspectives on the use of a continuous monitoring system for recognition of clinical decline three years after introduction and how it can be innovated to ensure sustainable use. The perspectives were structured by the four dimensions of Gagnon's list for adoption of ICT devices in healthcare. Generally, monitoring vital signs with the Visi Mobile enabled nurses to improve patient safety, because they could more frequently review vital signs to anticipate and act sooner on changes in patients' vital signs. Nurses gained knowledge and skills in using the system for measurement and interpretations over the three years. Patients felt safe while monitored, which seemed to overcome the physical concerns about the device. Although these findings are in line with multiple references [19,20,22,25,31,32], this is the first study that has performed a formal evaluation 3 years after initial introduction which also identifies four areas to ensure sustainable use.

First, the technical aspects of the device can be improved, such as the battery size, battery life, and Wi-Fi. These barriers were previously identified [20,25] and are also important factors for other devices [33]. The technical aspects of devices for vital signs measurement are important to address, with a priority regarding the reliability of measurements. Furthermore, the user-friendly technical aspects are important. Medical companies who produce the devices can now address these daily barriers for future innovation of their devices to improve adoption and the satisfaction of end-users [34,35].

The second opportunity concerns the nurses' interpretation of the data and alarms. First, false alarms can be reduced by preventing measurement errors. Although it appeared in our findings that nurses gained knowledge over the years, measurement errors leading to false alarms still occurred. This can provoke feelings of irritation and uncertainty towards the system [36]. It is unclear whether these measurement errors are caused by device-related factors or nurse-related factors. Further analysis is required on this topic. Secondly, effective interpretation of all available data and reporting of vital signs or MEWS using trends will enhance the value of the system, according to the nurses in our study. Nurses need to process all the data, which can be seen as overload. The use of algorithms may be a solution to support nurses in the interpretation of data [37,38]. Furthermore, nurses expressed in our study that integration of their clinical judgement into the recognition of clinical decline was pivotal to complementing the data assessed by the Visi Mobile. Nurses' feelings of worry must be recognized [11] and can be measured [39]. Future studies can address vital signs-based algorithms that are complemented by the nurses' worries and clinical judgement to improve recognition of clinical decline.

Thirdly, the perspectives of patients should be addressed in performing continuous vital signs monitoring. Patients appreciated interaction with their nurse, in line with previous research [40]. Nurse-patient interaction is the core of fundamental care [40,41], requiring attention in future studies, as remote monitoring might affect this. Furthermore, our results illustrate that the interpretation by patients of their clinical condition requires further attention. Patients expressed the need to be informed about the normal values of the vital signs. Therefore, future research should address the perspectives of patients, to ensure that patients with all levels of health literacy are kept informed and empowered [1]. Furthermore, although our patients felt safe with the device, future research can address the patients' responses towards the wide range of wireless devices. Finally, patients' perspectives were integrated as respondents in this study; we suggest, for future developments in continuous vital signs monitoring, partnering with patients in the research group [42].

Fourthly, continuous vital signs monitoring using a wearable, wireless device can be improved by defining and standardizing the use within nursing practice at general wards. In our study, nurses were not always in rooms with the monitors displaying vital signs data, which affected the reality of the term 'continuous'. Other studies did not use alarms [36], and vitals were interpreted differently [43]. Moreover, our respondents suggested training nurse assistants to administer the device, as they were part of the nursing staff, as well as developing clear guidelines on when to start or stop monitoring. Therefore, clear definition of the concept and practical guidance for these issues will enhance efficacy and prevent over-monitoring.

Our study must be interpreted in the light of several considerations. First, perspectives were explored in one setting using only one device, affecting the generalizability of the findings. Although research on technology in healthcare should address the context, other devices in other settings may lead to different long-term experiences. Secondly, cooperation between nurses and physicians has been previously identified, but not in our findings [11], suggesting that data saturation was not achieved in our study. Future studies must complement our findings regarding the sustainable use of innovations. Finally, we used Gagnon's list for data analysis, because previous interviews regarding the use of the Visi Mobile were also analysed with this list [20]. Another study in this field used the Behaviour Change Wheel as the theoretical basis of the analysis [44]. Our model enabled the analysis of the sustainable updating of the technology, while their aim was to assess nurses' behaviours regarding wireless monitoring.

5. Conclusions

Three years after the introduction of a continuous vital signs system on a general surgical ward, it enables nurses to ensure patient safety and provides feelings of safety for both nurses and patients. The nurses gained knowledge and skills to handle the system. Nurses and patients provided four opportunities to further improve the use of a continuous vital signs monitoring system. These concern the device itself, to make it more user-friendly, and the way nurses handle the output, including alarms and trends. Also, the patient's information and psychological needs regarding vital signs and the judgement of their clinical condition is important for nurses to address. Finally, it is important to outline what continuous monitoring is about, when it can be initiated, and what the responsibilities are for whom.

Supplementary Materials: The following supporting information can be downloaded at: https://www.mdpi.com/article/10.3390/jcm13020439/s1, Supplementary S1: Graphical presentation of the Visi Mobile; Supplementary S2: interview guide; Supplementary S3: Model of Gagnon.

Author Contributions: Conceptualization, H.H.J.v.N., F.L.B.-V., M.P., H.v.G. and G.H.-d.W.; methodology and investigation H.H.J.v.N., F.L.B.-V. and M.P.; formal analysis, H.H.J.v.N., F.L.B.-V., M.P. and W.B.-v.O.; writing—original draft preparation, H.H.J.v.N., F.L.B.-V. and W.B.-v.O.; writing—review and editing, H.H.J.v.N., F.L.B.-V., W.B.-v.O., H.v.G. and G.H.-d.W. All authors have read and agreed to the published version of the manuscript.

Funding: This research received no external funding.

Institutional Review Board Statement: This study was conducted in accordance with the Declaration of Helsinki. Ethical review and approval were waived for this study due to the Dutch law does not require formal ethical review for this type of study.

Informed Consent Statement: Informed consent was obtained from all subjects involved in this study.

Data Availability Statement: The data presented in this study are available on request from the corresponding author.

Acknowledgments: We thank the nurses and patients who participated in this study and shared their experience.

Conflicts of Interest: The authors declare no conflict of interest.

References

1. Kitson, A.L. The Fundamentals of Care Framework as a Point-of-Care Nursing Theory. *Nurs. Res.* **2018**, *67*, 99–107. [CrossRef] [PubMed]
2. Odell, M.; Victor, C.; Oliver, D. Nurses' role in detecting deterioration in ward patients: Systematic literature review. *J. Adv. Nurs.* **2009**, *65*, 1992–2006. [CrossRef]
3. Subbe, C.P.; Kruger, M.; Rutherford, P.; Gemmel, L. Validation of a modified Early Warning Score in medical admissions. *QJM* **2001**, *94*, 521–526. [CrossRef] [PubMed]
4. Jarvis, S.W.; Kovacs, C.; Briggs, J.; Meredith, P.; Schmidt, P.E.; Featherstone, P.I.; Prytherch, D.R.; Smith, G.B. Are observation selection methods important when comparing early warning score performance? *Resuscitation* **2015**, *90*, 1–6. [CrossRef]
5. Beaumont, K.; Luettel, D.; Thomson, R. Deterioration in hospital patients: Early signs and appropriate actions. *Nurs. Stand.* **2008**, *23*, 43–48. [CrossRef]
6. Kyriacos, U.; Jelsma, J.; Jordan, S. Monitoring vital signs using early warning scoring systems: A review of the literature. *J. Nurs. Manag.* **2011**, *19*, 311–330. [CrossRef]
7. Ludikhuize, J.; Smorenburg, S.M.; de Rooij, S.E.; de Jonge, E. Identification of deteriorating patients on general wards; measurement of vital parameters and potential effectiveness of the Modified Early Warning Score. *J. Crit. Care.* **2012**, *27*, 424.e7–424.e13. [CrossRef] [PubMed]

8. van Beuzekom, M.; Boer, F.; Akerboom, S.; Hudson, P. Patient safety in the operating room: An intervention study on latent risk factors. *BMC Surg.* **2012**, *12*, 10. [CrossRef]
9. Andersen, L.W.; Kim, W.Y.; Chase, M.; Berg, K.M.; Mortensen, S.J.; Moskowitz, A.; Novack, V.; Cocchi, M.C.; Donnino, M.W.; American Heart Association's Get With the Guidelines(®)—Resuscitation Investigators. The prevalence and significance of abnormal vital signs prior to in-hospital cardiac arrest. *Resuscitation* **2016**, *98*, 112–117. [CrossRef]
10. Kause, J.; Smith, G.; Prytherch, D.; Parr, M.; Flabouris, A.; Hillman, K.; Intensive Care Society (UK); Austrlian and New Zealand Intensive Care Society Clinical Trials Gropu. A comparison of antecedents to cardiac arrests, deaths and emergency intensive care admissions in Australia and New Zealand, and the United Kingdom-the ACADEMIA study. *Resuscitation* **2004**, *62*, 275–282. [CrossRef]
11. Peerboom, F.; Hafsteinsdottir, T.B.; Weldam, S.W.; Schoonhoven, L. Surgical nurses' responses to worry: A qualitative focus-group study in the Netherlands. *Intensive Crit. Care Nurs.* **2022**, *71*, 103231. [CrossRef] [PubMed]
12. Douw, G.; Huisman-de Waal, G.; van Zanten, A.R.; van der Hoeven, J.G.; Schoonhoven, L. Nurses' 'worry' as predictor of deteriorating surgical ward patients: A prospective cohort study of the Dutch-Early-Nurse-Worry-Indicator-Score. *Int. J. Nurs. Stud.* **2016**, *59*, 134–140. [CrossRef]
13. Bingham, G.; Fossum, M.; Barratt, M.; Bucknall, T. Clinical review criteria and medical emergency teams: Evaluating a two-tier rapid response system. *Crit. Care Resusc.* **2015**, *17*, 167–173. [CrossRef] [PubMed]
14. Bucknall, T.K.; Jones, D.; Bellomo, R.; Staples, M.; Investigators, R. Responding to medical emergencies: System characteristics under examination (RESCUE). A prospective multi-site point prevalence study. *Resuscitation* **2013**, *84*, 179–183. [CrossRef] [PubMed]
15. Ludikhuize, J.; de Jonge, E.; Goossens, A. Measuring adherence among nurses one year after training in applying the Modified Early Warning Score and Situation-Background-Assessment-Recommendation instruments. *Resuscitation* **2011**, *82*, 1428–1433. [CrossRef] [PubMed]
16. van Galen, L.S.; Struik, P.W.; Driesen, B.E.; Merten, H.; Ludikhuize, J.; van der Spoel, J.I.; Kramer, M.H.H.; Nanayakkara, P.W.B. Delayed Recognition of Deterioration of Patients in General Wards Is Mostly Caused by Human Related Monitoring Failures: A Root Cause Analysis of Unplanned ICU Admissions. *PLoS ONE* **2016**, *11*, e0161393. [CrossRef] [PubMed]
17. Yiu, C.J.; Khan, S.U.; Subbe, C.P.; Tofeec, K.; Madge, R.A. Into the night: Factors affecting response to abnormal Early Warning Scores out-of-hours and implications for service improvement. *Acute Med.* **2014**, *13*, 56–60. [CrossRef]
18. Breteler, M.J.M.; KleinJan, E.; Numan, L.; Ruurda, J.P.; Van Hillegersberg, R.; Leenen, L.P.H.; Hermans, M.; Kalman, C.J.; Blockhuis, T.J. Are current wireless monitoring systems capable of detecting adverse events in high-risk surgical patients? A descriptive study. *Injury* **2020**, *51* (Suppl. 2), S97–S105. [CrossRef]
19. Leenen, J.P.L.; Leerentveld, C.; van Dijk, J.D.; van Westreenen, H.L.; Schoonhoven, L.; Patijn, G.A. Current Evidence for Continuous Vital Signs Monitoring by Wearable Wireless Devices in Hospitalized Adults: Systematic Review. *J. Med. Internet Res.* **2020**, *22*, e18636. [CrossRef]
20. Weenk, M.; Bredie, S.J.; Koeneman, M.; Hesselink, G.; van Goor, H.; van de Belt, T.H. Continuous Monitoring of Vital Signs in the General Ward Using Wearable Devices: Randomized Controlled Trial. *J. Med. Internet Res.* **2020**, *22*, e15471. [CrossRef]
21. Watkins, T.; Whisman, L.; Booker, P. Nursing assessment of continuous vital sign surveillance to improve patient safety on the medical/surgical unit. *J. Clin. Nurs.* **2016**, *25*, 278–281. [CrossRef] [PubMed]
22. Stellpflug, C.; Pierson, L.; Roloff, D.; Mosman, E.; Gross, T.; Marsh, S.; Willis, V.; Gabrielson, D. Continuous Physiological Monitoring Improves Patient Outcomes. *Am. J. Nurs.* **2021**, *121*, 40–46. [CrossRef] [PubMed]
23. Eddahchouri, Y.; Peelen, R.V.; Koeneman, M.; Touw, H.R.W.; van Goor, H.; Bredie, S.J.H. Effect of continuous wireless vital sign monitoring on unplanned ICU admissions and rapid response team calls: A before-and-after study. *Br. J. Anaesth.* **2022**, *128*, 857–863. [CrossRef] [PubMed]
24. van Gemert-Pijnen, J.E.; Nijland, N.; van Limburg, M.; Ossebaard, H.C.; Kelders, S.M.; Eysenbach, G.; Seydel, E. A holistic framework to improve the uptake and impact of eHealth technologies. *J. Med. Internet Res.* **2011**, *13*, e111. [CrossRef] [PubMed]
25. Becking-Verhaar, F.L.; Verweij, R.P.H.; de Vries, M.; Vermeulen, H.; van Goor, H.; Huisman-de Waal, G.J. Continuous Vital Signs Monitoring with a Wireless Device on a General Ward: A Survey to Explore Nurses’ Experiences in a Post-Implementation Period. *Int. J. Environ. Res. Public Health* **2023**, *20*, 5794. [PubMed]
26. O'Brien, B.C.; Harris, I.B.; Beckman, T.J.; Reed, D.A.; Cook, D.A. Standards for reporting qualitative research: A synthesis of recommendations. *Acad. Med.* **2014**, *89*, 1245–1251. [CrossRef]
27. World Medical, A. World Medical Association Declaration of Helsinki: Ethical principles for medical research involving human subjects. *JAMA* **2013**, *310*, 2191–2194.
28. Elo, S.; Kyngas, H. The qualitative content analysis process. *J. Adv. Nurs.* **2008**, *62*, 107–115. [CrossRef]
29. Graneheim, U.H.; Lindgren, B.M.; Lundman, B. Methodological challenges in qualitative content analysis: A discussion paper. *Nurse Educ. Today* **2017**, *56*, 29–34. [CrossRef]
30. Gagnon, M.P.; Desmartis, M.; Labrecque, M.; Car, J.; Pagliari, C.; Pluye, P.; Fremont, P.; Gagnon, J.; Tremblay, N.; Legare, F. Systematic review of factors influencing the adoption of information and communication technologies by healthcare professionals. *J. Med. Syst.* **2012**, *36*, 241–277. [CrossRef]
31. Weller, R.S.; Foard, K.L.; Harwood, T.N. Evaluation of a wireless, portable, wearable multi-parameter vital signs monitor in hospitalized neurological and neurosurgical patients. *J. Clin. Monit. Comput.* **2018**, *32*, 945–951. [CrossRef]

32. Verrillo, S.C.; Cvach, M.; Hudson, K.W.; Winters, B.D. Using Continuous Vital Sign Monitoring to Detect Early Deterioration in Adult Postoperative Inpatients. *J. Nurs. Care Qual.* **2019**, *34*, 107–113. [CrossRef]
33. Haveman, M.E.; van Melzen, R.; Schuurmann, R.C.L.; Hermens, H.J.; Tabak, M.; de Vries, J.P.M. Feasibility and patient's experiences of perioperative telemonitoring in major abdominal surgery: An observational pilot study. *Expert. Rev. Med. Devices.* **2022**, *19*, 515–523. [CrossRef]
34. Schoville, R.R.; Titler, M.G. Guiding healthcare technology implementation: A new integrated technology implementation model. *Comput. Inform. Nurs.* **2015**, *33*, 99–107, quiz E1. [CrossRef]
35. Jeskey, M.; Card, E.; Nelson, D.; Mercaldo, N.D.; Sanders, N.; Higgins, M.S.; Shi, Y.; Michaels, D.; Miller, A. Nurse adoption of continuous patient monitoring on acute post-surgical units: Managing technology implementation. *J. Nurs. Manag.* **2011**, *19*, 863–875. [CrossRef]
36. Leenen, J.P.L.; Rasing, H.J.M.; van Dijk, J.D.; Kalkman, C.J.; Schoonhoven, L.; Patijn, G.A. Feasibility of wireless continuous monitoring of vital signs without using alarms on a general surgical ward: A mixed methods study. *PLoS ONE* **2022**, *17*, e0265435. [CrossRef]
37. Buchanan, C.; Howitt, M.L.; Wilson, R.; Booth, R.G.; Risling, T.; Bamford, M. Predicted Influences of Artificial Intelligence on the Domains of Nursing: Scoping Review. *JMIR Nurs.* **2020**, *3*, e23939. [CrossRef]
38. Van Bulck, L.; Couturier, R.; Moons, P. Applications of artificial intelligence for nursing: Has a new era arrived? *Eur. J. Cardiovasc. Nurs.* **2022**, *22*, e19–e20. [CrossRef]
39. Douw, G.; Huisman-de Waal, G.; van Zanten, A.R.H.; van der Hoeven, J.G.; Schoonhoven, L. Surgical ward nurses' responses to worry: An observational descriptive study. *Int. J. Nurs. Stud.* **2018**, *85*, 90–95. [CrossRef]
40. Downey, C.L.; Brown, J.M.; Jayne, D.G.; Randell, R. Patient attitudes towards remote continuous vital signs monitoring on general surgery wards: An interview study. *Int. J. Med. Inform.* **2018**, *114*, 52–56. [CrossRef]
41. Wiechula, R.; Conroy, T.; Kitson, A.L.; Marshall, R.J.; Whitaker, N.; Rasmussen, P. Umbrella review of the evidence: What factors influence the caring relationship between a nurse and patient? *J. Adv. Nurs.* **2016**, *72*, 723–734. [CrossRef] [PubMed]
42. Castro, E.M.; Van Regenmortel, T.; Vanhaecht, K.; Sermeus, W.; Van Hecke, A. Patient empowerment, patient participation and patient-centeredness in hospital care: A concept analysis based on a literature review. *Patient Educ. Couns.* **2016**, *99*, 1923–1939. [CrossRef] [PubMed]
43. van Goor, H.M.R.; Breteler, M.J.M.; Schoonhoven, L.; Kalkman, C.J.; van Loon, K.; Kaasjager, K.A.H. Interpretation of continuously measured vital signs data of COVID-19 patients by nurses and physicians at the general ward: A mixed methods study. *PLoS ONE* **2023**, *18*, e0286080. [CrossRef]
44. Leenen, J.P.L.; Dijkman, E.M.; van Hout, A.; Kalkman, C.J.; Schoonhoven, L.; Patijn, G.A. Nurses' experiences with continuous vital sign monitoring on the general surgical ward: A qualitative study based on the Behaviour Change Wheel. *BMC Nurs.* **2022**, *21*, 60. [CrossRef]

Disclaimer/Publisher's Note: The statements, opinions and data contained in all publications are solely those of the individual author(s) and contributor(s) and not of MDPI and/or the editor(s). MDPI and/or the editor(s) disclaim responsibility for any injury to people or property resulting from any ideas, methods, instructions or products referred to in the content.

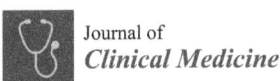

Article

Comparison of Fibrinogen Concentrate and Cryoprecipitate on Major Thromboembolic Events after Living Donor Liver Transplantation

Jae-Hwan Kim, Kyoung-Sun Kim, Hye-Mee Kwon, Sung-Hoon Kim, In-Gu Jun, Jun-Gol Song * and Gyu-Sam Hwang

Laboratory for Cardiovascular Dynamics, Department of Anesthesiology and Pain Medicine, Asan Medical Center, University of Ulsan College of Medicine, Seoul 05505, Republic of Korea; jaehwankim@amc.seoul.kr (J.-H.K.); kyoungsun.kim@amc.seoul.kr (K.-S.K.); hyemee.kwon@amc.seoul.kr (H.-M.K.); shkimans@amc.seoul.kr (S.-H.K.); igjun@amc.seoul.kr (I.-G.J.); kshwang@amc.seoul.kr (G.-S.H.)
* Correspondence: jungol.song@amc.seoul.kr; Tel.: +82-2-3010-3869

Abstract: (1) Background: Liver transplantation (LT) is associated with significant hemorrhage and massive transfusions. Fibrinogen replacement has a key role in treating massive bleeding during LT and hypofibrinogenemia is treated by fibrinogen concentrate or cryoprecipitate. However, these two products are known to be associated with major thromboembolism events (MTEs). We aimed to compare the effect of fibrinogen concentrate and cryoprecipitate on MTEs in living donor LT (LDLT) recipients. (2) Methods: We analyzed 206 patients who underwent LDLT between January 2021 and March 2022. The patients were divided into two groups according to fibrinogen concentrate or cryoprecipitate use. We compared the incidence of MTEs between the two groups. In addition, we performed multiple logistic regression analyses to identify the risk factors for MTEs. (3) Results: There was no significant difference in the incidence of MTEs (16 [14.7%] vs. 14 [14.4%], $p = 1.000$) between the cryoprecipitate group and fibrinogen concentrate group. In the multivariate analysis, cryoprecipitate (OR 2.09, 95%CI 0.85–5.11, $p = 0.107$) and fibrinogen concentrate (OR 2.05, 95%CI 0.82–5.12, $p = 0.126$) were not significantly associated with MTEs. (4) Conclusions: there was no significant difference in the incidence of MTEs between cryoprecipitate and fibrinogen concentrate in LDLT recipients.

Keywords: fibrinogen; liver transplantation; mortality; thromboembolism

1. Introduction

Patients undergoing liver transplantation (LT) are at risk of hemorrhage and receive massive transfusions if needed [1]. Hemostatic and coagulopathy related to cirrhotic liver disease are also known to cause massive bleeding in LT [2]. Fibrinogen has a key role in hemostasis and activates platelet aggregation by binding to glycoprotein IIb and IIIa receptors on platelet surfaces [3]. However, intraoperative fibrinogen levels are reduced because of hemorrhage followed by resuscitation with fluids and fibrinogen-poor blood products [4]. In cases of significant hemorrhage and hypofibrinogenemia, guidelines recommend treatment with either cryoprecipitate or fibrinogen concentrate [5].

Although cryoprecipitate and fibrinogen concentrate are used to treat hypofibrinogenemia, there is concern about thromboembolic risk in using two products. Thromboembolic complications including hepatic artery thrombosis are associated with a high rate of mortality and graft loss in LT [6,7].

In particular, cryoprecipitate is considered to have a higher thromboembolic risk than fibrinogen concentrate because cryoprecipitate is a non-purified product with platelet microparticles, fibronectin, factor VIII, and von Willebrand factor [8]. Previous studies on patients undergoing cardiac surgery have reported that the two products have similar thromboembolic risks [5,9]. However, a direct comparison of thromboembolic events between the two products in living donor LT (LDLT) is lacking in the literature.

Therefore, the aim of this study was to evaluate the effect of cryoprecipitate and fibrinogen concentrate on major thromboembolic events (MTEs) in patients undergoing LDLT. In addition, the incidence of 30-day major adverse cardiovascular events (MACEs), and 1-year graft failure and mortality were also compared between the two groups.

2. Materials and Methods

2.1. Study Design and Population

We analyzed LT recipients who underwent LDLT at our center between January 2021 and March 2022. Those who acquired hypofibrinogenemia were included and the following patients were excluded: age < 18 years, history of allergic reaction to fibrinogen concentrate or cryoprecipitate, did not receive any blood products transfusion, underwent multi-organ transplantation surgery, or those with missing data.

The Institutional Review Board of Asan Medical Center (protocol no. 2022-0724) approved the study design and waived the requirement for written informed consent based on the retrospective nature of the study. The research protocol followed the ethical guidelines of the 1975 Declaration of Helsinki reflected in the prior approval of the institution's human research committee. Each transplantation procedure was evaluated and approved by the local authorities and the Korean Network for Organ Sharing affiliated with the Ministry of Health and Welfare of the Republic of Korea.

2.2. Data Collection

Patient demographics and perioperative variables were collected using the electronic medical records of our institution. Patient characteristics included age, sex, diabetes mellitus (DM), hypertension (HTN), chronic kidney disease (CKD), coronary artery disease (CAD), cerebrovascular accident (CVA), Model for End-stage Liver Disease score (MELD-Na score), Child–Turcotte–Pugh score (CTP score), and causes for liver transplantation (i.e., HBV-related liver cirrhosis, HCV-related liver cirrhosis, alcoholic liver cirrhosis, hepatocellular carcinoma). Intraoperative laboratory values included hemoglobin, platelet, international normalized ratio (INR), creatinine, total bilirubin, albumin, aspartate transaminase (AST), alanine transaminase (ALT), and sodium. Variables related to intraoperative transfusion included massive transfusion, unit of transfused packed red blood cell (pRBC), fresh frozen plasma (FFP), platelet apheresis, cryoprecipitate, fibrinogen concentrate, baseline fibrinogen level in plasma, maximum amplitude at 10 min and maximum clot firmness in FIBTEM, and fibrinogen level in plasma after treatment protocol. Massive transfusion was defined as the use of more than 10 units of PRBCs within 24 h or more than 4 units within 1 h during surgery.

2.3. Transfusion Technique

Patients were divided into two groups according to whether they received fibrinogen concentrate or cryoprecipitate. The transfusion criterion for using fibrinogen concentrate or cryoprecipitate is fibrinogen < 80 mg or rotational thromboelastometry (ROTEM, Tem International GmbH, Munich, Germany) FIBTEM-maximum clot firmness (MCF) < 4 mm. Which blood product to use was determined by the anesthesiologist's discretion and the blood bank's inventory. Fibrinogen concentrate dose was approximated using the following formula [10]:

$$\text{Dose} = [\text{target FIBTEM-MCF (mm)} - \text{current FIBTEM-MCF (mm)}] \times \text{weight (kg)}/140$$

Fibrinogen content in the cryoprecipitate varies (150 mg–200 mg) depending on the manufacturer and blood donor. The U.S. Food and Drug Administration (FDA) for fibrinogen content in cryoprecipitate requires a minimum of 150 mg per unit [11,12]. Accordingly, we assumed that 1 unit of cryoprecipitate contained 200 mg of fibrinogen, and for a 70 kg adult, 2 g of fibrinogen or 10 units of cryoprecipitate was used because we targeted FIBTEM-MCF (mm) $\geq$ 8 mm. At our institution, intraoperative laboratory values and ROTEM were measured three times during the preanhepatic, anhepatic, and neohepatic periods.

2.4. Primary and Secondary Outcomes

The primary outcome was a composite of an MTE such as portal and hepatic vein thrombosis, hepatic artery thrombosis, intra-cardiac thrombus, pulmonary embolism, and ischemic stroke (by ultrasonography, transesophageal echocardiography, computed tomography) during 30 days after LDLT. Secondary outcomes were 30-day MACE, 1-year graft failure, and 1-year mortality.

A MACE was defined as the composite of postoperative cardiovascular mortality, atrial fibrillation, ventricular arrhythmias, ST-T wave changes with chest tightness, myocardial infarction [13].

2.5. Statistical Analysis

Data are presented as mean ± standard deviation, median (interquartile range [IQR]), or number (proportion), as appropriate. We used the chi-squared test or Fisher's exact test for categorical variables and Student's *t*-test or Mann–Whitney U test for continuous variables. Multivariable logistic regression analysis was applied to identify the risk factors for MTEs. We performed multiple logistic regression analysis including patients (n = 105) who did not receive cryoprecipitate and fibrinogen concentrate but received pRBC or FFP transfusion. All variables with p values < 0.1 in the univariate analysis were included in the multivariate analysis by backward elimination. Kaplan–Meier survival curve was used to depict the risk of 1-year mortality and graft failure. The log-rank test was used to evaluate differences between curves. All data were analyzed using SPSS Statistics for Windows, version 22.0 (IBM Corp., Armonk, NY, USA) or R version 3.1.2 (R Foundation for Statistical Computing, Vienna, Austria).

3. Results

Of the 570 patients who underwent LDLT at our institution during the study period, 364 patients were excluded according to the exclusion criteria. In total, 311 patients were divided into the cryoprecipitate group (n = 109), fibrinogen concentrate group (n = 97), and recipients who received a pRBC or FFP transfusion without cryoprecipitate or fibrinogen concentrate (n = 105). (Figure 1)

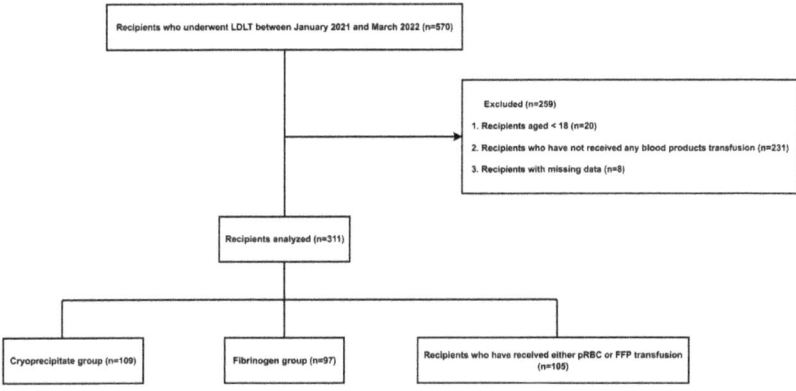

Figure 1. Study flow chart.

Table 1 shows the baseline characteristics and perioperative variables of the study patients. The median recipient age was 56 (50.0–62.0) years and 147 (71.4%) were men. Of the 206 recipients, 63 (30.6%) had DM, 45 (21.8%) had HTN, 8 (3.9%) had CKD, 5 (2.4%) had CAD, and 5 (2.4%) had CVA. Alcoholic liver cirrhosis (n = 89, 43.2%) was the most common cause of LT, followed by hepatocellular carcinoma (n = 80, 38.8%), HBV-related liver cirrhosis (n = 80, 38.8%), and HCV-related liver cirrhosis (n = 11, 5.3%).

Table 1. Baseline characteristics of the study population.

	Cryoprecipitate Group (n = 109)	Fibrinogen Group (n = 97)	Total (n = 206)	p-Value
Demographic data				
Age	55.0 (48.0–61.0)	58.0 (52.0–63.0)	56.0 (50.0–62.0)	0.046
Sex, male	75 (68.1)	72 (74.2)	147 (71.4)	0.481
BMI	22.9 (20.2–26.0)	23.7 (21.3–26.9)	23.2 (20.6–26.4)	0.101
Diabetes	32 (29.4)	31 (32.0)	63 (30.6)	0.800
Hypertension	23 (21.1)	22 (22.7)	45 (21.8)	0.916
CKD	5 (4.6)	3 (3.1)	8 (3.9)	0.847
CAD	3 (2.8)	2 (2.1)	5 (2.4)	1.000
CVA	3 (2.8)	2 (2.1)	5 (2.4)	1.000
MELD-Na score	18.0 (10.0–27.0)	15.0 (11.0–21.0)	17.0 (10.0–24.0)	0.368
CTP score	9.0 (7.0–11.0)	9.0 (7.0–10.0)	9.0 (7.0–11.0)	0.538
Cause for LT				
HBV LC	43 (39.5)	37 (38.1)	80 (38.8)	0.961
HCV LC	5 (4.6)	6 (6.2)	11 (5.3)	0.842
Alcoholic LC	50 (45.9)	39 (40.2)	89 (43.2)	0.497
HCC	40 (36.7)	40 (41.2)	80 (38.8)	0.600
HCC with HBV	27 (24.8)	23 (23.7)	50 (24.3)	0.989
HCC with HCV	4 (3.7)	6 (6.2)	10 (4.9)	0.521
HCC with Alcoholic LC	7 (6.4)	12 (12.4)	19 (9.2)	0.218
Laboratory variables				
Hemoglobin, g/dL	9.3 (8.2–11.0)	10.2 (8.4–12.0)	9.9 (8.3–11.7)	0.052
Platelet, 10^9/L	59.0 (42.0–88.0)	58.0 (38.0–79.0)	58.0 (38.0–82.0)	0.462
INR	1.49 (1.23–1.86)	1.38 (1.24–1.65)	1.42 (1.23–1.75)	0.110
AST	38.0 (28.0–56.0)	37.0 (26.0–52.0)	38.0 (27.0–54.0)	0.347
ALT	21.0 (15.0–34.0)	21.0 (14.0–28.0)	21.0 (15.0–32.0)	0.369
Total bilirubin	2.9 (1.2–7.7)	2.0 (1.2–3.4)	2.2 (1.2–5.2)	0.082
Albumin, g/dL	3.0 (2.6–3.4)	2.9 (2.5–3.4)	2.9 (2.6–3.4)	0.496
Sodium	138.0 (134.0–140.0)	138.0 (134.0–141.0)	138.0 (134.0–141.0)	0.850
Creatinine, mg/dL	0.85 (0.72–1.15)	0.78 (0.61–0.98)	0.82 (0.66–1.06)	0.036
Intraoperative variables				
Operation time, hour	12.5 ± 2.2	12.6 ± 1.9	12.6 ± 2.1	0.816
Crystalloid, mL	6200.0 (4400.0–8900.0)	7200.0 (5200.0–9700.0)	6450.0 (4700.0–9050.0)	0.187
Colloid, mL	3600.0 (2800.0–4800.0)	4000.0 (2800.0–5600.0)	3600.0 (2800.0–5200.0)	0.190
Urine output, mL	1570.0 (1010.0–2350.0)	2000.0 (1400.0–2690.0)	1755.0 (1200.0–2580.0)	0.006

Note: values are expressed as the mean ± SD, number (%), or median (1Q, 3Q). Abbreviations: BMI, body mass index; CKD, chronic kidney disease; CAD, coronary artery disease; CVA, cerebrovascular accident; MELD-Na, Model for End-stage Liver Disease-Sodium; CTP, Child–Turcotte–Pugh; LT, liver transplantation; LC, liver cirrhosis; HCC, hepatocellular carcinoma; INR, international normalized ratio; AST, aspartate aminotransferase; ALT, alanine aminotransferase.

Except for the older age in the fibrinogen group (55.0 vs. 58.0, p = 0.046), the two groups did not show significant differences in patient-related variables such as sex, DM, HTN, CKD, CAD, CVA, MELD-Na score, CTP score, and cause for LT. The two groups did not show significant differences in the laboratory variables except for higher preoperative creatinine levels in the cryoprecipitate group (0.85 [0.72–1.15] vs. 0.78 [0.61–0.98], p = 0.036). With regard to the intraoperative variables, the two groups did not show significant differences in the operation time (p = 0.816), total use of crystalloid (p = 0.187), and total use of synthetic colloid (p = 0.190). The fibrinogen group had more urine output than the cryoprecipitate group (1570.0 [1010.0–2350.0] vs. 2000.0 [1400.0–2690.0], p = 0.006).

Table 2 shows the variables for the intraoperative transfusion and fibrinogen levels and ROTEM values before and after intervention. The intraoperative transfusion variables (massive transfusion, pRBC, FFP, platelet apheresis) were not significantly different between the two groups. The baseline fibrinogen levels of the cryoprecipitate group and the fibrinogen concentrate group were 75.0 (60.0–86.0) and 78.0 (62.0–96.0) ($p = 0.206$), respectively. Also, the results of the baseline MA10 (4.0 [3.0–6.0] vs. 4.0 [3.0–6.0], $p = 0.521$) and MCF (4.0 [3.0–7.0] vs. 5.0 [4.0–7.0], $p = 0.479$) of the FIBTEM and fibrinogen levels after intervention (97.0 [78.0–120.0] vs. 100.0 [81.0–116.0], $p = 0.838$) were not significantly different between the two groups. However, in ROTEM, the fibrinogen group had a significantly higher MA 10 (4.0 [3.0–6.0] vs. 5.0 [3.0–6.0], $p = 0.033$) and MCF (4.0 [3.0–6.0] vs. 5.0 [4.0–7.0], $p = 0.019$) after intervention. (Table 2).

Table 2. Details of intraoperative transfusion and intervention.

	Cryoprecipitate Group ($n = 109$)	Fibrinogen Group ($n = 97$)	Total ($n = 206$)	p-Value
Intraoperative transfusion				
pRBC (unit)	10.0 (6.0–18.0)	10.0 (5.0–17.0)	10.0 (6.0–18.0)	0.757
FFP (unit)	10.0 (4.0–14.0)	10.0 (6.0–18.0)	10.0 (5.0–16.0)	0.461
Platelet apheresis (unit)	1.0 (0.0–1.0)	1.0 (0.0–1.0)	1.0 (0.0–1.0)	0.990
Fibrinogen (g)	0.0 (0.0–0.0)	2.0 (2.0–4.0)	0.0 (0.0–2.0)	<0.001
Cryoprecipitate (unit)	10.0 (10.0–10.0)	0.0 (0.0–0.0)	5.0 (0.0–10.0)	<0.001
Massive transfusion	57 (52.3)	54 (55.7)	111 (53.9)	0.730
Baseline				
Fibrinogen in plasma (mg/dL)	75.0 (60.0–86.0)	78.0 (62.0–96.0)	77.0 (60.0–91.0)	0.206
FIBTEM				
MA 10 (mm)	4.0 (3.0–6.0)	4.0 (3.0–6.0)	4.0 (3.0–6.0)	0.521
MCF (mm)	4.0 (3.0–7.0)	5.0 (4.0–7.0)	5.0 (3.0–7.0)	0.479
After treatment for acquired hypofibrinogenemia				
Fibrinogen in plasma (mg/dL)	97.0 (78.0–120.0)	100.0 (81.0–116.0)	98.0 (80.0–118.0)	0.838
FIBTEM				
MA 10 (mm)	4.0 (3.0–6.0)	5.0 (3.0–6.0)	5.0 (3.0–6.0)	0.033
MCF (mm)	4.0 (3.0–6.0)	5.0 (4.0–7.0)	5.0 (3.0–7.0)	0.019
Fibrinogen administered				
Preanhepatic	21 (19.3)	25 (25.8)	46 (22.3)	
Anhepatic	12 (11.0)	2 (2.1)	14 (6.8)	1.000
Postreperfusion	76 (69.7)	70 (72.2)	146 (70.9)	

Note: values are expressed as median (1Q, 3Q) or number (%). Abbreviations: pRBC, packed red blood cell; FFP, fresh frozen plasma; FIBTEM, assay for tissue factor activation and platelet inhibition; MA 10, maximum amplitude at 10 min; MCF, maximum clot firmness.

3.1. Primary Outcome

There were no significant differences in the incidence of MTEs between the cryoprecipitate group and the fibrinogen concentrate group (16 [16.7%] vs. 14 [14.4%], $p = 1.000$; Table 3). MTEs occurred in three cases, which were hepatic artery thrombosis in two patients (1.8%) in the cryoprecipitate group and ischemic stroke in one patient (1.0%) in the fibrinogen group. There were no cases of intra-cardiac thrombus or pulmonary embolism. Multivariate analysis demonstrated that the duration of surgery (hour, OR 1.22, 95% CI 1.04–1.44, $p = 0.014$) was significantly associated with an MTE (Table 4).

To determine the impact of cryoprecipitate and fibrinogen concentrate on thromboembolism, we compared the incidence of MTEs in patients ($n = 105$) who did not receive cryoprecipitate and fibrinogen concentrate but received either a pRBC or FFP transfusion with patients ($n = 206$) who received either cryoprecipitate or fibrinogen concentrate during LDLT. There was no statistical difference in MTEs between the two groups (Supplemental Table S1).

Table 3. Primary and secondary outcomes.

	Cryoprecipitate Group (n = 109)	Fibrinogen Group (n = 97)	Total (n = 206)	p-Value
MTE	16 (14.7)	14 (14.4)	30 (14.6)	1.000
Portal and hepatic vein thrombosis	14 (12.8)	13 (13.4)	27 (13.1)	1.000
Hepatic artery thrombosis	2 (1.8)	0 (0)	2 (1.0)	0.529
Ischemic stroke	0 (0)	1 (1.0)	1 (0.5)	0.953
30-day MACE	24 (22.0)	13 (13.4)	37 (18.0)	0.154
1-year mortality	10 (9.2)	7 (7.2)	17 (8.3)	0.798
1-year graft failure	16 (14.7)	8 (8.3)	24 (11.7)	0.223

Note: values are presented as number (%). Abbreviations: MTE, major thromboembolic event; MACE, major adverse cardiovascular event.

Table 4. Multivariate logistic regression analyses of major thromboembolic events.

	Univariate Analysis			Multivariate Analysis		
	OR	95% CI	p Value	OR	95% CI	p Value
Age (yr)	0.99	0.96–1.02	0.540			
Male sex	2.71	1.09–6.92	0.031	2.43	0.97–6.11	0.058
Diabetes	1.85	0.92–3.71	0.083	1.79	0.88–3.66	0.110
Hypertension	1.36	0.64–2.89	0.427			
Coronary artery disease	1.32	0.28–6.21	0.723			
Cerebral vascular disease	1.20	0.14–10.27	0.866			
Chronic kidney disease	0.64	0.08–5.13	0.677			
Massive transfusion	1.38	0.69–2.73	0.358			
MELD-Na score	0.99	0.95–1.03	0.678			
Duration of surgery (hour)	1.22	1.05–1.43	0.012	1.22	1.04–1.44	0.014
Cause for LT						
HBV LC	0.86	0.43–1.71	0.662			
HCV LC	3.09	0.92–10.41	0.068			
Alcoholic LC	0.95	0.47–1.91	0.881			
HCC	1.53	0.77–3.01	0.223			
Blood products						
[a] No transfusion	(reference)					
Cryoprecipitate	2.09	0.85–5.11	0.107			
Fibrinogen concentrate use	2.05	0.82–5.12	0.126			

Abbreviations: OR, odds ratio; CI, confidence interval; HCC, hepatocellular carcinoma; MELD-Na, Model for End-stage Liver Disease-Sodium; LT, liver transplantation; LC, liver cirrhosis. [a] Patients who did not receive cryoprecipitate and fibrinogen concentrate but received pRBC or FFP transfusion.

3.2. Secondary Outcomes

There were no significant differences in the incidence of 30-day MACE (24 [22.0%] vs. 13 [13.4%], $p = 0.154$), 1-year mortality (10 [9.2%] vs. 7 [7.2%], $p = 0.798$), and 1-year graft failure (16 [14.7%] vs. 8 [8.3%], $p = 0.223$) between the cryoprecipitate group and the fibrinogen concentrate group (Table 3).

Figure 2 shows the Kaplan–Meier curves of 1-year mortality and 1-year graft failure in the two groups. One-year mortality (log-rank test; $p = 0.6$) and graft failure (log-rank test; $p = 0.2$) were not significantly different between the two groups.

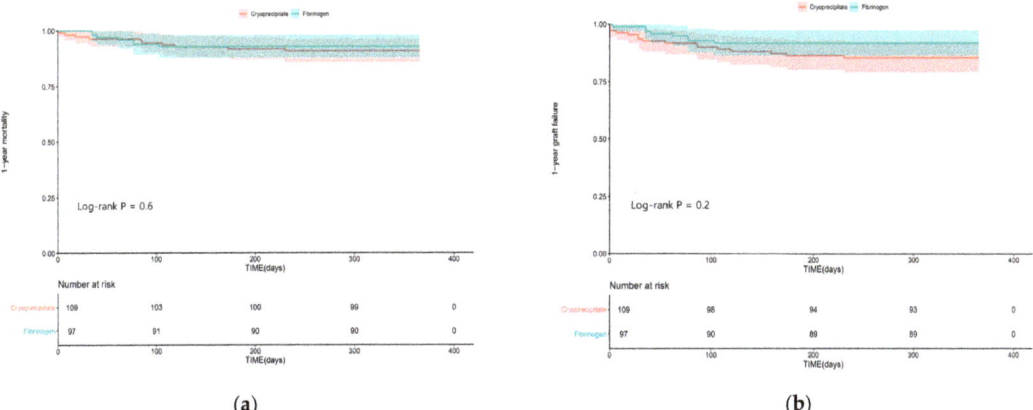

Figure 2. Kaplan–Meier curves of (**a**) 1-year mortality; (**b**) 1-year graft failure in the cryoprecipitate group and fibrinogen concentrate group.

4. Discussion

In this retrospective study, we found that there was no significant difference in MTEs between LDLT patients using cryoprecipitate and those using fibrinogen concentrate. Moreover, there were no significant differences in the incidences of 30-day MACE, 1-year graft failure, and mortality between the two groups.

Fibrinogen is a plasma glycoprotein synthesized in the liver. It transforms into fibrin by thrombin, playing a crucial role in clot formation, platelet activation, and aggregation [14]. While cryoprecipitate and fibrinogen concentrate are both plasma-derived, fibrinogen concentrate has a standardized concentration, leading to a predictable hemostatic effect; moreover, fibrinogen concentrate is purified, pasteurized, and filtered, which results in lower risks of viral transmission and immunological transfusion reaction [8,9]. Additionally, fibrinogen concentrate is easily reconstituted in sterile water and has a low administration volume and short administration time; after reconstitution, fibrinogen concentrate has a long shelf life of up to 24 h, thus reducing wastage [8]. Cryoprecipitates are allogenic blood products that are non-purified and contain various coagulation factors in addition to fibrinogen such as factor VIII, factor XIII, and von Willebrand factor [11]. The variability of fibrinogen contents in cryoprecipitate hinders an accurate prediction of its hemostatic effect; however, various coagulation factors have a positive impact on hemostasis in patients with hemodilution or massive blood loss [8,11].

Despite advances in surgical techniques, understanding of the pathophysiology of coagulation in end-stage liver disease patients, and point-of-care treatment, LT is still expected to cause massive bleeding and require a massive transfusion [1]. Acquired hypofibrinogenemia is followed by fluid resuscitation and fibrinogen-poor blood transfusion in surgery, and dysfibrinogenemia is common in LT recipients [15]. In our study, a massive transfusion was observed whether fibrinogen concentrate or cryoprecipitate was administered for acquired hypofibrinogenemia.

Before treatment for acquired hypofibrinogenemia, the baseline plasma fibrinogen levels (mg/dL) for the two groups were 75.0 in the cryoprecipitate group and 78.0 in the fibrinogen concentrate group. The American Society of Anesthesiologists task force for perioperative blood management recommends fibrinogen replacement in patients with bleeding when the plasma fibrinogen level is less than 80–100 mg/dL [16]. In our study, although there were no differences in the baseline fibrinogen levels, MA10, and MCF of FIBTEM between the two groups, the fibrinogen group showed a significantly higher MA 10 (4.0 [3.0–6.0] vs. 5.0 [3.0–6.0], $p = 0.033$) and MCF (4.0 [3.0–6.0] vs. 5.0 [4.0–7.0], $p = 0.019$) in ROTEM after intervention (Table 2). However, no significant difference was found in the fibrinogen levels between the two groups after intervention. In a systematic review comparing cryoprecipitate and fibrinogen concentrate in bleeding patients, it was also reported that there was no significant difference in the increased plasma fibrinogen levels between the two groups after intervention [17]. To assess clot strength, FIBTEM MCF in ROTEM is employed. In a study utilizing a trauma-induced coagulopathy model, it was found that after administration, fibrinogen concentrate resulted in a stronger FIBTEM MCF value compared to cryoprecipitate [18]. However, in a randomized controlled trial conducted by Galas et al. in pediatric cardiac surgery, there was no significant difference in FIBTEM MCF between cryoprecipitate and fibrinogen concentrate after intervention [9]. We presume that this discrepancy in the viscoelastic coagulation test is due to the variability of fibrinogen levels in cryoprecipitate [11,12]. In our study, we assumed that one unit of cryoprecipitate contained 200 mg of fibrinogen; however, as the volume of one unit of cryoprecipitate varies from 15 mL to 20 mL, the fibrinogen content also varies from 150 mg to 200 mg, in which the fibrinogen concentrate is standardized. Our study also demonstrated results similar to a previous study. However, considering the weak coagulation balance in patients with ESLD and the occurrence of massive bleeding during surgery and hemodilution, we believe that further clinical research is needed in this context.

The currently recommended treatment for hypofibrinogenemia is fibrinogen concentrate or cryoprecipitate [19]. Fibrinogen administration in LT for hypofibrinogenemia reduces surgical bleeding [20]; however, fibrinogen concentrate and cryoprecipitate carry thromboembolic risks. A previous study reported that cryoprecipitate is associated with a major thromboembolic risk [6], but did not make a direct comparison between cryoprecipitate and fibrinogen concentrate, and there are only a few studies comparing the thromboembolic risk of the two products. Recent randomized trials of adult [5] and children [9] patients undergoing cardiac surgery demonstrated that there was no significant difference in the thromboembolic risk between fibrinogen concentrate and cryoprecipitate. A systematic review also showed that the two products had no significant difference in thromboembolic risk and did not mention whether one product was superior to the other [17]. Especially in patients with end-stage liver disease, the decrease in both procoagulant and anticoagulant factors can lead to a weak rebalanced hemostasis, making them susceptible to both hemorrhagic and thrombotic complications [21]. Notably, several studies have suggested that fibrinogen supplementation does not increase thromboembolic risk [20,22]. This supports our current findings that fibrinogen replacement using cryoprecipitate or fibrinogen concentrate does not increase thromboembolic risk, emphasizing the safety of fibrinogen administration in the setting of coagulopathy during LT.

In our study, the incidence of any adverse outcomes including 1-year mortality was not significantly different between the two groups. Several studies comparing the two products were conducted in various clinical settings, such as cardiac surgery [5,9,23], obstetric bleeding [24], and trauma [25] in which acquired hypofibrinogenemia frequently appears. A recent randomized clinical trial on patients undergoing cardiac surgery demonstrated that no statistically significant difference was found in the mortality rate between the fibrinogen concentrate group and the cryoprecipitate group [5]. In addition, postoperative mortality in pediatric cardiac surgery was also not significantly different between the two products [9,23].

In our study, there were no statistically significant differences in the incidence of 1-year graft failure (14.7% vs. 8.3%, $p = 0.223$) and MACE (22.0% vs. 13.4%, $p = 0.154$) between the two groups, although the incidences were numerically higher in the cryoprecipitate group. We speculate that the small sample size of our study might be one of the reasons that a significant difference between the two groups was not found in the secondary outcomes. Moreover, while HBV-related LC is the most common cause of LT in South Korea [26], alcoholic LC was the most common etiology in our study patients. This suggests that alcoholic LC and HCC are accompanied by other etiologies including viral hepatitis. Further studies with larger sample sizes are needed to compare the incidences of graft failure and MACE between these two groups in LDLT.

In our study, the duration of surgery was associated with MTEs. In the same manner, T. Maeda et al. demonstrated that the duration of surgery was a risk factor for thrombosis in a multicenter cardiovascular surgery study [27]. Since thromboembolism in LT has multifactorial causes, further studies are needed.

This study has several limitations. Firstly, as our study was retrospective and based on a single center, unmeasured confounding factors may exist. Secondly, as our study only included patients undergoing LT with hypofibrinogenemia, these findings may not be generalized to other clinical settings that require fibrinogen replacement. In addressing these limitations, it is necessary to conduct future studies with multicenter studies and a prospective design. A larger sample size will improve the statistical power, aiding in reliable conclusions and revealing subtle associations. In addition, exploring subgroups, including disease severity and treatment regimens, is crucial for in-depth insights. Moreover, incorporating diagnostic tools in future research will provide a current evaluation of fibrinogen replacement therapy's effect on thromboembolic risks. Despite these limitations, our data are meaningful in that the outcomes of fibrinogen concentrate and cryoprecipitate in patients undergoing LDLT were directly compared.

In conclusion, there was no significant difference in MTEs between LDLT patients receiving fibrinogen concentrate and those receiving cryoprecipitate. Fibrinogen concentrate may be used as an alternative to cryoprecipitate in the treatment of acquired hypofibrinogenemia in LDLT.

Supplementary Materials: The following supporting information can be downloaded at: https://www.mdpi.com/article/10.3390/jcm12237496/s1, Table S1: demographic feature between no transfusion and fibrinogen products transfusion group.

Author Contributions: Conceptualization, J.-G.S. and G.-S.H.; methodology, I.-G.J.; formal analysis, H.-M.K. and S.-H.K.; writing—original draft preparation, J.-H.K.; funding acquisition, S.-H.K.; writing—review and editing, K.-S.K. and J.-G.S.; supervision, G.-S.H. All authors have read and agreed to the published version of the manuscript.

Funding: This research was supported by a grant of the Korea Health Technology R&D Project through the Korea Health Industry Development Institute (KHIDI), funded by the Ministry of Health & Welfare, Republic of Korea (grant number: HR20C0026), and was also supported by grants (2023IE0008 and 2023IP0134) from the Asan Institute for Life Sciences, Asan Medical Center, Seoul, Korea.

Institutional Review Board Statement: The research protocol followed the ethical guidelines of the 1975 Declaration of Helsinki reflected in the prior approval of the institution's human research committee. Each transplantation procedure was evaluated and approved by the local authorities and the Korean Network for Organ Sharing affiliated with the Ministry of Health and Welfare of the Republic of Korea. The Institutional Review Board of Asan Medical Center (protocol no. 2022-0724) approved the study design.

Informed Consent Statement: Patient consent was waived due to the retrospective nature of the study.

Data Availability Statement: The data presented in this study are available on request from the corresponding author. The data are not publicly available due to privacy.

Conflicts of Interest: The authors declare no conflict of interest.

References

1. Pandey, C.K.; Singh, A.; Kajal, K.; Dhankhar, M.; Tandon, M.; Pandey, V.K.; Karna, S.T. Intraoperative blood loss in orthotopic liver transplantation: The predictive factors. *World J. Gastrointest. Surg.* **2015**, *7*, 86–93. [CrossRef]
2. Cleland, S.; Corredor, C.; Ye, J.J.; Srinivas, C.; McCluskey, S.A. Massive haemorrhage in liver transplantation: Consequences, prediction and management. *World J. Transplant.* **2016**, *6*, 291–305. [CrossRef]
3. Levy, J.H.; Szlam, F.; Tanaka, K.A.; Sniecienski, R.M. Fibrinogen and hemostasis: A primary hemostatic target for the management of acquired bleeding. *Anesth. Analg.* **2012**, *114*, 261–274. [CrossRef] [PubMed]

4. Chow, J.H.; Lee, K.; Abuelkasem, E.; Udekwu, O.R.; Tanaka, K.A. Coagulation Management During Liver Transplantation: Use of Fibrinogen Concentrate, Recombinant Activated Factor VII, Prothrombin Complex Concentrate, and Antifibrinolytics. *Semin. Cardiothorac. Vasc. Anesth.* **2018**, *22*, 164–173. [CrossRef] [PubMed]
5. Callum, J.; Farkouh, M.E.; Scales, D.C.; Heddle, N.M.; Crowther, M.; Rao, V.; Hucke, H.P.; Carroll, J.; Grewal, D.; Brar, S.; et al. Effect of Fibrinogen Concentrate vs Cryoprecipitate on Blood Component Transfusion After Cardiac Surgery: The FIBRES Randomized Clinical Trial. *JAMA* **2019**, *322*, 1966–1976. [CrossRef] [PubMed]
6. Nguyen-Buckley, C.; Gao, W.; Agopian, V.; Wray, C.; Steadman, R.H.; Xia, V.W. Major Thromboembolic Complications in Liver Transplantation: The Role of Rotational Thromboelastometry and Cryoprecipitate Transfusion. *Transplantation* **2021**, *105*, 1771–1777. [CrossRef]
7. Mourad, M.M.; Liossis, C.; Gunson, B.K.; Mergental, H.; Isaac, J.; Muiesan, P.; Mirza, D.F.; Perera, M.T.; Bramhall, S.R. Etiology and management of hepatic artery thrombosis after adult liver transplantation. *Liver Transpl.* **2014**, *20*, 713–723. [CrossRef]
8. Hensley, N.B.; Mazzeffi, M.A. Pro-Con Debate: Fibrinogen Concentrate or Cryoprecipitate for Treatment of Acquired Hypofibrinogenemia in Cardiac Surgical Patients. *Anesth. Analg.* **2021**, *133*, 19–28. [CrossRef]
9. Galas, F.R.; de Almeida, J.P.; Fukushima, J.T.; Vincent, J.L.; Osawa, E.A.; Zeferino, S.; Camara, L.; Guimaraes, V.A.; Jatene, M.B.; Hajjar, L.A. Hemostatic effects of fibrinogen concentrate compared with cryoprecipitate in children after cardiac surgery: A randomized pilot trial. *J. Thorac. Cardiovasc. Surg.* **2014**, *148*, 1647–1655. [CrossRef]
10. Tanaka, K.A.; Bader, S.O.; Gorlinger, K. Novel approaches in management of perioperative coagulopathy. *Curr. Opin. Anaesthesiol.* **2014**, *27*, 72–80. [CrossRef]
11. Nascimento, B.; Goodnough, L.T.; Levy, J.H. Cryoprecipitate therapy. *Br. J. Anaesth.* **2014**, *113*, 922–934. [CrossRef] [PubMed]
12. Curry, N.; Wong, H. Cryoprecipitate transfusion: Current perspectives. *Int. J. Clin. Transfus. Med.* **2016**, *4*, 89–97. [CrossRef]
13. Kim, K.S.; Kwon, H.M.; Jung, K.W.; Sang, B.H.; Moon, Y.J.; Kim, B.; Jun, I.G.; Song, J.G.; Hwang, G.S. Markedly prolonged QTc interval in end-stage liver disease and risk of 30-day cardiovascular event after liver transplant. *J. Gastroenterol. Hepatol.* **2021**, *36*, 758–766. [CrossRef] [PubMed]
14. Franchini, M.; Lippi, G. Fibrinogen replacement therapy: A critical review of the literature. *Blood Transfus.* **2012**, *10*, 23–27. [CrossRef] [PubMed]
15. Kujovich, J.L. Hemostatic defects in end stage liver disease. *Crit. Care Clin.* **2005**, *21*, 563–587. [CrossRef] [PubMed]
16. American Society of Anesthesiologists Task Force on Perioperative Blood Management. Practice guidelines for perioperative blood management: An updated report by the American Society of Anesthesiologists Task Force on Perioperative Blood Management. *Anesthesiology* **2015**, *122*, 241–275. [CrossRef]
17. Jensen, N.H.; Stensballe, J.; Afshari, A. Comparing efficacy and safety of fibrinogen concentrate to cryoprecipitate in bleeding patients: A systematic review. *Acta Anaesthesiol. Scand.* **2016**, *60*, 1033–1042. [CrossRef]
18. Whyte, C.S.; Rastogi, A.; Ferguson, E.; Donnarumma, M.; Mutch, N.J. The Efficacy of Fibrinogen Concentrates in Relation to Cryoprecipitate in Restoring Clot Integrity and Stability against Lysis. *Int. J. Mol. Sci.* **2022**, *23*, 2944. [CrossRef]
19. Spahn, D.R.; Bouillon, B.; Cerny, V.; Duranteau, J.; Filipescu, D.; Hunt, B.J.; Komadina, R.; Maegele, M.; Nardi, G.; Riddez, L.; et al. The European guideline on management of major bleeding and coagulopathy following trauma: Fifth edition. *Crit. Care* **2019**, *23*, 98. [CrossRef]
20. Sabate, A.; Dalmau, A. Fibrinogen: A Clinical Update on Liver Transplantation. *Transplant. Proc.* **2015**, *47*, 2925–2928. [CrossRef]
21. Lisman, T.; Porte, R.J. Rebalanced hemostasis in patients with liver disease: Evidence and clinical consequences. *Blood* **2010**, *116*, 878–885. [CrossRef] [PubMed]
22. Caballero, M.; Sabate, A.; Gutierrez, R.; Beltran, J.; Perez, L.; Pujol, R.; Viguera, L.; Costa, M.; Reyes, R.; Martinez, A.; et al. Blood component requirements in liver transplantation: Effect of 2 thromboelastometry-guided strategies for bolus fibrinogen infusion-the TROMBOFIB randomized trial. *J. Thromb. Haemost.* **2023**, *21*, 37–46. [CrossRef] [PubMed]
23. Downey, L.A.; Andrews, J.; Hedlin, H.; Kamra, K.; McKenzie, E.D.; Hanley, F.L.; Williams, G.D.; Guzzetta, N.A. Fibrinogen Concentrate as an Alternative to Cryoprecipitate in a Postcardiopulmonary Transfusion Algorithm in Infants Undergoing Cardiac Surgery: A Prospective Randomized Controlled Trial. *Anesth. Analg.* **2020**, *130*, 740–751. [CrossRef] [PubMed]
24. Ahmed, S.; Harrity, C.; Johnson, S.; Varadkar, S.; McMorrow, S.; Fanning, R.; Flynn, C.M.; JM, O.R.; Byrne, B.M. The efficacy of fibrinogen concentrate compared with cryoprecipitate in major obstetric haemorrhage—An observational study. *Transfus. Med.* **2012**, *22*, 344–349. [CrossRef] [PubMed]
25. Obaid, O.; Anand, T.; Nelson, A.; Reina, R.; Ditillo, M.; Stewart, C.; Douglas, M.; Friese, R.; Gries, L.; Joseph, B. Fibrinogen Supplementation for the Trauma Patient: Should You Choose Fibrinogen Concentrate Over Cryoprecipitate? *J. Trauma. Acute Care Surg.* **2022**, *93*, 453–460. [CrossRef]
26. Choi, H.J. Current status and outcome of liver transplantation in South Korea. *Clin. Mol. Hepatol.* **2022**, *28*, 117–119. [CrossRef]
27. Maeda, T.; Miyata, S.; Usui, A.; Nishiwaki, K.; Tanaka, H.; Okita, Y.; Katori, N.; Shimizu, H.; Sasaki, H.; Ohnishi, Y.; et al. Safety of Fibrinogen Concentrate and Cryoprecipitate in Cardiovascular Surgery: Multicenter Database Study. *J. Cardiothorac. Vasc. Anesth.* **2019**, *33*, 321–327. [CrossRef]

Disclaimer/Publisher's Note: The statements, opinions and data contained in all publications are solely those of the individual author(s) and contributor(s) and not of MDPI and/or the editor(s). MDPI and/or the editor(s) disclaim responsibility for any injury to people or property resulting from any ideas, methods, instructions or products referred to in the content.

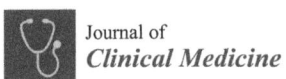

Article

Younger Age and Parenchyma-Sparing Surgery Positively Affected Long-Term Health-Related Quality of Life after Surgery for Pancreatic Neuroendocrine Neoplasms

Anna Caterina Milanetto [1,*], Claudia Armellin [1], Gloria Brigiari [2], Giulia Lorenzoni [2] and Claudio Pasquali [1]

[1] Chirurgia Generale 3, Pancreatic and Digestive Endocrine Surgery Research Group, Department of Surgery, Oncology and Gastroenterology, University of Padova, 35128 Padova, Italy
[2] Unit of Biostatistics, Epidemiology and Public Health, Department of Cardiac, Thoracic, Vascular Sciences and Public Health, University of Padova, 35128 Padova, Italy
* Correspondence: acmilanetto@unipd.it; Tel.: +39-049-8218831

Abstract: (1) Background: Patients with pancreatic Neuroendocrine Neoplasms (PanNENs) often have a long overall survival. We evaluated determinants of quality of life (QoL) after surgery for PanNENs. (2) Methods: Patients operated on for a PanNEN in our center (1990–2021) received three EORTC QoL questionnaires (QLQ-C30, QLQ-GI.NET21, QLQ-PAN26). Six domains were selected as outcome variables (global QoL, physical function -PF, social function -SF, disease-related worries -DRWs, pain, upper-gastrointestinal (GI) symptoms) and evaluated in relation to the clinical variables. Statistical analysis was performed using R software v 4.2.2. (3) Results: One hundred and four patients enrolled showed a good global QoL (median 83.3). Old age was a determinant of worse global QoL (p 0.006) and worse PF (p 0.003). Multiple comorbidities (p 0.002) and old age (p 0.034) were associated with pain, while male gender was related to better PF (p 0.007) and less pain (p 0.012). Patients who had undergone parenchyma-sparing surgery demonstrated better PF (p 0.037), better SF (p 0.012), and less upper-GI symptoms (p 0.047). At multivariable analysis, age (p 0.005) and type of surgery (p 0.028) were confirmed as determinants of global QoL. (4) Conclusions: In patients operated on for a PanNEN, a good HRQoL is generally reported; notably, younger age and parenchyma-sparing surgery seem to positively affect HRQoL.

Keywords: pancreas; neuroendocrine neoplasm; health-related quality of life; EORTC questionnaire; pancreatic surgery; parenchyma-sparing surgery

1. Introduction

Neuroendocrine neoplasms of the pancreas (PanNENs) are a heterogeneous group of neoplasms arising from cells in the diffuse neuroendocrine system located in the islets of Langerhans [1]. According to the Surveillance Epidemiology and End Results (SEERs) program, their incidence is currently estimated at 0.7 per 100,000, with a slight increase during the last years [2]. While a part of PanNENs produce biologically active peptides and are usually associated with distinct clinical syndromes (Functioning, F-PanNENs), most PanNENs are not related to a clinically significant hormone hyperproduction and are referred to as Non-Functioning (NF-PanNENs) [3]. According to their histopathological features, PanNENs are divided into well-differentiated neuroendocrine tumors (NETs) and poorly differentiated neuroendocrine carcinomas (NECs), with the latter having the worst prognosis and thus avoiding surgical resection. Surgery is the only curative treatment for PanNENs and is the best choice when tumors are localized to the pancreas, varying from enucleation to major pancreatic resections.

Patients with a PanNET usually show a favorable prognosis once operated on and a long survival when compared to other abdominal neoplasms [2], even if presenting with distant metastases at diagnosis. In the case of metastatic disease, other treatments may be required: loco-regional treatment (i.e., trans-arterial embolization for liver metastases) and systemic treatments, such as somatostatin analogues (SSAs), peptide receptor radionuclide therapy (PRRT), targeted therapy (i.e., Everolimus, Sunitinib), and chemotherapy, depending on tumor differentiation and grade.

Health-related quality of life (HRQoL) is an outcome of paramount importance in PanNEN patients, and it is a multidimensional construct that needs to be assessed as a patient-reported outcome [4]. The European Organization for Research and Treatment of Cancer (EORTC) is a leading association in determining HRQoL, and it constructed several questionnaires to assess that outcome in different neoplastic settings. The quality of life of NEN patients has been investigated in several recent studies [5–13], mentioning the impact of medical treatments in HRQoL, and using EORTC questionnaires as reference tools. Caplin et al. [5] in a study about the effect of SSAs on metastatic gastro-entero-pancreatic (GEP)-NETs demonstrated comparable levels of global QoL between the treatment and the placebo groups; Jimenez-Fonseca [6] confirmed the clinical benefit of SSA and also sunitinib, clearly supported by HRQoL assessment. Pavel et al. [7] reported that everolimus was associated with a worsening of HRQoL for GEP-NET patients, and Ramage et al. [8] showed that HRQoL is maintained in patients with PanNENs during treatment with everolimus, even if disease progression or death were recorded in 44% of patients during follow-up. An improvement in global QoL was reported after PRRT by Teunissen et al. [9] and Marinova et al. [10] in terms of increasing global health and the mitigation of physical complaints, whereas Martini et al. [11] showed in GEP-NET patients an overall stable HRQoL under PRRT but significant HRQoL impairments compared with the general population. Finally, in a recent systematic review and metanalysis by Ronde et al. [12], all treatments considered for GEP-NENs (SSA, PRRT, targeted therapies, and chemotherapy) appeared beneficial for disease stabilization while maintaining stable global health status, even if high-quality HRQoL reporting was lacking.

Most of the published studies about HRQoL in NEN patients involved not only pancreatic NENs but GEP-NEN patients globally, as it was also reported in a recent systematic review by Watson et al. [13], that a heterogeneous group of NENs consists of neoplasms arising from different organs which show different biological behavior and prognosis, thus the patients' outcomes are not comparable. To the best of our knowledge, this is the first study reporting about HRQoL determinants only in surgically treated PanNENs.

The primary endpoint of our study was to investigate HRQoL in patients who had already undergone a previous surgery for a PanNEN using the EORTC QoL questionnaires, and to verify if patients operated on for a PanNEN have an HRQoL of more than 66/100 in the functional scale and less than 33/100 in the symptoms scale. A secondary endpoint was to evaluate determinants of HRQoL, and to verify if patient-related (i.e., age, gender, other diseases, postoperative pancreatic function), disease-related (i.e., tumor grade and symptoms, tumor burden), or treatment-related (i.e., type of surgery, SSAs, systemic treatments) factors may influence the HRQoL. Another secondary endpoint was to compare the HRQoL of PanNEN patients with the HRQoL of the general population and of all cancer and hepato-pancreato-biliary (HPB) cancer populations, as reported in the EORTC reference values manual, and to verify if patients operated on for a PanNEN have a better HRQoL than the people affected by all/HPB cancer, and a slightly worse HRQoL than the general population.

2. Materials and Methods

2.1. Study Population

Patients who underwent surgery for a PanNEN between 1st January 1990 and 31st December 2021 in our Pancreatic Surgical Unit were identified from hospital computerized systems. Inclusion criteria were histologically confirmed diagnosis of PanNEN, and at least six months of follow-up after surgery. The majority of patients were enrolled during a routinely outpatient clinic follow-up, while the others were contacted by phone, were sent the questionnaires, and they returned the completed consent forms and questionnaires by mail. Clinical records of the included patients were retrieved (gender, age, other diseases, MEN-1 diagnosis, tumor functional state, tumor grade, type of surgery, tumor burden, SSA therapy, systemic/loco-regional treatment, further pancreatic surgery, and pancreatic function) and entered into an anonymized database. Written informed consent was obtained from all the patients. The study was approved by the local Ethical Committee (reference number 5091/AO/21). Enrollment of patients, questionnaire administration, and clinical data collection were carried out from 1 January 2022 to 31 December 2022.

2.2. HRQoL Assessment

To assess HRQoL in PanNEN patients, we used the Italian version of three different questionnaires from the EORTC website: EORTC QLQ-C30, EORTC QLQ-GI.NET21, and EORTC QLQ-PAN26 [14]. The EORTC Core Quality of Life Questionnaire (EORTC QLQ-C30) is a generic questionnaire which measures cancer patients' physical, psychological, and social functions, and it consists of 30 items divided into 16 functional scales, 12 symptom scales, and 2 global health and QoL items [15]. The EORTC gastro-intestinal NET questionnaire (EORTC QLQ-GINET21) is a specific questionnaire for gastro-intestinal (GI) NEN patients, and it includes 21 items (10 functional and 11 symptom scales) [16,17], and the EORTC pancreatic cancer questionnaire (EORTC QLQ-PAN26) is a specific questionnaire for pancreatic cancer patients, and it consists of 26 items (11 functional and 15 symptom scales) [18]. The scores for each item were first standardized to a 0–100 linear scale according to the EORTC QLQ Scoring Manual [19]. For the functional scales and global QoL, a high score represents a high level of functioning (i.e., better HRQoL), whereas for the symptom scales, a high score indicates a high level of symptomatology (i.e., worse HRQoL).

The three different questionnaires may include similar domains of HRQoL; for example, the domain "social functioning", is called "SF" in QLQ-C30, "SF21" in QLQ-GINET21, and "SF26" in QLQ-PAN26. Therefore, we created global domains consisting of all the items describing the same functioning or symptom scale among the three questionnaires (Table 1).

Table 1. Domain creation (all items included). In blue, items from EORTC-QLQ-C30. In yellow, items from EORTC-PAN26. In orange, items from EORTC-GiNET21. QoL, quality of life. PF, physical functioning. EF, emotional functioning. SX, sexuality. SF, social functioning. RF, role functioning. HCS, healthcare satisfaction. CF, cognitive functioning. PA, pain. TR, treatment-related symptoms. LGI, lower gastrointestinal symptoms. OS, other symptoms. UGI, upper-gastrointestinal symptoms. FI, financial difficulties. ED, endocrine symptoms. DRWs, disease-related worries. BI, body image.

Global QoL											
29	30										
Functional Scales											
		PF				EF				SX	
1	2	3	4	5	42	21	22	23	24	55	56	51
		SF				RF		HCS		CF	
26	27	42	44	49	52	6	7	53	54	50	20	25
Symptom Scales											
		PA						TR			
9	19	31	33	34	35	48	38	43	50	39	40
		LGI						OS			
16	17	35	36	32	40	46	47	8	10	11	12	18
		UGI								FI	
13	14	15	34	37	38	36	37	39	44	45	28
ED				DRWs					BI		
31	32	33	41	43	47	41	51	48	49	45	46

Finally, we selected the domains to be considered for the subsequent data analyses according to the current literature and to their relevance in the specific field of PanNENs.

The following HRQoL domains were considered as outcome variables and evaluated in relation to the clinical predictive variables: global QoL, physical functioning (PF), social functioning (SF), disease-related worries (DRWs), pain (PA, including pancreatic and bone–muscle pain), and upper-gastrointestinal symptoms (upper-GI, including appetite, nausea/vomiting, abdominal discomfort, acid ingestion/heartburn, difficulties with eating, restrictions in type and quantity of food, indigestion, itching, and jaundice).

Every chosen domain was first elaborated on separately, and a weighted average of the scores of each item grouped in each domain was calculated for every patient. Missing data were managed following indications reported in the EORTC QLQ-C30 Scoring Manual [19]: if at least half of the items of every single domain reported a valid score, the average score was considered valid. We considered as "missing data" all the missed answers due to a non-pertinent question (expressed as "NA" in the questionnaires, i.e., questions regarding systemic treatments' side effects for patients who did not receive any of those treatments) and all the missed answers due to a non-given answer. Median values (with interquartile ranges) were calculated.

Clinical predictive variables were considered binary whenever possible, as follows: gender (male vs. female), age (65–90 years vs. 20–64 years), MEN1 diagnosis (yes vs. no), PanNEN type (non-functioning vs. functioning), tumor grade (G2 vs. G1), surgery (parenchyma-sparing vs. standard resection), other treatments after surgery (SSA therapy, systemic/locoregional treatment, and/or redo surgery: yes vs. no), and postoperative pancreatic function (normal vs. exocrine insufficiency and/or new-onset diabetes). In the other cases, we established cut-off values as follows: comorbidities (no vs. single vs. multiple), and tumor burden (no evidence of disease vs. local recurrence vs. distant metastases).

2.3. Statistical Analysis

Descriptive statistics were reported as median (I–III quartiles) for continuous variables and percentages (absolute numbers) for categorical variables. The association between baseline characteristics and QoL scores was evaluated using the univariable Gamma model to account for the non-normal distribution of the outcomes. The marginal effect was computed considering the partial derivatives of the marginal expectation. Results were reported as average marginal effect (AME), 95% CI, and p-value. The AME should be interpreted as the mean change in the outcome variables (functional or symptom scales) per unit increase in the independent variable. Analyses were performed with R software v 4.2.2 [20] together with the package margins.

3. Results

In total, 112 patients operated on for a PanNEN in our Pancreatic Surgical Unit between 1990 and 2021 met the inclusion criteria, and 104 patients provided all the questionnaires needed and were enrolled in the study (response rate 92.9%). The median time from surgery to questionnaire completion was 109 (range, 6–384) months. Clinical data of the study population are reported in Table 2.

There were 41 men and 63 women, with a mean age of 63 (SD 13.5) years. Among them, 58% had non-functioning PanNEN (75% G1), 64% had multiple comorbidities, 54% had undergone a standard pancreatic resection, and 83% of patients showed a normal (or not impaired) pancreatic function at the time of the study. As reported in Table 3, patients showed good global QoL results (median 83.3; IQR 58.3–100) and reported low DRWs (median 26.7; IQR 13.3–33.3). Physical (median 94.4; IQR 77.8–100) and social (median 88.9; IQR 77.8–94.4) functions were modestly affected. Pain (median 9.2; IQR 0–19.1) and upper-GI symptoms (median 3.9; IQR 0–9.1) were rarely reported.

Distribution of EORTC scores according to the variables of interest are reported in Figure 1 and also detailed in the Supplementary Materials. Then, in Table 4, we have detailed the results of the univariable analysis.

Table 2. Clinical features of the study population (n = 104).

	At the Time of Surgery	
Gender, n (%)	Male	41 (39.4)
	Female	63 (60.6)
Type of NEN, n (%)	Functioning [1]	44 (42.3)
	Nonfunctioning	60 (57.7)
Tumor grade, n (%)	G1	73 (75.3)
	G2	24 (24.7)
	N/A	7
Type of surgery, n (%)	Parenchyma-sparing resection [2]	48 (46.1)
	Standard resection [3]	56 (53.9)
MEN-1 syndrome, n (%)	Yes	18 (17.3)
	No	86 (82.7)
	At the time of the study	
Age (years)	median (range)	63 (20–90)
	Under 65	53 (51.0)
	More/equal 65	51 (49.0)
Comorbidities, n (%)	No	13 (12.6)
	Single	24 (23.3)
	Multiple	66 (64.1)
	N/A	1
Tumor burden, n (%)	NED	91 (87.5)
	LR	6 (5.8)
	DM	7 (6.7)
Systemic and/or locoregional treatments, n (%)	Current	5 (4.8)
	Previous	2 (1.9)
	No	97 (93.3)
SSA therapy, n (%)	Current	10 (9.6)
	Previous	2 (1.9)
	No	92 (88.5)
New surgery, n (%)	Yes [4]	6 (5.8)
	No	98 (94.2)
Pancreatic function, n (%)	New onset diabetes mellitus	5 (4.8)
	Exocrine insufficiency	5 (4.8)
	Exocrine/Endocrine insufficiency	8 (7.7)
	Normal	86 (82.7)

Legend. NEN, neuroendocrine neoplasm. MEN, multiple endocrine neoplasia. SS-A, somatostatin analogues. N/A, missing data. NED, no evidence of disease. LR, local recurrence. DM, distant metastases. [1] In total, 34 insulinoma, 7 gastrinoma, 2 VIPoma, 1 glucagonoma. [2] In total, 33 enucleation, 11 central pancreatectomy, 4 duodenum-preserving pancreatic head resection. [3] In total, 1 total pancreatectomy, 9 pancreato-duodenectomy, 34 distal pancreatectomy, 12 spleen-preserving distal pancreatectomy. All results are reported as number of patients (apart from age). [4] In MEN1 patients.

Table 3. Preliminary analysis of questionnaires' data.

Outcome Variable (Missing Data) [1]	Median Value	IQR	Min	Max
Global QoL	83.3	58.3–100	5.6	100
Functional scales				
Physical functioning (0.2%)	94.4	77.8–100	5.6	100
Role functioning (0.5%)	100	83.3–100	0.0	100
Emotional functioning (1.2%)	91.7	75.0–100	25.0	100
Cognitive functioning	100	83.3–100	16.7	100
Social functioning (2.9%)	88.9	77.8–94.4	27.8	100
Healthcare satisfaction (8.3%)	77.8	66.7–100	0.0	100
Sexuality (23.7%)	100	100–100	0.0	100
Symptomatic scales				
Disease-related worries (10.2%)	26.7	13.3–33.3	8.0	80.0
Body image (8.4%)	8.3	0.0–16.7	0.0	66.7
Financial difficulties (1%)	0.0	0.0–0.0	0.0	100
Pain (1%)	9.2	0.0–19.0	0.0	80.9
Endocrine symptoms (1.3%)	0.0	0.0–16.7	0.0	88.9
Treatment-related symptoms (35.6%)	0.0	0.0–11.1	0.0	44.4
Lower-GI symptoms (0.4%)	8.3	4.2–20.8	0.0	62.5
Upper-GI symptoms (1%)	3.9	0.0–9.1	0.0	66.7
Other symptoms [2] (0.2%)	13.3	0.0–26.7	0.0	73.3

Legend. QoL, quality of life. GI, gastrointestinal. IQR, interquartile range. [1] The percentage of missing data is reported in brackets. [2] Fatigue, dyspnea, and sleep disorders.

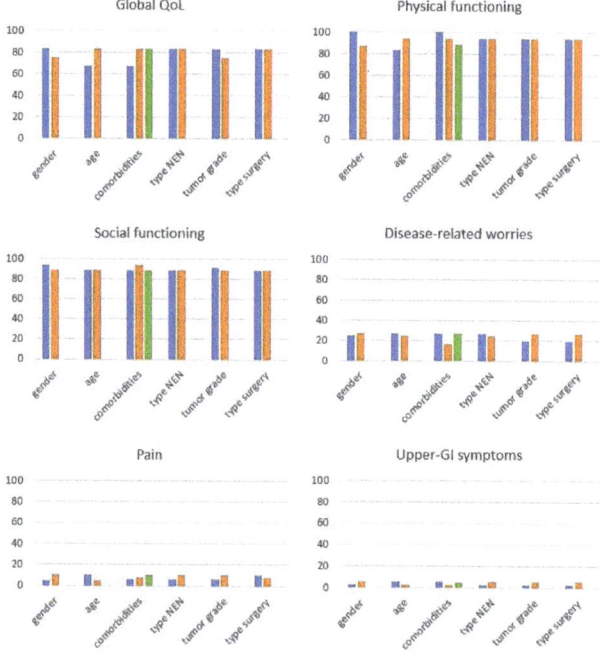

Figure 1. Distribution of EORTC scores according to the variables of interest. Data are median. **Legend.** Gender (male, in blue vs. female, in orange), age (65–90 years, in blue vs. 20–64 years, in orange), comorbidities (no, in blue vs. single, in orange vs. multiple, in green), type of pancreatic neuroendocrine neoplasm (non-functioning, in blue vs. functioning, in orange), tumor grade (G2, in blue vs. G1, in orange), surgery (parenchyma-sparing, in blue vs. standard resection, in orange). QoL, quality of life. GI, gastrointestinal.

Table 4. Results of the gamma regression. Data are reported as average marginal effect, 95% CI, and p-value.

	Functional Scales								Symptomatic Scales			
	Global QoL		Physical Functioning		Social Functioning		Disease-Related Worries		Pain		Upper-GI Symptoms	
	AME (95% CI)	p Value	AME (95% CI)	p Value	AME (95% CI)	p Value	AME (95% CI)	p Value	AME (95% CI)	p Value	AME (95% CI)	p Value
Gender												
Male	0.08 (−0.01, 0.17)	0.082	**0.11 (0.03, 0.19)**	**0.007**	0.05 (−0.02, 0.12)	0.17	−0.05 (−0.12, 0.03)	0.211	**−0.08 (−0.14, −0.02)**	**0.012**	−0.02 (−0.06, 0.02)	0.351
Female												
Age												
>/=65 y	**−0.12 (−0.21, −0.03)**	**0.006**	**−0.12 (−0.2, −0.04)**	**0.003**	−0.06 (−0.13, 0.01)	0.1	0.05 (−0.02, 0.13)	0.149	**0.07 (0.01, 0.14)**	**0.034**	0.04 (−0.01, 0.09)	0.082
<65 y												
Comorbidities												
No												
Single	0.06 (−0.1, 0.23)	0.44	−0.03 (−0.18, 0.12)	0.712	0.02 (−0.11, 0.15)	0.792	−0.05 (−0.16, 0.06)	0.352	0.03 (−0.03, 0.09)	0.304	−0.01 (−0.06, 0.04)	0.607
Multiple	−0.05 (−0.19, 0.09)	0.499	−0.11 (−0.24, 0.02)	0.105	−0.07 (−0.18, 0.04)	0.236	0.05 (−0.05, 0.16)	0.331	**0.1 (0.04, 0.15)**	**0.002**	0.03 (−0.02, 0.08)	0.223
Type of NEN												
NF	−0.02 (−0.11, 0.07)	0.718	0 (−0.08, 0.08)	0.989	−0.03 (−0.1, 0.04)	0.399	0.03 (−0.04, 0.11)	0.381	−0.01 (−0.08, 0.06)	0.737	0.02 (−0.02, 0.06)	0.346
F												
Tumor grade												
G2	0.06 (−0.05, 0.17)	0.267	−0.01 (−0.11, 0.08)	0.794	0 (−0.08, 0.08)	0.963	−0.02 (−0.1, 0.66)	0.65	−0.03 (−0.11, 0.04)	0.339	−0.01 (−0.06, 0.03)	0.61
G1												
Type of surgery												
Limited	0.07 (−0.02, 0.16)	0.141	**0.09 (0.01, 0.17)**	**0.037**	**0.09 (0.02, 0.16)**	**0.012**	−0.06 (−0.13, 0.01)	0.108	−0.01 (−0.08, 0.05)	0.693	**−0.04 (−0.08, 0)**	**0.047**
Standard												

Legend. QoL, quality of life. GI, gastrointestinal. AME, average marginal effect. NEN, neuroendocrine neoplasm. NF, nonfunctioning. F, functioning.

First, a worse global QoL was found to be significantly associated with older age (AME = −0.12; 95% CI = −0.21, −0.03; p value 0.006). No association was detected between global QoL and gender, comorbidities, type of NEN, tumor grade, or type of surgery.

Among the functional scales considered, a worse PF was found to be significantly associated with older age (AME −0.12; 95% CI −0.2, −0.04; p 0.003), whereas a significantly better PF was observed in male patients (AME 0.11; 95% CI 0.03, 0.19; p 0.007) and in patients who had undergone parenchyma-sparing surgery (AME 0.09; 95% CI 0.01, 0.17; p 0.037). Parenchyma-sparing surgery was also associated with a better SF (AME 0.09; 95% CI 0.02, 0.16; p 0.012).

In the analysis of symptomatic scales, pain was less complained by male patients (AME −0.08; 95% CI −0.14, −0.02; p 0.012), while it scored worse results both in older age (AME 0.07; 95% CI 0.01, 0.14; p 0.034) and in the case of multiple comorbidities (AME 0.10; 95% CI 0.04, 0.15; p 0.002). The presence of a single comorbidity was not related to significant changes in pain; this was also independent from tumor type, tumor grade, and type of surgery. Type of surgery showed a correlation with upper-GI symptoms, with better results in case of parenchyma-sparing surgery (AME −0.04; 95% CI −0.08, 0, p 0.047). Finally, DRWs showed no statistically significant correlations at all.

Within the multivariable analysis, three clinical variables were finally chosen in relation to global QoL depending on their theoretical meaningfulness for the study of NENs and on the significance of univariable analysis results: age, gender, and type of surgery. Data confirmed the significance of age (AME −0.12; 95% CI −0.22, −0.04; p 0.005) and type of surgery (AME 0.10; 95% CI 0.01, 0.19; p 0.028) in the determination of global QoL, while gender was not substantially related to QoL in this population (AME 0.07; 95% CI −0.02, 0.17; p 0.12).

4. Discussion

In this observational single-center study, 104 patients showed a good global QoL (median 83.3; IQR 58.3–100) after pancreatic surgery for a PanNEN. Despite the need for a pancreatic resection, a correct diagnosis and several treatment options may provide an excellent quality of life. The major long-term HRQoL determinants for those patients were found to be gender, age, and type of surgery, with age and surgery confirmed also as determinants of global QoL at multivariable analysis.

The male gender was related to a better PF (AME 0.11; p 0.007), and to a higher tolerance for pain (AME −0.08; p 0.012). In a similar study regarding HRQoL in patients operated on for a small intestinal NEN [21], the female gender and old age were found to be associated with worse outcomes. Then, treatment with SSAs and non-symptomatic NENs were associated with a better QoL, but those statistically significant results could not be verified in the present study due to biological and clinical differences existing between pancreatic and small intestinal NENs, and thus in the variables investigated.

In our study, men showed modestly increased scores for social relations and globally lower rates of DRWs; however, when comparing men and women, no significant implications can be suggested in the relation and attitude of both genders toward their neoplasm. In a recent study, Pijnappel et al. [22] investigated the experience of fear of tumor recurrence or progression in patients with pancreatic cancer treated with surgical resection, palliative systemic treatment, or best supportive care. In that study, and also according to our results, even if overall survival was not directly related to QoL, patients need to be guided by healthcare professionals through their treatment journey to deal with the internal distress caused by the fear of disease.

A globally worse QoL may be reasonably assumed in elderly people, and lower scores were also confirmed in our study, where at the time of questionnaire completion, PanNEN patients had a mean age of 63 years. Notably, 75% of patients underwent surgery for a grade 1 PanNET, a histological feature harboring a low risk of tumor recurrence, and patients' long survival. Old age was a determinant of a worse global QoL, confirmed at multivariable analysis (AME −0.13; p 0.005). In a recent study, Okuyama et al. [23] showed a general deterioration of the activities of daily living (ADL) among older patients after surgery for cancers of the GI and HPB tracts. However, the heterogeneity of the tumors included in that study does not make any comparison made with our results reliable.

As might be expected, in the present study, old age played a crucial role in the impairment of PF (AME −0.12; p 0.003), with a progressively increasing incidence of chronic diseases (multiple comorbidities in 64% of patients), and thus of soreness and pain complaints, as confirmed by the significant correlation between pain and both old age (AME 0.07; p 0.034) and multiple comorbidities (AME 0.1; p 0.002). A recent longitudinal study by Modica et al. [24] analyzed HRQoL in 39 patients with a GEP-NEN, with about half of them diagnosed with a PanNEN. HRQoL was assessed in relation to clinical severity and heterogeneity of NENs, as well as resilience. A higher number of therapies and lower levels of resilience were associated with lower global QoL scores and higher levels of symptomatic scales, while patients with a GEP-NEN showed higher HRQoL scores in many HRQoL domains; then, no statistically significant differences were highlighted between patients who underwent surgery and those who did not. Unfortunately, the global data reported for all GEP-NENs patients made a comparison with the present study unfeasible.

In our study, 54% of patients underwent a standard pancreatic resection, and 83% maintained normal (or not impaired) pancreatic function after surgery. Concerning parenchyma-sparing resections for PanNEN and benign neoplasms, the reported incidence of new onset/worsening diabetes mellitus and of exocrine insufficiency is 1–8% and 2–8%, respectively [25,26]. In our population, parenchyma-sparing resections were related to better PF (AME 0.09; p 0.037) and SF (AME 0.09; p 0.012), and they ensured a lower risk of developing upper-GI symptoms (AME −0.04; p 0.047), and the HRQoL domain that no other tumor nor patients' features seemed to affect. Short- and long-term outcomes, including QoL, were also assessed in a recent series of 81 patients surgically treated by pancreatic enucleation [27]; despite significant postoperative morbidity rates, those patients reported excellent long-term outcomes and a QoL being comparable to the general population.

The EORTC QLQ-C30 Manual [28] includes reference values for QLQ-C30, and it has a specific section for QoL in the general population and in different groups of cancer patients. Notably, in that manual, an HPB cancer patients' group is analyzed, consisting mainly of men aged more than 50 years and of 298 pancreatic cancer patients (out of 750 total HPB cancer patients). Those patients showed a scarce global QoL (median value 58.3, IQR 41.7–75.0) with good functional results (both PF and SF) but high rates regarding fatigue, insomnia, and appetite loss symptoms [28]. All cancer patients globally reported a discrete global QoL (median value 66.7, IQR 50.0–83.3), with functional scales median values over 80.0, and complaining above all about fatigue, pain, and insomnia (median values more than 25.0) [28]. Our study population of surgically treated PanNEN patients showed excellent outcomes (median global QoL over 83.0 and median values of functional and symptoms scales ranging between 80.0 and 100 and 4.0 and 27.0, respectively) when compared to HPB and all cancer patients. Moreover, PanNEN patients' outcomes are similar to the results reported in the EORTC manual for the general population, with a median global QoL of 75.0 (IQR 58.3–83.3), functional scales with a median of 100 in both PF and SF, and symptomatic scales' rates globally less than 25.0 [27].

Our study has some strengths and limitations.

Regarding the strengths, this study reports a single-center case series of high numerosity when considering that PanNENs represent a rare disease. This is the first study reporting about HRQoL determinants only in patients who were surgically treated for a PanNEN. All enrolled patients were operated on and followed-up at the same pancreatic surgical center, so treatment choices appear homogeneous over the years. Patients were followed-up regularly in the postoperative period and were examined for HRQoL after a long-term follow-up, with a median time of nine years after surgery. Finally, among the patients in regular follow-up first asked to join the study, we observed a very high response rate (93%) to the questionnaires.

Regarding the limitations, the research planning started in 2020, and we decided to administer to pancreatic NEN patients the three validated EORTC questionnaires, which could better investigate HRQoL in that peculiar study population. In fact, specific EORTC questionnaires for functioning and/or NF-PanNENs were not available at that time. Patients made a great effort to answer all the questions of the three questionnaires, which sometimes were not applicable to their personal experience, and we also had to merge all the items of similar domains among the different questionnaires to ensure a proper data analysis with reliable results. In the spring of 2023, EORTC released two new questionnaires regarding PanNETs (QLQ-P.NET15 for gastrinoma/nonfunctioning and QLQ-PNET19 for insulinoma) which are still in the validation phase.

5. Conclusions

This is the first study evaluating long-term HRQoL after surgery in patients with a PanNEN. In this subset of patients, younger age and parenchyma-sparing surgery seem to positively affect HRQoL, and a good global QoL is reported even when compared to the general population. Elderly women who have undergone a standard pancreatic resection and are affected by multiple comorbidities show the worst HRQoL outcomes and may be the subset of operated PanNEN patients who need more support by the healthcare system and healthcare professionals.

Supplementary Materials: The following supporting information can be downloaded at: https://www.mdpi.com/article/10.3390/jcm12206529/s1, Table S1. Distribution of EORTC scores according to the variables of interest. Data are median [I quartile-III quartile].

Author Contributions: Conceptualization, A.C.M. and C.P.; formal analysis, C.A., G.L. and G.B.; writing—original draft preparation, A.C.M. and C.A.; writing—review and editing, A.C.M., G.L., G.B. and C.P. All authors have read and agreed to the published version of the manuscript.

Funding: This research was partially financially supported by IPSEN SpA, but they had no input into the content.

Institutional Review Board Statement: The study was conducted according to the guidelines of the Declaration of Helsinki and approved by the Ethics Committee of Azienda Ospedale-Università di Padova (protocol code 5091/AO/21).

Informed Consent Statement: Written informed consent has been obtained from the patients to publish this paper.

Data Availability Statement: The data presented in this study are available on request from the corresponding author. The data are not publicly available due to privacy.

Conflicts of Interest: The sponsors had no role in the design, execution, interpretation, or writing of the study.

References

1. Khanna, L.; Prasad, S.R.; Sunnapwar, A.; Kondapaneni, S.; Dasyam, A.; Tammisetti, V.S.; Salman, U.; Nazarullah, A.; Katabathina, V.S. Pancreatic Neuroendocrine Neoplasms: 2020 Update on Pathologic and Imaging Findings and Classification. *Radiographics* **2020**, *40*, 1240–1262. [CrossRef] [PubMed]
2. Dasari, A.; Shen, C.; Halperin, D.; Zhao, B.; Zhou, S.; Xu, Y.; Shih, T.; Yao, J.C. Trends in the Incidence, Prevalence, and Survival Outcomes in Patients with Neuroendocrine Tumors in the United States. *JAMA Oncol.* **2017**, *3*, 1335–1342. [CrossRef] [PubMed]
3. Öberg, K.; Knigge, U.; Kwekkeboom, D.; Perren, A.; ESMO Guidelines Working Group. Neuroendocrine gastro-entero-pancreatic tumors: ESMO Clinical Practice Guidelines for diagnosis, treatment and follow-up. *Ann. Oncol.* **2012**, *23* (Suppl. 7), vii124–vii130. [CrossRef] [PubMed]
4. Cella, D.F. Measuring quality of life in palliative care. *Semin. Oncol.* **1995**, *22*, 73–81. [PubMed]
5. Caplin, M.E.; Pavel, M.; Ćwikła, J.B.; Phan, A.T.; Raderer, M.; Sedláčková, E.; Cadiot, G.; Wolin, E.M.; Capdevila, J.; Wall, L.; et al. Lanreotide in metastatic enteropancreatic neuroendocrine tumors. *N. Engl. J. Med.* **2014**, *371*, 224–233. [CrossRef]

6. Jiménez-Fonseca, P.; Carmona-Bayonas, A.; Martín-Pérez, E.; Crespo, G.; Serrano, R.; Llanos, M.; Villabona, C.; García-Carbonero, R.; Aller, J.; Capdevila, J.; et al. Health-related quality of life in well-differentiated metastatic gastroenteropancreatic neuroendocrine tumors. *Cancer Metastasis Rev.* **2015**, *34*, 381–400. [CrossRef]
7. Pavel, M.; Unger, N.; Borbath, I.; Ricci, S.; Hwang, T.L.; Brechenmacher, T.; Park, J.; Herbst, F.; Beaumont, J.L.; Bechter, O. Safety and QOL in Patients with Advanced NET in a Phase 3b Expanded Access Study of Everolimus. *Target. Oncol.* **2016**, *11*, 667–675. [CrossRef]
8. Ramage, J.K.; Punia, P.; Faluyi, O.; Frilling, A.; Meyer, T.; Saharan, R.; Valle, J.W. Observational Study to Assess Quality of Life in Patients with Pancreatic Neuroendocrine Tumors Receiving Treatment with Everolimus: The OBLIQUE Study (UK Phase IV Trial). *Neuroendocrinology* **2019**, *108*, 317–327. [CrossRef]
9. Teunissen, J.J.; Kwekkeboom, D.J.; Krenning, E.P. Quality of life in patients with gastroenteropancreatic tumors treated with [177Lu-DOTA0, Tyr3]octreotate. *J. Clin. Oncol.* **2004**, *22*, 2724–2729. [CrossRef]
10. Marinova, M.; Mücke, M.; Mahlberg, L.; Essler, M.; Cuhls, H.; Radbruch, L.; Conrad, R.; Ahmadzadehfar, H. Improving quality of life in patients with pancreatic neuroendocrine tumor following peptide receptor radionuclide therapy assessed by EORTC QLQ-C30. *Eur. J. Nucl. Med. Mol. Imaging* **2018**, *45*, 38–46. [CrossRef]
11. Martini, C.; Buxbaum, S.; Rodrigues, M.; Nilica, B.; Scarpa, L.; Holzner, B.; Virgolini, I.; Gamper, E.M. Quality of Life in Patients with Metastatic Gastroenteropancreatic Neuroendocrine Tumors Receiving Peptide Receptor Radionuclide Therapy: Information from a Monitoring Program in Clinical Routine. *J. Nucl. Med.* **2018**, *59*, 1566–1573. [CrossRef]
12. Ronde, E.M.; Heidsma, C.M.; Eskes, A.M.; Schopman, J.E.; Nieveen van Dijkum, E.J.M. Health-related quality of life and treatment effects in patients with well-differentiated gastroenteropancreatic neuroendocrine neoplasms: A systematic review and meta-analysis. *Eur. J. Cancer Care* **2021**, *30*, e13504. [CrossRef] [PubMed]
13. Watson, C.; Tallentire, C.W.; Ramage, J.K.; Srirajaskanthan, R.; Leeuwenkamp, O.R.; Fountain, D. Quality of life in patients with gastroenteropancreatic tumours: A systematic literature review. *World J. Gastroenterol.* **2020**, *26*, 3686–3711. [CrossRef]
14. EORTC Quality of Life. Available online: https://qol.eortc.org/questionnaires/ (accessed on 23 July 2023).
15. Aaronson, N.K.; Ahmedzai, S.; Bergman, B.; Bullinger, M.; Cull, A.; Duez, N.J.; Filiberti, A.; Flechtner, H.; Fleishman, S.B.; de Haes, J.C.; et al. The European Organization for Research and Treatment of Cancer QLQ-C30: A quality-of-life instrument for use in international clinical trials in oncology. *J. Natl. Cancer Inst.* **1993**, *85*, 365–376. [CrossRef] [PubMed]
16. Yadegarfar, G.; Friend, L.; Jones, L.; Plum, L.M.; Ardill, J.; Taal, B.; Larsson, G.; Jeziorski, K.; Kwekkeboom, D.; Ramage, J.K.; et al. Validation of the EORTC QLQ-GINET21 questionnaire for assessing quality of life of patients with gastrointestinal neuroendocrine tumours. *Br. J. Cancer* **2013**, *108*, 301–310. [CrossRef]
17. Davies, A.H.; Larsson, G.; Ardill, J.; Friend, E.; Jones, L.; Falconi, M.; Bettini, R.; Koller, M.; Sezer, O.; Fleissner, C.; et al. Development of a disease-specific Quality of Life questionnaire module for patients with gastrointestinal neuroendocrine tumours. *Eur. J. Cancer* **2006**, *42*, 477–484. [CrossRef]
18. Eaton, A.; Karanicolas, P.; Mchir, J.; Bottomley, A.; Allen, P.; Gonen, M. Psychometric validation of the EORTC QLQ-PAN26 pancreatic cancer module for assessing health related quality of life after pancreatic resection. *JOP* **2017**, *18*, 19–25.
19. Fayers, P.M.; Aaronson, N.K.; Bjordal, K.; Groenvold, M.; Curran, D.; Bottomley, A. Scoring procedures. In *The EORTC QLQ-C30 Scoring Manual*, 3rd ed.; EORTC Quality of Life Group Publications: Brussels, Belgium, 2001; pp. 6–14.
20. R Core Team. *R: A Language and Environment for Statistical Computing*; R Foundation for Statistical Computing: Vienna, Austria, 2022; Available online: https://www.R-project.org/ (accessed on 1 September 2023).
21. Milanetto, A.C.; Nordenström, E.; Sundlöv, A.; Almquist, M. Health-Related Quality of Life After Surgery for Small Intestinal Neuroendocrine Tumours. *World J. Surg.* **2018**, *42*, 3231–3239. [CrossRef]
22. Pijnappel, E.N.; Dijksterhuis, W.P.M.; Sprangers, M.A.G.; Augustinus, S.; de Vos-Geelen, J.; de Hingh, I.H.J.T.; Molenaar, I.Q.; Busch, O.R.; Besselink, M.G.; Wilmink, J.W.; et al. The fear of cancer recurrence and progression in patients with pancreatic cancer. *Support. Care Cancer* **2022**, *30*, 4879–4887. [CrossRef]
23. Okuyama, A.; Kosaka, H.; Kaibori, M.; Higashi, T.; Ogawa, A. Activities of daily living after surgery among older patients with gastrointestinal and hepatobiliary-pancreatic cancers: A retrospective observational study using nationwide health services utilisation data from Japan. *BMJ Open* **2023**, *13*, e070415. [CrossRef]
24. Modica, R.; Scandurra, C.; Maldonato, N.M.; Dolce, P.; Dipietrangelo, G.G.; Centello, R.; Di Vito, V.; Giannetta, E.; Isidori, A.M.; Lenzi, A.; et al. Health-related quality of life in patients with neuroendocrine neoplasms: A two-wave longitudinal study. *J. Endocrinol. Investig.* **2022**, *45*, 2193–2200. [CrossRef] [PubMed]
25. Crippa, S.; Boninsegna, L.; Partelli, S.; Falconi, M. Parenchyma-sparing resections for pancreatic neoplasms. *J. Hepato-Biliary-Pancreatic Sci.* **2010**, *17*, 782–787. [CrossRef] [PubMed]
26. Beger, H.G.; Mayer, B.; Vasilescu, C.; Poch, B. Long-term Metabolic Morbidity and Steatohepatosis Following Standard Pancreatic Resections and Parenchyma-sparing, Local Extirpations for Benign Tumor: A Systematic Review and Meta-analysis. *Ann. Surg.* **2022**, *275*, 54–66. [CrossRef]

27. Giuliani, T.; De Pastena, M.; Paiella, S.; Marchegiani, G.; Landoni, L.; Festini, M.; Ramera, M.; Marinelli, V.; Casetti, L.; Esposito, A.; et al. Pancreatic Enucleation Patients Share the Same Quality of Life as the General Population at Long-Term Follow-Up: A Propensity Score-Matched Analysis. *Ann. Surg.* **2023**, *277*, e609–e616. [CrossRef] [PubMed]
28. Scott, N.W.; Fayers, P.M.; Aaronson, N.K.; Bottomley, A.; de Graeff, A.; Groenvold, M.; Gundy, C.; Koller, M.; Petersen, M.A.; Sprangers, M.A.G.; et al. EORTC QLQC30 tables of reference values. In *The EORTC QLQ-C30 Reference Values Manual*; EORTC Quality of Life Group Publications: Brussels, Belgium, 2008; pp. 14–294.

Disclaimer/Publisher's Note: The statements, opinions and data contained in all publications are solely those of the individual author(s) and contributor(s) and not of MDPI and/or the editor(s). MDPI and/or the editor(s) disclaim responsibility for any injury to people or property resulting from any ideas, methods, instructions or products referred to in the content.

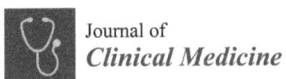

Article

Comparison of Two Techniques Performing the Supine-to-Sitting Postural Change in Patients with Sternotomy

Marica Giardini [1], Marco Guenzi [2], Ilaria Arcolin [1,*], Marco Godi [1], Massimo Pistono [2] and Marco Caligari [3]

[1] Istituti Clinici Scientifici Maugeri IRCCS, Division of Physical Medicine and Rehabilitation of Veruno Institute, 28013 Gattico-Veruno, Italy; marica.giardini@icsmaugeri.it (M.G.); marco.godi@icsmaugeri.it (M.G.)

[2] Istituti Clinici Scientifici Maugeri IRCCS, Division of Cardiac Rehabilitation of Veruno Institute, 28103 Gattico-Veruno, Italy; marco.guenzi@icsmaugeri.it (M.G.); massimo.pistono@icsmaugeri.it (M.P.)

[3] Istituti Clinici Scientifici Maugeri IRCCS, Integrated Laboratory of Assistive Solutions and Translational Research (LISART), Scientific Institute of Pavia, 27100 Pavia, Italy; marco.caligari@icsmaugeri.it

* Correspondence: ilaria.arcolin@icsmaugeri.it; Tel.: +39-0322-884906

Abstract: Patients with sternotomy are advised to follow sternal precautions to avoid the risk of sternal complications. However, there are no standard recommendations, in particular to perform the supine-to-sitting postural change, where sternal asymmetrical force may be applied. The aim of this study was to compare the rotational movement and the use of a tied rope (individual device for supine-to-sitting, "IDSS") to perform the supine-to-sitting postural change. A total of 92 patients (26% female) admitted to a rehabilitative post-surgery ward with sternotomy were assessed for sternal instability. Levels of pain and perceived effort during the two modalities of postural change and at rest were assessed. Patients reported higher values of pain and perceived effort (both $p < 0.0005$) during rotational movement with respect to the use of the IDSS. Moreover, patients with sternal instability (14%) and female patients with macromastia (25%) reported higher pain than those stable or without macromastia (both $p < 0.05$). No other risk factors were associated with pain. Thus, the IDSS seems to reduce the levels of pain and perceived effort during the supine-to-sitting postural change. Future studies with quantitative assessments are required to suggest the adoption of this technique, mostly in patients with high levels of pain or with sternal instability.

Keywords: perceived effort; pain; postural change; rehabilitation; sternal instability; sternotomy; supine-to-sitting

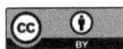

Citation: Giardini, M.; Guenzi, M.; Arcolin, I.; Godi, M.; Pistono, M.; Caligari, M. Comparison of Two Techniques Performing the Supine-to-Sitting Postural Change in Patients with Sternotomy. *J. Clin. Med.* **2023**, *12*, 4665. https://doi.org/10.3390/jcm12144665

Academic Editor: Dimitrios E. Magouliotis

Received: 20 May 2023
Revised: 7 July 2023
Accepted: 11 July 2023
Published: 13 July 2023

Copyright: © 2023 by the authors. Licensee MDPI, Basel, Switzerland. This article is an open access article distributed under the terms and conditions of the Creative Commons Attribution (CC BY) license (https://creativecommons.org/licenses/by/4.0/).

1. Introduction

Median sternotomy is the gold standard in cardiac surgery incisions for the treatment of all congenital and acquired heart diseases [1]. It is performed on about one million patients every year all over the world [2]. However, sternotomy is not immune from complications, such as dehiscence, mediastinitis, osteomyelitis, and sternal displacements [3]. Sternal displacements are the most common sternal complication following cardiac surgery [4]. This is due to micromotion between the two halves of the wired sternum [5]. Sternal displacements have an underestimated incidence of about 1–8% [6–8], which causes an increased mortality of 10–40% in patients. It should therefore be clinical practice to prompt the patient to avoid sudden movements during the acute phase, which may result in high traction forces to the sternal edges [9]. Additionally, repetitive inadequate movements can cause a gradual gliding trauma in the post-acute phase. This can develop into a sternal separation produced mainly by lateral distraction forces, usually accompanied by pain syndromes [10].

Cough and asymmetrical movements with upper limbs and trunk are the main risk factors for sternal displacement [4,11–14]. Thus, optimising timely intervention and providing the patient with detailed indications on how to perform daily life activities might reduce pain, morbidity, mortality, and total cost of care [1,2,15–18]. These indications are called "sternal precautions" [19]. However, in recent years, some studies agreed that this term is excessively restrictive. It was suggested to adopt pain and/or sternum discomfort as a marker to identify the possible presence of sternal instability; in this view, patients should be instructed to perform daily life activities within a pain-free range [17,20]. Recent studies showed that providing patients with instructions to encourage the use of upper limbs within pain limit or discomfort during daily activities did not increase the risk of sternal complications with respect to conventional "restrictive" precautions [17,21]. Moreover, it did seem that restrictive guidelines could induce self-efficacy in patients, promoting anxiety and depression [22].

Although the health facilities affect how indications are provided, 90% of the physiotherapists offered pre- and post-operative information, such as early mobilisation, post-sternotomy restrictions, techniques for bed/chair mobility, breathing exercises, coughing techniques, and information about exercising the lower extremities [23,24]. While exercises, such as cardiopulmonary and general mobility, are usually performed for a few minutes a day, and with the assistance or supervision of the physiotherapist, postural changes are the most common movements, repeated several times in the day. The postural change that particularly urges with shear forces to the sternum is the "supine-to-sit" [24]. The two most common methods to perform this postural change are (1) the "rotational" one (with the indication: "Keep your move into the tube" by Adams et al. [25]), i.e., passage from the supine position to the lateral decubitus position and then, pushing with the arms on the bed, to the sitting position [26]; and (2) the use of a rope (which will be called individual device for supine-to-sitting "IDSS") tied to the bottom of the bed, to be pulled symmetrically with the upper limbs in order to reach the sitting position. Although the second modality is quite usual in post-operative settings in improving autonomy and in reducing the risks, there is lack of evidence in literature. Up to now, no studies investigated implications for the sternal wound, and apparently no comparison study between the two methods exists.

Thus, the aim of the present study was to evaluate which of the two postural change modalities, through a rotational movement or performed using the IDSS, was less painful and evoked less perceived effort, in order to identify which modality should be recommended to patients with sternotomy.

2. Materials and Methods

2.1. Participants

This observational study was conducted between April and October 2022, at the Istituti Clinici Scientifici Maugeri IRCCS, Institute of Veruno, Italy. Patients were recruited among those admitted to the Cardiac Rehabilitation ward, those of which underwent surgery with median sternotomy under general anesthesia. All subjects met the following inclusion criteria: (1) presence of pain due to the sternotomy, defined as a score of at least 1 point on the numeric rating scale (NRS), during the postural change supine-to-sitting; (2) normal cognitive functioning (maximum of 0–2 errors in the Short Portable Mental State Questionary [27]); (3) ability to provide informed consent; (4) ability to get out of bed autonomously; and (5) stable clinical parameters. Exclusion criteria were other important comorbidities (i.e., orthopedic surgery < 6 months before, neurological disease, etc.), the presence of medical devices that limit movement (i.e., drainage) or the medical prescription of wearing sternal support harness.

The study protocol was approved by the Ethics Committee of the Istituti Clinici Scientifici Maugeri, Italy (approval number #2448 CE) and all participants signed the informed consent.

2.2. Assessment and Data Collection

All subjects were evaluated the day of admission by a physiotherapist with at least ten years of experience in cardiac rehabilitation. Age, sex, height, weight, smoking history, comorbidities, presence of macromastia in women (EU bra size > 80), and measurement of chest circumference in an upright position, at the mamillar line with the use of a tape measure, were recorded. The following evaluations were used:

2.2.1. Sternal Instability Scale (SIS)

SIS is a 4-point scale that aims to assess the stability of the sternum and assign a corresponding grade to the findings of examination as follows: 0, clinically stable sternum (no detectable motion)—normal; 1, minimally separated sternum (slight increase in motion upon special testing—upper limbs, trunk); 2, partially separated sternum—regional (moderate increase in motion upon special testing); and 3, completely separated sternum—entire length (marked increase in motion upon special testing) [14].

2.2.2. Numerical Rating Scale (NRS)

The patient's pain assessment was conducted via a self-reported NRS of 11 points, where 0 means no pain and 10 means worst pain [28]. The NRS can be verbally administered without the use of physical materials. NRS showed evidence of acceptability, reliability, and validity [29,30]. NRS values of 1–3 indicate mild pain, 4–6 moderate pain, and ≥ 7 severe pain [31].

Moreover, the perceived level of effort during postural changes was rated using the NRS (0–10).

2.3. Procedure

After recording the subjects' anthropometric data and evaluating sternal stability with the SIS scale, subjects were asked to perform the postural change from the supine to the sitting position. The postural change was carried out with two distinct techniques: (a) rotational postural change [18] and (b) postural change using IDSS. The IDSS was a simple durable strip of inelastic fabric, soft to the touch, washable, 390 cm long, and 10 cm wide. Folded in two, it was tied to the foot of the patient's bed by means of a lark's head knot (see the Supplementary Materials).

For both techniques, before performing the postural change, patients were in the semi-Fowler's position, lying on the bed with a trunk inclination of 30° [32], while at the end of the postural change they reached the sitting position on the bed with their feet on the floor. One familiarization trial for each modality was allowed and the instructions were standardized as follows:

- Rotational postural change [18]: (a) move your feet towards the edge of the bed; (b) roll on the side; (c) lower the legs from the edge of the bed; and (d) reach the sitting position by helping yourself with the arms (pushing to the side), trying to keep them as close as possible to the trunk.
- Postural change using IDSS: (a) move the legs towards the edge of the bed, putting them diagonally; (b) tighten the IDSS with one hand, turning the palm upwards; (c) with the other hand, always with the palm facing upwards, grab the hand that already holds the IDSS; (d) pull the IDSS by bending the elbows and, at the same time, activate the abdominal muscles, bringing the trunk to 90° with respect to the bed plane; and (e) place your legs completely outside the bed top and settle in a sitting position.

During this procedure, a dynamometer was placed between the IDSS and the footboard of the bed in order to measure the peak force, expressed in kilograms–weight, exerted by the patient on the IDSS.

2.4. Follow-Up

At discharge from the cardiac rehabilitation ward, patients were instructed to use the learnt sternal precautions, such as performing the supine-to-sitting postural change with their most pain-free modality. Patients were interviewed through a follow-up call after 6 months from the discharge in order to report if they had serious complications, as would infection or sternal instability, that required other medical interventions.

2.5. Statistical Analysis

Mean ± standard deviation (SD) values were used for descriptive statistics and figures.

A test for normality (Shapiro–Wilk) was performed in all recorded variables. Comparisons of mean pain levels during the three postural conditions (at rest, rotational postural change, and IDSS) were made by one-way repeated-measure ANOVA tests. When ANOVA gave a significant result, the post-hoc Tukey test was conducted to assess differences between postural conditions. To detect differences in perceived level of effort between the two postural conditions (rotational postural change and IDSS) a paired Student's t-tests was performed.

The clinical meaning of differences between the two modalities of postural change was assessed through the calculation of the Cohen's d effect size, with the commonly used interpretation that refers to effect sizes as small ($d = 0.2$), medium ($d = 0.5$), and large ($d = 0.8$) based on benchmarks suggested by Cohen [33].

Then, to evaluate the effect of each risk factor (sternal instability, smoking history, presence of macromastia (only women), chronic obstructive pulmonary disease (COPD), obesity, and diabetes) on pain, a subgroup analysis was performed with patients divided for the presence/absence of the main factor risk. Sternal instability was defined as a score ≥ 1 on SIS, while the presence of macromastia as an EU bra size > 80. For each risk factor, a 2-way repeated-measures ANOVA was conducted with the groups (with or without each factor risk) as independent factors and within the three postural conditions (at rest, during rotational and IDSS postural change). When ANOVA gave a significant result, the post-hoc Tukey test was conducted to assess differences between postural conditions.

Spearman's rank correlation was used to evaluate correlation among variables. Correlation coefficients (ρ) were interpreted as follows: strong correlation if the coefficient value lies between 0.50 and 1; moderate if the value lies between 0.30 and 0.49; and fair if the value lies below 0.29 [34].

Sample size was calculated from El-Ansary et al. [35]; in this study, patients who underwent cardiac surgery via median sternotomy reported a mean pain of about 3.1 points (SD = 2.3) during the supine-to-sitting postural change two weeks after surgery. Since a change of 2 points on NRS was found to be clinically meaningful [36], we expected a difference in pain between the rotational postural change and IDSS postural change of about a 0.5 effect size. Therefore, a sample size of at least 84 patients was required to detect differences between the two postural changes with 90% power (alpha = 0.05, 2-tailed).

Statistical analysis was performed using Statistica software (version 7.1, StatSoft Inc., Tulsa, OK, USA).

3. Results

Of 181 patients admitted to our cardiac rehabilitation ward with median sternotomy, 92 patients (51%) met the inclusion criteria. The participants' demographic and clinical data are reported in Table 1.

Patients were admitted and assessed between the fifth and the fifteenth day after surgery, with a mean time of 8.14 ± 2.62 days. The mean traction force exerted on IDSS during the postural change was 10.13 ± 4.20 kg.

On the SIS, 79 patients (86%) reported a score of 0 (stable, no sternal movements), 7 (8%) a score of 1 (minimally separated sternum), 5 (5%) a score of 2 (partially separated sternum), and only 1 (1%) the worst score of 3 (completely separated sternum).

Table 1. Characteristics of enrolled patients (*n* = 92).

	Mean	SD
Age (years)	66.37	12.05
Sex (M/F)	68/24	
Height (cm)	167.14	8.31
Weight (kg)	73.66	13.35
BMI index	26.25	3.52
Obesity (yes, no)	13/79	
Thorax size (cm)	99.70	8.29
Macromastia (yes/no, only women)	6/18	
Diabetes (yes/no)	16/76	
COPD (yes/no)	2/90	
Smoking history (yes/no)	22/70	
Time from surgery (days)	8.14	2.62

Abbreviations: BMI, body mass index; COPD, chronic obstructive pulmonary disease; F, female; and M, male.

3.1. Pain and Perceived Level of Effort

The mean values of pain and perceived level of effort during the three postural conditions are shown in Figure 1. The mean pain on NRS was 0.73 ± 1.44 points at rest, 5.34 ± 2.32 points during the rotational postural change, and 1.04 ± 1.40 points when performing the postural change with the IDSS. Pain was significantly different between the conditions (ANOVA, F(2,91) = 250.70; $p < 0.0005$). Post-hoc analysis showed that pain was significantly higher during the rotational postural change with respect to the other two conditions ($p < 0.0005$). No difference in pain was found between rest and IDSS. The difference of pain during rotational postural change and the other two conditions showed a large effect size (d = 2.2 when compared to rest, d = 2.3 when compared to IDSS). When analyzing the distribution of pain during the three different postural conditions, it emerged that patients experienced severe pain only in the rotational condition (Figure 2).

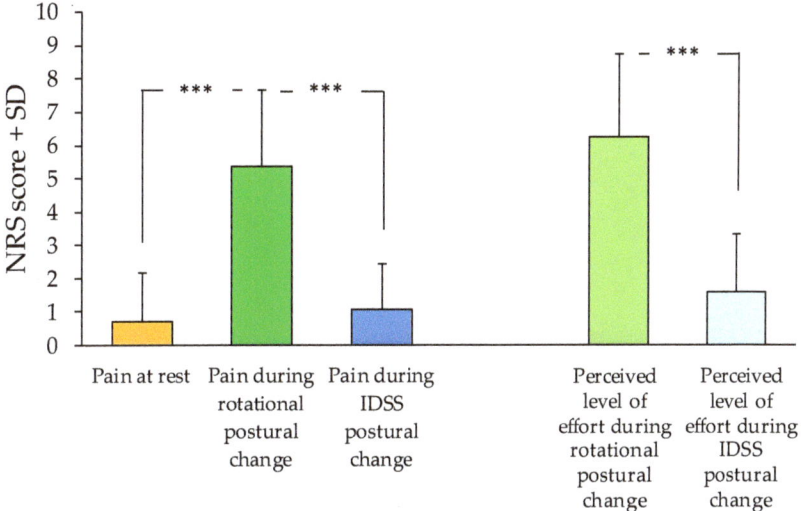

Figure 1. Comparison between pain at rest and across both postural changes, and between perceived level of effort during rotational and IDSS postural change; *** $p < 0.0005$.

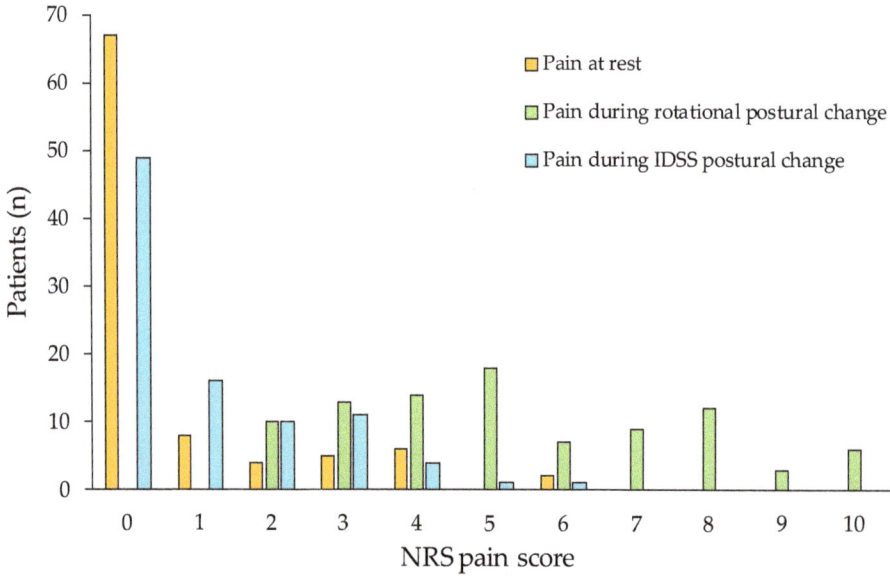

Figure 2. Frequency of pain distribution, assessed by NRS, at rest, during rotational and IDSS postural changes in the whole sample ($n = 92$).

Patients reported a mean perceived level of effort on NRS of 6.2 ± 2.5 points during the rotational movement and of 1.6 ± 1.7 points when using the IDSS. The difference between the two modalities of postural change was significant (t-test, $p < 0.0005$) and large, with an effect size of 1.84.

Subgroup analysis revealed that subjects with sternal instability showed more pain than stable patients (ANOVA, $F(1,90) = 4.79$, $p < 0.05$), but there was no interaction between pain and conditions. Moreover, female patients with macromastia had higher pain value than those without macromastia (ANOVA, $F(1,22) = 7.21$, $p < 0.05$), even if there was no interaction between pain and conditions. No differences were found in the other subgroup analyses.

Pain at rest did not correlate with other clinical parameters, such as the time from surgical intervention ($\rho = 0.001$). A strong correlation was found between pain and perceived level of effort during the rotational postural change ($\rho = 0.64$, $p < 0.0005$), while a moderate correlation emerged during the IDSS postural change ($\rho = 0.42$, $p < 0.0005$). No other correlations were found between the remaining clinical variables and the assessment data.

3.2. Follow-Up Call

The 100% of the sample went home with the indication to use the IDSS to perform the supine-to-sitting postural change, as 93% of them reported less pain with respect to the rotational movement and the 7% reported equal pain. At the 6-month follow-up, no patients reported wound infection and no patients with a sternal instability at the previous clinical assessment (SIS > 0 points) reported sternal complications that required rehospitalization. Only a patient (1.1% of the whole sample), a woman without sternal instability during the rehabilitation recovery, had a subsequent sternal displacement.

4. Discussion

The aim of this study was to assess which modality of supine-to-sitting postural change, through a rotational movement or performed using the IDSS, induced lower levels of pain and perceived effort in post-operative patients with sternotomy. The results show that the postural change performed using the IDSS was less painful compared to the rotational modality. The level of pain reported by patients during the resting position and in performing the postural change using the IDSS was mild and almost similar between the two conditions. On the contrary, patients reported moderate levels of pain in performing the rotational postural change.

The risk of sternal complications following median sternotomy is frequently reported in literature, suggesting that it would be customary to instruct patients to adopt sternal precautions in order to reduce the incidence of complications [37,38]. Nevertheless, only few studies are available in the literature supporting or refuting the usefulness of sternal precautions [19,25,37,38]. Despite this, lack of literature led to adopting precautions that appear to vary from facility-to-facility; these measures generally include a restriction on upper extremity movements and lifting limitations [19].

Although these hindrances appear to be important, they seem not to be sufficient in order to reduce the risk of complications. Recent studies showed that in the same way, transfers and elevating both arms simultaneously overhead creates the greatest sternal separation [35,39]. In particular, small magnitude of multi-planar motion at the sternal edges occurs during both dynamic upper limb and trunk tasks in patients over the first 3 postoperative months post-sternotomy [39]. In addition, Irion et al. [37,38] measured supra-sternal skin movement during a variety of daily activities, finding that the greatest skin movement occurred during supine-to-sitting using upper extremities, while the least movement occurred when lifting containers up to 5 kg of water (approximately 8 lbs). Moreover, patients with chronic sternal instability experienced the greatest amount of pain during transitions from supine to short sitting. In fact, not surprisingly, in our study, the higher levels of pain (7–10 on NRS) were reported by patients only during the rotational postural change, which is the most common way of performing the supine-to-sitting movement.

Therefore, addressing limitations of the supine-to-sitting transfer seems to be important following median sternotomy. Although modifications to supine-to-sitting postural change using the technique encouraged as part of sternal precautions were shown to decrease stress compared to a typically discouraged method [37,38], these modifications still produced more stress than lifting 5 kg, which is the maximum load allowed to raise for patients [37,38]. As a consequence, since modifications proposed until now in the literature to the supine-to-sitting transfer do not seem sufficient, the results concerning pain of our study may be of considerable importance in the clinical practice for the management of patients with sternotomy.

In fact, finding alternative solutions appears to be essential for guaranteeing the safety of patients. Our work confirmed that more than 50% of patients who undergo sternotomy surgery report persistent pain in the sternum. These findings are superimposable to the study of Moore et al. [40], who found that chest incisional pain was reported by 60% of subjects 3 weeks after cardiac surgery. However, in comparison to the rotational postural change, the use of IDSS in performing the supine-to-sitting postural change resulted in a reduction in the level of pain in our post-operative patients with sternotomy, associated with a decrease in perceived level of effort. Although we never directly measured the forces acting on the sternotomy, we believe that the reduction in the levels of pain and perceived level of effort using the IDSS may indirectly reflect a reduction in the forces acting to the sternum. Indeed, patients used a traction force of about 10 kg for IDSS postural change, which may be comparable to that commonly produced by opening a door, and which was well below the forces occurring during a sneeze or cough [25].

Moreover, the use of IDSS seems especially important in the elderly who are accustomed to carrying out the supine-to-sitting transfer using the rotational pattern compared to younger adults who preferred to perform the postural change through the long sitting position [41]. This behaviour could be due to the fact that older individuals may have decreased abdominal strength and postural stability with an increased fear of falling, and the rotational strategy allowed them to keep an elbow on the mat and maintain a larger base of support [42]. Since patients are often already accustomed in daily pre-surgery for carrying out the rotational movement, they may instinctively continue with the same modality even after the surgical operation, despite the fact that it makes them feel pain.

Among risk factors associated with mechanical forces acting upon the sternotomy site, some were identified also in our sample: chronic obstructive lung disease [17,43], macromastia [8,44], and obesity [16,17,45]. However, maybe due to the small sample, we found higher perceived levels of pain and effort only in patients with macromastia. This supports the hypothesis that women with larger breasts are subjected to increased inferolateral tension across their sternotomy [46], with higher perception of pain caused by the stress force. On the other hand, the presence of diabetes and smoking history did not influence the perception of pain and effort.

Indeed, patient-reported pain was cited as being the main restriction used to guide exercise prescription and progression in the return to daily living movements [47]. In the present study, no patient reported levels of pain and/or perceived effort that were higher in using IDSS compared to performing the rotational postural change. By using IDSS in the correct way, forces exercised by the upper limbs and the abdominal muscles acted symmetrically on the chest, avoiding those asymmetrical forces that are produced during the rotational postural change. As a matter of fact, in reaching the sitting position from the lateral decubitus, the upper limbs produce thrust forces with different intensities and directions, which may impact asymmetrically on the ribcage, placing under stress the sternal wound [39,48].

The good correlation found between pain and perceived level of effort, in both the modalities of postural change, may suggest that weaker patients experienced a higher level of effort in the strain, and consequently, more pain. However, this hypothesis needs to be verified.

Finally, only the 1.1% of the total sample reported a complication, i.e., sternal instability, 6 months after hospital discharge. This result is in line with the noted cases of complications in literature (1–8% [14]). Thus, it is possible to suppose that the precautions given at the discharge, such as the use of IDSS, were opportune for the safety of the patients.

Limitations

Results of our study are based only on patient-reported outcome measures (pain and perceived effort). One of the limitations was the lack of other types of measure, such as ultrasound. This useful technique might be use in future research to provide valuable real-time feedback regarding sternal healing in patients following cardiac surgery via median sternotomy and may allow for quantitatively assessing motion at the sternal edges. Another limitation was the simple follow-up call at 6 months after hospital discharge; since it is known that sternal healing continues beyond the first three post-operative months [49], we might expect that using a monthly follow-up could allow to find the differences in pain during the two postural steps. Moreover, the heterogeneous but limited sample size did not allow for obtaining solid conclusions about differences in pain and perceived effort in each subgroup of patients stratified by risk factors.

Future research should implement the actual results measuring the motion at the sternal edges during the supine-to-sitting postural change, following patients over a post-operative period of at least 3 months, and assessing the supine-to-sitting abdominal muscles activation and the use of upper limbs to verify the relationship existing between pain, perceived effort, and level of effort in the strain. Moreover, future studies might stratify the population with sternotomy by clinical characteristics in order to give appropriate instructions for each subgroup.

5. Conclusions

Sternal displacement is associated with unilateral and rotational movements and the supine-to-sitting postural change is one of the most challenging because of the force applied to the sternum. Thus, since the use of the IDSS seems to reduce the levels of pain and perceived effort during the supine-to-sitting postural change, future studies with quantitative assessments are required to verify its effectiveness and to suggest the adoption of this technique, mostly in patients with high levels of pain and in those with sternal instability.

Supplementary Materials: The following supporting information can be downloaded at: https://www.mdpi.com/article/10.3390/jcm12144665/s1, Video S1: Postural change modalities.

Author Contributions: Conceptualization, M.P. and M.C.; data curation, M.G. (Marica Giardini) and M.G. (Marco Guenzi); formal analysis, M.G. (Marica Giardini), I.A. and M.G. (Marco Godi); funding acquisition, M.C.; investigation, M.G. (Marco Guenzi); methodology, M.C.; project administration, M.C.; supervision, M.G. (Marco Godi); visualization, M.P.; writing—original draft, M.G. (Marica Giardini) and M.G. (Marco Guenzi); writing—review and editing, I.A. and M.G. (Marco Godi). All authors have read and agreed to the published version of the manuscript.

Funding: This research received no external funding.

Institutional Review Board Statement: The study was conducted in accordance with the Declaration of Helsinki, and approved by the Ethics Committee of Istituti Clinici Scientifici Maugeri (approval number #2448 CE, 6 October 2020).

Informed Consent Statement: Informed consent was obtained from all subjects involved in the study, along with the consent to publish this paper.

Data Availability Statement: The data presented in this study are available on request from the corresponding author. The data are not publicly available due to privacy restrictions.

Acknowledgments: The authors would like to express their sincere gratitude to all the people who participated in this study. This work was supported by the "Ricerca Corrente" funding scheme of the Ministry of Health, Italy.

Conflicts of Interest: The authors declare no conflict of interest.

References

1. Bonow, R.O.; Carabello, B.A.; Chatterjee, K.; De Leon, A.C.; Faxon, D.P.; Freed, M.D.; Gaasch, W.H.; Lytle, B.W.; Nishimura, R.A.; O'Gara, P.T.; et al. ACC/AHA 2006 guidelines for the management of patients with valvular heart disease: A report of the American College of Cardiology/American Heart Association Task Force on Practice Guidelines (writing Committee to Revise the 1998 guidelines for the management of patients with valvular heart disease) developed in collaboration with the Society of Cardiovascular Anesthesiologists endorsed by the Society for Cardiovascular Angiography and Interventions and the Society of Thoracic Surgeons. *J. Am. Coll. Cardiol.* **2006**, *48*, e1–e148. [PubMed]
2. Go, A.S.; Mozaffarian, D.; Roger, V.L.; Benjamin, E.J.; Berry, J.D.; Blaha, M.J.; Dai, S.; Ford, E.S.; Fox, C.S.; Franco, S.; et al. American Heart Association Statistics Committee and Stroke Statistics Subcommittee. Heart disease and stroke statistics—2014 update: A report from the American Heart Association. *Circulation* **2014**, *129*, e28–e292. [PubMed]
3. Pradeep, A.; Rangasamy, J.; Varma, P.K. Recent developments in controlling sternal wound infection after cardiac surgery and measures to enhance sternal healing. *Med. Res. Rev.* **2021**, *41*, 709–724. [CrossRef] [PubMed]
4. Schiraldi, L.; Jabbour, G.; Centofanti, P.; Giordano, S.; Abdelnour, E.; Gonzalez, M.; Raffoul, W.; Di Summa, P.G. Deep sternal wound infections: Evidence for prevention, treatment, and reconstructive surgery. *Arch. Plast. Surg.* **2019**, *46*, 291–302. [CrossRef] [PubMed]
5. Sidhu, V.P.S.; Towler, M.R.; Papini, M. Measurement of Adhesion of Sternal Wires to a Novel Bioactive Glass-Based Adhesive. *J. Funct. Biomater.* **2019**, *10*, 37. [CrossRef]
6. Robicsek, F.; Fokin, A.; Cook, J.; Bhatia, D. Sternal Instability After Midline Sternotomy. *Thorac. Cardiovasc. Surg.* **2000**, *48*, 1–8. [CrossRef]
7. Gummert, J.F.; Barten, M.J.; Hans, C.; Kluge, M.; Doll, N.; Walther, T.; Hentschel, B.; Schmitt, D.V.; Mohr, F.W.; Diegeler, A. Mediastinitis and cardiac surgery--an updated risk factor analysis in 10,373 consecutive adult patients. *Thorac. Cardiovasc. Surg.* **2002**, *50*, 87–91. [CrossRef]
8. Salehi Omran, A.; Karimi, A.; Ahmadi, S.H.; Davoodi, S.; Marzban, M.; Movahedi, N.; Abbasi, K.; Boroumand, M.A.; Davoodi, S.; Moshtaghi, N. Superficial and deep sternal wound infection after more than 9000 coronary artery bypass graft (CABG): Incidence, risk factors and mortality. *BMC Infect. Dis.* **2007**, *7*, 112. [CrossRef]
9. Rupprecht, L.; Schmid, C. Deep sternal wound complications: An overview of old and new therapeutic options. *Open J. Cardiovasc. Surg.* **2013**, *6*, 9–19. [CrossRef]

10. McGregor, W.E.; Trumble, D.R.; Magovern, J.A. Mechanical analysis of midline sternotomy wound closure. *J. Thorac. Cardiovasc. Surg.* **1999**, *117*, 1144–1150. [CrossRef]
11. Savage, E.B.; Grab, J.D.; O'Brien, S.M.; Ali, A.; Okum, E.J.; Perez-Tamayo, R.A.; Eiferman, D.S.; Peterson, E.D.; Edwards, F.H.; Higgins, R.S. Use of both internal thoracic arteries in diabetic patients increases deep sternal wound infection. *Ann. Thorac. Surg.* **2007**, *83*, 1002–1006. [CrossRef] [PubMed]
12. Ariyaratnam, P.; Bland, M.; Loubani, M. Risk factors and mortality associated with deep sternal wound infections following coronary bypass surgery with or without concomitant procedures in a UK population: A basis for a new risk model? *Interact. Cardiovasc. Thorac. Surg.* **2010**, *11*, 543–546. [CrossRef] [PubMed]
13. Careaga Reyna, G.; Aguirre Baca, G.G.; Medina Concebida, L.E.; Borrayo Sánchez, G.; Prado Villegas, G.; Argüero Sáncheza, R. Risk Factors for Mediastinitis and Sternal Dehiscence After Cardiac Surgery. *Rev. Esp. Cardiol.* **2006**, *59*, 130–135. [CrossRef]
14. El-Ansary, D.; Waddington, G.; Denehy, L.; McManus, M.; Fuller, L.; Katijjahbe, A.; Adams, R. Physical Assessment of Sternal Stability Following a Median Sternotomy for Cardiac Surgery: Validity and Reliability of the Sternal Instability Scale (SIS). *Int. J. Phys. Ther. Rehab.* **2018**, *4*, 140. [CrossRef] [PubMed]
15. Gregory, A.J.; Noss, C.D.; Chun, R.; Gysel, M.; Prusinkiewicz, C.; Webb, N.; Raymond, M.; Cogan, J.; Rousseau-Saine, N.; Lam, W.; et al. Perioperative optimization of the cardiac surgical patient. *Can. J. Cardiol.* **2023**, *39*, 497–514. [CrossRef] [PubMed]
16. Satsangi, D.K. Search for the best heart valve—From replacement to repair. *Ind. J. Thorac. Cardiovasc. Surg.* **2011**, *27*, 152–160. [CrossRef]
17. Tuyl, L.J.; Mackney, J.H.; Johnston, C.L. Management of sternal precautions following median sternotomy by physical therapists in Australia: A web-based survey. *Phys. Ther.* **2012**, *92*, 83–97. [CrossRef]
18. Katijjahbe, M.A.; Denehy, L.; Granger, C.L.; Royse, A.; Royse, C.; Bates, R.; Logie, S.; Clarke, S.; El-Ansary, D. The Sternal Management Accelerated Recovery Trial (S.M.A.R.T)—Standard restrictive versus an intervention of modified sternal precautions following cardiac surgery via median sternotomy: Study protocol for a randomised controlled trial. *Trials* **2017**, *18*, 290. [CrossRef]
19. Cahalin, L.P.; LaPier, T.K.; Shaw, D.K. Sternal precautions: Is it time for change? Precautions versus restrictions-a review of literature and recommendations for revision. *Cardiopulm. Phys. Ther. J.* **2011**, *22*, 5–15. [CrossRef]
20. Brocki, B.C.; Thorup, C.B.; Andreasen, J.J. Precautions related to midline sternotomy in cardiac surgery: A review of mechanical stress factors leading to sternal complications. *Eur. J. Cardiovasc. Nurs.* **2010**, *9*, 77–84. [CrossRef]
21. McKenna, H.; Jones, J.; Harmon, E.Y. Move in the tube sternal precautions: A retrospective analysis of a single inpatient rehabilitation facility. *Cardiopulm. Phys. Ther. J.* **2022**, *33*, 108–115. [CrossRef]
22. Vitomskyi, V. Critical review of the justification of limitations in physical therapy and activities of daily living in cardiac surgery patients. *Physiother. Q.* **2022**, *30*, 51–58. [CrossRef]
23. Tucker, B.; Jenkins, S.; Davies, K.; McGann, R.; Waddell, J.; King, R. The physiotherapy management of patients undergoing coronary artery surgery: A questionnaire survey. *Aust. J. Physiother.* **1996**, *42*, 129–137. [CrossRef] [PubMed]
24. Westerdahl, E.; Möller, M. Physiotherapy-supervised mobilization and exercise following cardiac surgery: A national questionnaire survey in Sweden. *J. Cardiothorac. Surg.* **2010**, *5*, 67. [CrossRef]
25. Adams, J.; Lotshaw, A.; Exum, E.; Campbell, M.; Spranger, C.B.; Beveridge, J.; Baker, S.; McCray, S.; Bilbrey, T.; Shock, T.; et al. An alternative approach to prescribing sternal precautions after median sternotomy, "Keep Your Move in the Tube". *Bayl. Univ. Med. Cent. Proc.* **2016**, *29*, 97–100. [CrossRef]
26. Katijjahbe, A.; Granger, C.L.; Denehy, L.; Royse, A.; Royse, C.; Bates, R.; Logie, S.; Ayub, A.N.; Clarke, S.; El-Ansary, D. Standard restrictive sternal precautions and modified sternal precautions had similar effects in people after cardiac surgery via median sternotomy ('SMART' Trial): A randomised trial. *J. Physiother.* **2018**, *64*, 97–106. [CrossRef]
27. Malhotra, C.; Chan, A.; Matchar, D.; Seow, D.; Chuo, A.; Do, Y.K. Diagnostic performance of short portable mental status questionnaire for screening dementia among patients attending cognitive assessment clinics in Singapore. *Ann. Acad. Med. Singap.* **2013**, *42*, 315–319. [CrossRef]
28. Jensen, M.P.; Turner, J.A.; Romano, J.M. What is the maximum number of levels needed in pain intensity measurement? *Pain* **1994**, *58*, 387–392. [CrossRef]
29. Bijur, P.E.; Latimer, C.T.; Gallagher, E.J. Validation of a verbally administered numerical rating scale of acute pain for use in the emergency department. *Acad. Emerg. Med.* **2003**, *10*, 390–392. [CrossRef]
30. Williamson, A.; Hoggart, B. Pain: A review of three commonly used pain rating scales. *J. Clin. Nurs.* **2005**, *14*, 798–804. [CrossRef]
31. Hetmann, F.; Kongsgaard, U.E.; Sandvik, L.; Schou-Bredal, I. Prevalence and predictors of persistent post-surgical pain 12 months after thoracotomy. *Acta Anaesthesiol. Scand.* **2015**, *59*, 740–748. [CrossRef]
32. Zhu, Q.; Huang, Z.; Ma, Q.; Wu, Z.; Kang, Y.; Zhang, M.; Gan, T.; Wang, M.; Huang, F. Supine versus semi-Fowler's positions for tracheal extubation in abdominal surgery-a randomized clinical trial. *BMC Anesthesiol.* **2020**, *20*, 185. [CrossRef] [PubMed]
33. Cohen, J. A power primer. *Psychol. Bull.* **1992**, *112*, 155. [CrossRef] [PubMed]
34. Akoglu, H. User's guide to correlation coefficients. *Turk. J. Emerg. Med.* **2018**, *18*, 91–93. [CrossRef] [PubMed]
35. El-Ansary, D.; Waddington, G.; Adams, R. Measurement of nonphysiological movement in sternal instability by ultrasound. *Ann. Thorac. Surg.* **2007**, *83*, 1513–1516. [CrossRef]
36. Walton, D.M.; Elliott, J.M.; Salim, S.; Al-Nasri, I. A reconceptualization of the pain numeric rating scale: Anchors and clinically important differences. *J. Hand Ther.* **2018**, *31*, 179–183. [CrossRef]
37. Irion, G. Effect of upper extremity movement on sternal skin stress. *Acute Care Perspect.* **2006**, *15*, 3–6. [CrossRef]

38. Irion, G.; Boyte, B.; Ingram, J.; Kirchem, C.; Weathers, J. Sternal skin stress produced by functional upper extremity movements. *Acute Care Perspect.* **2007**, *16*, 1–5.
39. Balachandran, S.; Denehy, L.; Lee, A.; Royse, C.; Royse, A.; El-Ansary, D. Motion at the sternal edges during upper limb and trunk tasks in-vivo as measured by real-time ultrasound following cardiac surgery: A three-month prospective, observational study. *Heart Lung Circ.* **2019**, *28*, 1283–1291. [CrossRef] [PubMed]
40. Moore, S.M. A comparison of women's and men's symptoms during home recovery after coronary artery bypass surgery. *Heart Lung* **1995**, *24*, 495–501. [CrossRef]
41. Alexander, N.B.; Fry-Welch, D.K.; Marshall, L.M.; Chung, C.C.; Kowalski, A.M. Healthy Young and Old Women Differ in Their Trunk Elevation and Hip Pivot Motions When Rising from Supine to Sitting. *J. Am. Geriatr. Soc.* **1995**, *43*, 338–343. [CrossRef] [PubMed]
42. Mount, J.; Kresge, L.; Klaus, G.; Mann, L.; Palomba, C. Movement patterns used by the elderly when getting out of bed. *Phys. Occup. Ther. Geriatr.* **2006**, *24*, 27–43. [CrossRef]
43. Orhan, S.N.; Ozyazicioglu, M.H.; Colak, A. A biomechanical study of 4 different sternum closure techniques under different deformation modes. *Interact. Cardiovasc. Thorac. Surg.* **2017**, *25*, 750–756. [CrossRef] [PubMed]
44. Parker, R.; Adams, J.L.; Ogola, G.; McBrayer, D.; Hubbard, J.M.; McCullough, T.L.; Hartman, J.M.; Cleveland, T. Current Activity Guidelines for CABG Patients are too Restrictive: Comparison of the Forces Exerted on the Median Sternotomy during a Cough vs. Lifting Activities Combined with Valsalva Maneuver. *Thorac. Cardiovasc. Surg.* **2008**, *56*, 190–194. [CrossRef]
45. Losanoff, J.E.; Richman, B.W.; Jones, J.W. Disruption and infection of median sternotomy: A comprehensive review. *Eur. J. Cardiothorac. Surg.* **2002**, *21*, 831–839. [CrossRef]
46. Balachandran, S.; Lee, A.; Denehy, L.; Lin, K.Y.; Royse, A.; Royse, C.; El-Ansary, D. Risk factors for sternal complications after cardiac operations: A systematic review. *Ann. Thorac. Surg.* **2016**, *102*, 2109–2117. [CrossRef]
47. Balachandran, S.; Lee, A.; Royse, A.; Denehy, L.; El-Ansary, D. Upper limb exercise prescription following cardiac surgery via median sternotomy: A web survey. *J. Cardiopulm. Rehabil. Prev.* **2014**, *34*, 390–395. [CrossRef]
48. El-Ansary, D.; Adams, R.; Waddington, G. Sternal instability during arm elevation observed as dynamic, multiplanar separation. *Int. J. Ther. Rehabil.* **2009**, *16*, 609–614. [CrossRef]
49. Wang, B.; He, D.; Wang, M.; Qian, Y.; Lu, Y.; Shi, X.; Liu, Y.; Zhan, X.; Di, D.; Zhu, K.; et al. Analysis of sternal healing after median sternotomy in low risk patients at midterm follow-up: Retrospective cohort study from two centres. *J. Cardiothorac. Surg.* **2019**, *14*, 193. [CrossRef]

Disclaimer/Publisher's Note: The statements, opinions and data contained in all publications are solely those of the individual author(s) and contributor(s) and not of MDPI and/or the editor(s). MDPI and/or the editor(s) disclaim responsibility for any injury to people or property resulting from any ideas, methods, instructions or products referred to in the content.

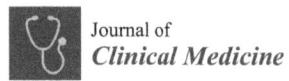

Article

The Impact of Bariatric Surgery on Quality of Life in Patients with Obesity

Radu Petru Soroceanu [1,2,†], Daniel Vasile Timofte [1,2,*,†], Radu Danila [1,2,†], Sergiu Timofeiov [1,2,*,†], Roxana Livadariu [1,2,†], Ancuta Andreea Miler [1,2,†], Bogdan Mihnea Ciuntu [1,2,†], Daniela Drugus [3,†], Laura Elisabeta Checherita [4,†], Ilie Cristian Drochioi [5,†], Mihai Liviu Ciofu [5,†] and Doina Azoicai [3,†]

[1] Department of Surgery, "Grigore T. Popa" University of Medicine and Pharmacy, 700115 Iasi, Romania; petru.soroceanu@umfiasi.ro (R.P.S.); radu.danila@umfiasi.ro (R.D.); roxana.livadariu@umfiasi.ro (R.L.); ancuta-andreea_a_miler@d.umfiasi.ro (A.A.M.); bogdan-mihnea.ciuntu@umfiasi.ro (B.M.C.)
[2] Department of Surgery, "St. Spiridon" County Clinical Emergency Hospital, 700111 Iasi, Romania
[3] Department of Preventive Medicine and Interdisciplinarity, "Grigore T. Popa" University of Medicine and Pharmacy, 700115 Iasi, Romania; daniela.drugus@umfiasi.ro (D.D.); doina.azoicai@umfiasi.ro (D.A.)
[4] Dental Medicine Department, "Grigore T. Popa" University of Medicine and Pharmacy, 700115 Iasi, Romania; checherita.laura@gmail.com
[5] Department of Oral and Maxillofacial Surgery, "Grigore T. Popa" University of Medicine and Pharmacy, 700115 Iasi, Romania; ilie-cristian.drochioi@umfiasi.ro (I.C.D.); mihai.ciofu@umfiasi.ro (M.L.C.)
* Correspondence: daniel.timofte@umfiasi.ro (D.V.T.); tudose.timofeiov@umfiasi.ro (S.T.)
† These authors contributed equally to this work.

Citation: Soroceanu, R.P.; Timofte, D.V.; Danila, R.; Timofeiov, S.; Livadariu, R.; Miler, A.A.; Ciuntu, B.M.; Drugus, D.; Checherita, L.E.; Drochioi, I.C.; et al. The Impact of Bariatric Surgery on Quality of Life in Patients with Obesity. *J. Clin. Med.* 2023, 12, 4225. https://doi.org/10.3390/jcm12134225

Academic Editor: Dimitrios E. Magouliotis

Received: 20 May 2023
Revised: 16 June 2023
Accepted: 20 June 2023
Published: 23 June 2023

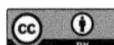

Copyright: © 2023 by the authors. Licensee MDPI, Basel, Switzerland. This article is an open access article distributed under the terms and conditions of the Creative Commons Attribution (CC BY) license (https://creativecommons.org/licenses/by/4.0/).

Abstract: Obesity has become a widespread health problem influencing people's health, general well-being, and healthcare costs. It also represents an important risk factor for multiple comorbidities and malignancies. Objectives: the primary objective of this study was to provide notable insights to healthcare professionals regarding the management of patients with obesity, to highlight the effectiveness of bariatric surgical methods in losing excess weight, and to establish the relationship between weight loss and changes in quality of life (QoL). Material and methods: our study evaluated the QoL of 76 patients following bariatric surgery at different postoperative stages using the 36-Item Short Form Survey (SF-36) and The World Health Organization Quality of Life—BREF (WHOQOL-BREF) questionnaires. Results: regarding the type of bariatric procedure performed, out of the 76 respondents, 39.47% underwent gastric bypass surgery (RYGB), 56.57% underwent sleeve gastrectomy (LSG), and only 3.94% underwent single anastomosis duodeno-ileal switch (SADI-S). Pertaining to the SF-36 questionnaire, the lowest average scores were found in the energy/fatigue subscales and in the limitations due to mental health, which remained consistent across surgery types with a significant decrease in the SADI-S group. Concerning the WHOQOL-BREF questionnaire, the lowest mean scores were found in the environment (15.03 ± 2.37) and social relations (16.08 ± 2.22) subscales, whilst the highest average scores were in physical health (16.30 ± 2.03) and mental health (16.57 ± 2.16). Conclusions: the findings revealed that whilst bariatric surgery significantly improved physical health, it resulted in a decrease in mental health scores. Consequently, the study emphasizes the importance of adopting a holistic approach to managing obesity that considers improving both physical and mental health outcomes.

Keywords: obesity; bariatric surgery; quality of life; questionnaire; clinical outcomes; LSG; RYGB

1. Introduction

Obesity has emerged as a pandemic and a serious public health issue due to its high prevalence and detrimental effects on mortality, morbidity, healthcare costs, and QoL [1]. It is now considered a chronic disease [2], and scientific interest in the QoL of individuals with obesity has surged in the past decade. According to estimates, by 2030, over one billion people worldwide will suffer from obesity, affecting one in five women and one in seven men [3]. The most significant population affected by obesity resides in countries with low to middle standards of living, with a predicted twofold increase in obesity rates in low and middle-income countries and a threefold increase in low-income states compared with 2010 reports. This dramatic rise in the prevalence of obesity has prompted global public health research. Current studies demonstrate that QoL decreases inversely proportional to the body mass index (BMI), and individuals with advanced stages of obesity experience more severe declines [4,5]. Regardless of the therapeutic approach, weight loss can improve the QoL in individuals affected by obesity.

Excess body weight is known to substantially diminish the QoL, especially through its impact on overall health and by directly impeding daily activities, resulting in decreased well-being [6]. Furthermore, research on the topic has established that individuals with obesity also experience social stigmatization in addition to physical health consequences [7].

Although public health campaigns are crucial in preventing obesity through initiatives such as dietary changes and lifestyle modifications, their effectiveness may be limited for individuals who already have obesity, particularly in severe and complex cases (with a BMI of ≥ 40 kg/m^2 or BMI of 35–40 kg/m^2 accompanied by significant health issues related to excess weight) [8,9]. In such situations, bariatric surgery is considered an optimal treatment option. Research has shown that bariatric surgery not only leads to more substantial weight loss, but also offers better management of type 2 diabetes compared with lifestyle interventions or medication alone [10–12]. The two most commonly performed types of bariatric surgery are LSG and RYGB [13].

While recent studies indicate comparable long-term results for both LSG and RYGB, the recurrence of weight gain and comorbidity symptoms in some patients have prompted bariatric surgeons to explore modifications to existing techniques or introduce new ones [14,15]. Among these options, the SADI-S procedure has demonstrated superior effectiveness in achieving long-term weight loss and in remitting comorbidities. However, its technical complexity and potential for adverse events have constrained its widespread adoption [16].

Although multiple studies highlight the positive impact of weight loss on obesity-related comorbidities (both through conservative and surgical means), there are no specific tools, analyses, or questionnaires specifically designed for assessing QoL in patients with obesity [10,17–20].

Therefore, the objectives of our study were to evaluate the overall QoL in patients who underwent different bariatric surgical interventions, to assess specific QoL domains (e.g., physical functioning, mental health, social functioning), to compare the impact of specific bariatric procedures on QoL, and to identify potential predictors or factors associated with significant improvements in QoL following these procedures (such as patient demographics, preoperative conditions, or surgical technique) using the SF-36 and WHOQOL-BREF questionnaires.

2. Materials and Methods

2.1. Study Design

The present study was designed as a cross-sectional, non-randomized, and anonymized study based on two commonly used questionnaires used in assessing QoL. The questionnaires were transferred to "Google Forms". The link was distributed to each individual patient online by email or by telephone. Contact details of our patients were extracted from the database in our bariatric surgery center.

2.2. Inclusion Criteria

The study was implemented in our bariatric surgery center based in the 3rd Surgical Unit at "St. Spiridon" County Clinical Emergency Hospital, Iasi, Romania. Invitations for the survey were sent to 130 patients who underwent a bariatric procedure within the previous 12 months. Incomplete answers or sections of the questionnaires led to the exclusion from the study. Only 76 patients, which included women and men, in various postoperative stages (following LSG, RYGB, or SADI-S) were included in the study. All participants voluntarily completed the questionnaires between 4 January 2023 and 28 February 2023.

2.3. The Questionnaires Used

Typically, only a few standardized instruments are used to examine QoL in obese patients. The SF-36 is a self-reported questionnaire that assesses QoL in patients across 8 subscales: physical functionality (PF), limitations in usual role activities (RP), bodily pain (BP), general health (GH), vitality (VT), social functioning (SF), limitations in usual role activities because of emotional problems (RE), and general mental health (MH). The WHOQOL-BREF questionnaire was created by the World Health Organization for the cross-cultural examination of subjective elements related to QoL as an alternative research tool. The 26 items that make up this instrument are divided into 4 categories: physical health (7 items), mental health (6 items), social relationships (3 items), and environmental health (8 items). The physical health domain consists of several items assessing mobility, daily activities, functional capacity, energy, pain, and sleep, while the psychological domain takes into account the perceived self-image, negative thoughts, positive attitudes, self-esteem, mindset, learning ability, memory, concentration, and mental state. The social relationships domain looks at personal relationships, social support, and sex life, while the environmental health field covers financial resources, safety, social and health services, the physical living environment, opportunities for learning and personal development, recreation, noise and pollution, and transportation.

For our cohort, we used the two stated instruments, SF-36 and WHOQOL-BREF, for simultaneous data analysis. The items in the SF-36 questionnaire were translated from English. The patients included in our study speak Romanian as their native language; subsequently, the original questionnaire was compared with its translated version. All translations were performed by two independent certified translators. The questionnaires were finalized and distributed to the patients.

2.4. Data Collection and Statistical Methods

Data obtained from the questionnaires were transferred to MS Excel 2010, sourced from Iași, România, "Grigore T. Popa" University of Medicine and Pharmacy. The respondents were classified based on the surgical procedure used (LSG, RYGB, or SADI-S).

The data were then uploaded and processed using the statistical functions in SPSS v. 26.0. All patient data protection provisions were enforced, as the medical team in the teaching hospital was well informed on data and patients' rights protection. The confidence interval was set at 95% and a *p*-value < 0.05 (two-sided) was considered statistically significant.

In calculating the differences between two or more groups at the 95% significance threshold, depending on the distribution of the value series, descriptive statistics, the Pearson correlation coefficient (r), and the Cronbach α coefficient for internal consistency were used.

3. Results

3.1. Demographic Characteristics

In our study, the distribution of respondents according to sex indicated an increased frequency of female respondents. Female respondents represented 69.74% and male respondents represented 30.26%.

The study group presented a normal distribution of respondents regarding age, with a maximum frequency of 30.26% corresponding to the 30–39 age group (Table 1).

Regarding the type of bariatric procedure performed, out of the 76 respondents, 39.47% underwent RYGB, 56.57% underwent LSG, and only 3.94% underwent SADI-S. In the group of patients with RYGB (30 respondents), the age ranged from 23 to 69 years, with an average age of 39.47 years (standard deviation = 14.31). Male respondents had a slightly higher average age than female respondents (48.55 vs. 36.47 years) (Table 1). In the group of respondents with LSG (43 respondents), the age ranged from 20 to 69 years, with an average age of 39.97 years (standard deviation = 10.73). Male and female respondents had no significant differences in the mean age. The group of respondents who underwent SADI-S had an average age of 41.33 years (standard deviation = 5.13). The average age was significantly higher among respondents who underwent SADI-S compared with those who underwent RYGB or LSG (41.33 vs. 40.10 vs. 39.97 years).

Table 1. Descriptive characteristics regarding the age of respondents according to the type of surgical procedure and sex.

	Sex	n	%	Mean Age	Std. Dev.	Min. Age	Max. Age	p
RYGB	Women	21	27.63	36.47	13.01	23	65	0.269
	Men	9	11.84	48.55	14.31	26	69	
	Total	30	39.47	40.10	14.31	23	69	
LSG	Women	31	40.79	39.35	10.22	20	69	0.441
	Men	12	15.78	41.58	12.28	27	69	
	Total	43	56.57	39.97	10.73	20	69	
SADI-S	Women	1	1.31	-	-	-	-	-
	Men	2	2.63	42.00	7.07	37	47	
	Total	3	3.94	41.33	5.13	36	47	

Out of all the respondents in the study, 39.47% underwent RYGB. Breaking down this percentage by sex, with respect to all respondents, results in 27.63% female and 11.84% male respondents. Among the aforementioned male respondents, 96.66% were under the age of 65.

Out of all the respondents in the study, 56.57% underwent LSG. Breaking down this percentage by sex, with respect to all respondents, results in 40.79% female and 15.78% male respondents. Among the male respondents, 96.66% were under the age of 65.

Regarding BMI evolution, the obtained results reveal that preoperatively 92.11% of the respondents presented a BMI $\geq$ 35 kg/m2, and post-operatively only 23.68% presented a BMI $\geq$ 35 kg/m^2, finding a correction of the BMI in all groups of patients included in the study (Figure 1).

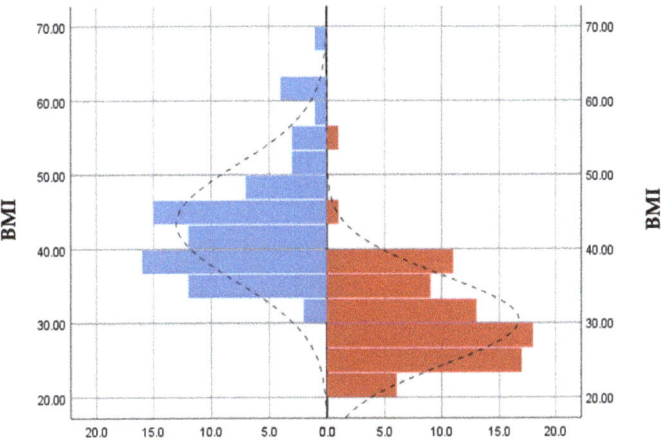

Figure 1. Preoperative (blue) and postoperative (red) BMI distribution.

3.2. Socio-Economic Aspects

Socio-economic aspects can have a major impact on stress and anxiety levels. They can also significantly interfere with lifestyle choices (such as smoking) and have major effects on health, as well as income levels. Regarding income, 50% of patients earn between 2500 and 5000 RON monthly, 27.63% earn more than 5000 RON monthly, and 22.36% earn less than 2500 RON.

3.3. Quality of Life Aspects

The SF-36 questionnaire scores (Table 2), along with the Cronbach α coefficient for each subscale, ranged from 0.664 (SF) to 0.704 (PF and MH), indicating good internal consistency. The lowest average scores were found in the vitality subscales (61.13 ± 15.20) and limitations due to mental health (65.78 ± 13.30), which remained consistent across surgery types, with a significant decrease in the SADI-S group (Tables 2 and 3). Social functioning (89.14 ± 14.76) and self-reported bodily pain (90.49 ± 14.44) had high mean scores (with items related to daily work interference and sickness) compared with others. The general state of health was also assessed.

Table 2. Statistical indicators regarding the SF-36 questionnaire score for each subscale.

Subscale	Avg.	SD	Mean	Min.	Max.	Q25	Q75	Cronbach α
PF	84.01	25.82	95.00	0.00	100.00	82.50	100.00	0.704
RP	85.85	30.09	100.00	0.00	100.00	100.00	100.00	0.667
RE	65.78	13.30	66.66	33.33	100.00	66.66	66.66	0.672
VT	61.13	15.20	65.00	15.00	100.00	52.50	75.00	0.674
MH	68.65	16.92	76.00	32.00	100.00	60.00	88.00	0.704
SF	89.14	14.76	100.00	37.50	100.00	87.50	100.00	0.664
BP	90.49	14.44	100.00	45.00	100.00	78.75	100.00	0.688
GH	76.52	16.22	80.00	31.25	100.00	65.00	90.00	0.685

Physical functionality (PF), limitations in usual role activities (RP), limitations in usual role activities because of emotional problems (RE), vitality (VT), general mental health (MH), social functioning (SF), bodily pain (BP) and general health (GH)

Table 3. Mean values of the SF-36 questionnaire score according to each subscale and type of surgical intervention.

	RYGB	LSG	SADI-S	p
PF	82.33 ± 26.21	84.41 ± 26.48	95.00 ± 8.66	0.717
RP	82.50 ± 31.58	87.20 ± 30.06	100.00 ± 0.00	0.577
RE	66.66 ± 15.16	65.11 ± 12.50	66.67 ± 0.00	0.884
VT	63.50 ± 15.81	65.81 ± 15.11	58.33 ± 11.54	0.631
MH	71.33 ± 14.78	74.79 ± 17.55	52.00 ± 18.33	0.068
SF	88.75 ± 14.06	89.53 ± 15.65	87.50 ± 12.50	0.958
BP	87.41 ± 14.30	92.73 ± 14.23	89.16 ± 18.76	0.302
GH	70.12 ± 17.07	75.94 ± 15.96	80.00 ± 13.22	0.652

Physical functionality (PF), limitations in usual role activities (RP), limitations in usual role activities because of emotional problems (RE), vitality (VT), general mental health (MH), social functioning (SF), bodily pain (BP) and general health (GH)

Table 3 highlights a weak correlation between the mental health subscale (MH) and the SF-36 questionnaire subscales for various surgical procedures. However, a strong correlation exists between the SF (social functionality) subscales and RP (limitations due to physical health), with coefficients of 0.958 and 0.884, respectively. The SADI-S procedure had an average value of 52.00, with a high standard deviation of ±18.33, indicating that the data is scattered from the average.

The subscales with the highest mean values for a particular surgical intervention are physical pain (92.73 ± 14.23), social functionality (89.53 ± 15.65), and limitations due to physical health (87.20 ± 30.06), which are linked to the LSG procedure. The highest mean scores associated with the RYGB procedure are also included in Table 3.

The WHOQOL-BREF questionnaire had good consistency with Cronbach α coefficients ranging from 0.781 (environment) to 0.845 (social relations). The lowest mean scores were found in the environment (15.03 ± 2.37) and social relations (16.08 ± 2.22) subscales, while the highest average scores were in physical health (16.30 ± 2.03) and mental health

(16.57 ± 2.16). Each subscale had similar average and median scores, implying an even distribution (Table 4).

Table 4. Descriptive statistics of the score obtained from the WHOQOL-BREF questionnaire based on each domain.

Domains	Avg.	SD	Mean	Min.	Max.	Q25	Q75	Cronbach α
Physical health	16.30	2.03	16.57	12.00	20.00	14.85	17.71	0.835
Mental health	16.57	2.16	16.66	10.00	20.00	15.33	18.33	0.782
Social relationships	16.08	2.22	16.00	12.00	20.00	14.66	17.33	0.845
Environment	15.03	2.37	15.00	8.00	20.00	13.50	17.00	0.781

The multivariate analysis of risk factors associated with self-reported QoL on the subscales assessed with the SF-36 questionnaire and the domains of QoL assessed with the WHOQOL-BREF indicates a strong correlation between physical functioning (PF) scores and limitations due to physical health status (RP) (0.000). A significant correlation is also observed between limitations due to physical health status (RP) and social functioning (SF) (0.000) and pain (P) (0.018). Last but not least, physical functionality is closely related to the level of quality of life, with a significant correlation of 0.041.

Regarding the limitations due to emotional problems (RE), they are strongly associated with the level of vitality (VT) with a significant correlation (0.022). At the same time, the data also shows an association between perceived limitations due to emotional problems with social functioning (SF) (0.005) and the domains of social relations (SR) (0.079) and physical health (PH) (0.002).

Mental health (MH) significantly correlates with general health (GH) (0.12) and social functioning (SF) (0.29). At the same time, mental health is significantly correlated with environmental health, measured as a domain of quality of life (E) (0.016).

The overall trend of mental health (MH) scores compared with the trend of vitality (VT) scores, physical health (PH) scores compared with social functioning (SF) scores, and environmental scores (E) compared with the general trend of scores for social functioning (SF) are illustrated below (Figures 2–4).

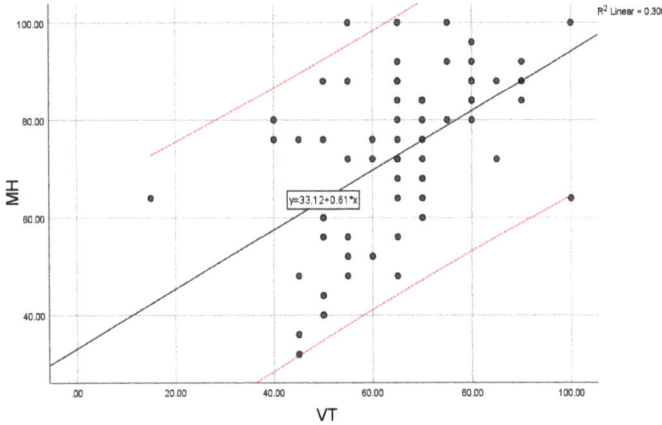

Figure 2. Mental health (MH) compared with the general trend for vitality (VT) scores; "y" indicates the overall trend of the scores.

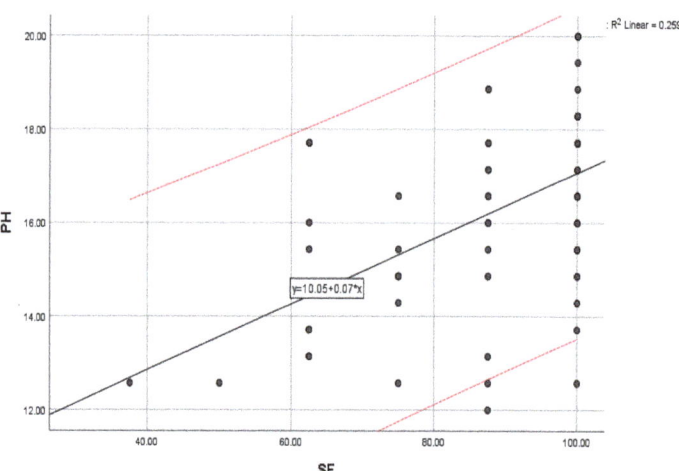

Figure 3. Physical health scores (PH) compared with the general trend for social functioning (SF) scores; "y" indicates the overall trend of the scores.

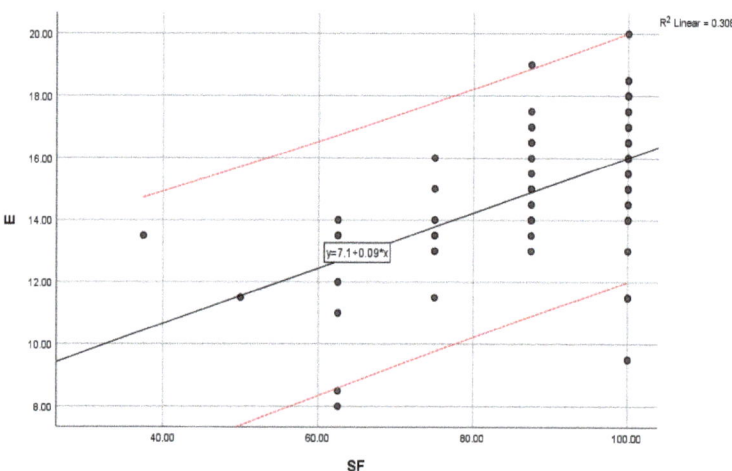

Figure 4. Environmental scores (E) compared with the general trend for social functioning (SF) scores; "y" indicates the overall trend of the scores.

4. Discussion

Recent studies regarding bariatric surgery and its impact on post-surgical patient QoL have primarily focused on biomedical aspects, such as weight loss and improvement of associated pathologies. However, as the amount of such surgical procedures performed worldwide continues to rise, it is crucial to holistically assess the QoL of the patients, including physical and mental performance [21]. Investigations on the topic use the SF-36 instrument to assess these dimensions, but the interpretation of the results is still a matter of debate among experts. In addition, evaluating the QoL for surgical patients may require more specific instruments tailored to certain pathologies, as the SF-36 questionnaire is considered generic and has limitations [22].

A recent study by de Vries (2022) suggests various ways to evaluate post-surgery bariatric patients, both from a clinical and QoL perspective [23]. However, our study also highlighted that scores for physical functionality based on daily activities may not accurately reflect a patient's QoL. To address these limitations, future research should consider utilizing more specific alternative QoL assessment tools taking into account the specific needs of bariatric patients. Thus, we can better assess the impact of bariatric surgery on the QoL of our patients and identify areas for improvement in post-surgical care.

Bariatric surgery typically leads to pronounced weight loss and improvement of pre-existing diseases, and it can positively affect the QoL of patients, particularly in terms of physical performance, according to a recent study by Albarrán-Sánchez et al. [24]. However, the study also found that mental health scores may decline post-surgery due to factors such as depression, anxiety, eating disorders, unrealistic expectations, low self-esteem, or personality traits. Our study did not focus on these factors, but we did observe low scores in mental health domains similar to the Albarrán-Sánchez study. Upon analyzing the SF-36 scores, we found that the most significant improvements in a patient's QoL were related to their physical health rather than their mental health.

The Albarrán-Sánchez study also highlighted several factors that may contribute to mental health issues after surgery. First, patients may have a lower sense of overall well-being due to feeling like they are still dealing with a chronic illness, even if they have regained physical function [24]. Our study found that physical function is closely linked to social and emotional well-being. The authors of the study noted that patients may still feel inadequate after surgery, especially because they will continue to have periodic follow-up appointments and may find the lifestyle changes required post-surgery stressful. Additionally, research indicates that accepting morphological changes regarding body image can also cause stress [25].

After undergoing bariatric surgery, it is common for patients to experience micronutrient deficiencies. As a result, many patients require regular supplementation of vitamins and minerals, particularly in the case of vitamin B12, which is only obtained from external sources. These deficiencies can be attributed to reduced dietary intake and structural and functional alterations in the gastrointestinal tract, especially in procedures involving malabsorption. However, the occurrence of vitamin and mineral deficiencies following sleeve gastrectomy (LSG) compared with Roux-en-Y gastric bypass (RYGB) has not been documented yet. In a previous study monitoring bariatric patients through the course of 12 months, the authors highlight that the levels of vitamin B12 show a significant decrease, underscoring the importance of long-term supplementation with iron, vitamin B12, and other multivitamins and essential minerals [26]. It should be noted that patients who are not closely monitored may develop anemia due to changes in gastrointestinal absorption [27].

Vitamin D deficiency is also very common among bariatric patients. In a clinical study involving patients with obesity, altered basal blood glucose, and hypovitaminosis D, it was observed that correcting vitamin D deficiency through supplementation improves insulin resistance, reduces the risk of developing type 2 diabetes (T2DM), prevents sarcopenia, and regulates adipocyte differentiation [28,29]. Numerous studies have demonstrated the role of vitamin D in modulating the immune system. The low levels of vitamin D in the general population of Europe pose a public health concern, as they have been associated with increased susceptibility to infections and chronic diseases [30]. A recent study found that individuals with low vitamin D levels have an 80% higher likelihood of acquiring a COVID-19 infection compared with a control group with normal levels.

In addition, regarding mental health and emotional well-being, multiple studies closely link depression and obesity. Both pathologies are considered risk factors for one another and tend to associate within individuals. They also seem to have shared biological mechanisms [31]. Recent scientific research, as demonstrated by studies conducted by Robinson et al. and Sullivan et al., provides evidence supporting the influence of genetic factors on both obesity and depression [32,33]. These studies indicate that there is an estimated 40% heritability for major depressive disorder (MDD) and BMI. Furthermore, through genome-wide association analyses, Pigeyre et al. identified over 200 genomic regions associated with BMI, obesity status, and fat distribution. It seems that the genes located in proximity to BMI-associated loci show significant expression in the hypothalamus and pituitary gland [34]. These brain regions are responsible for regulating both mood and energy homeostasis. Additionally, more than 50 genetic loci associated with depression phenotypes, specifically related to MDD genetics, have been identified [35]. Wheeler and Pierce note that the genes exhibiting the strongest signals were previously linked to severe early-onset obesity and are situated in close proximity or even have overlapping positions [36].

The results of a study published in the Journal of the American Medical Association (JAMA) indicate that a substantial number of young individuals with severe obesity who underwent bariatric surgery reported a reduction of over 50% in their excess body weight, resulting in significant improvements in health and QoL compared with young individuals who were engaged in an intensive lifestyle modification program [37]. Obesity is a major but manageable risk factor for many diseases. Additionally, current research consistently demonstrates that obesity has a negative impact on QoL, and the severity of these effects escalates proportionally with the level of obesity, which aligns with the findings of our study [38].

Patients with severe obesity have been reported to have a lower QoL, particularly in regard to mental health, compared with normal-weight patients [39]. However, physical functionality has the greatest impact on perceived QoL [40]. Bariatric surgery has been found to improve various aspects of QoL, including patient satisfaction, self-esteem, body perception, and social interaction, in addition to weight loss [39]. Our study found a close relationship between physical and mental health. The latter (MH) significantly correlates with general health (GH). Despite the significant weight loss in the first year following bariatric surgery, few prospective studies have evaluated the long-term effect of depression, anxiety, and QoL, as well as their effects on weight loss recovery [24].

A recent meta-analysis indicates that RYGB and LSG may improve the post-operative QoL of the patients. The study assesses patients at various time points, from one up to five years after surgery [40]. Our study found that patients who underwent RYGB or LSG reported a higher self-perceived QoL when compared with those who underwent SADI-S, as measured using the SF-36 questionnaire. The meta-analysis also suggests that more complex or invasive procedures may result in lower QoL in the short and medium term, but improvement is seen after nine years.

Our study also found that evaluating the QoL of bariatric surgery patients is challenging, despite the weight loss and improvement of coexisting illnesses. Research in the literature emphasizes the importance of including patient-reported QoL assessment in the therapeutic approach, as it provides valuable data for evaluating the success of surgery beyond clinical evaluation. Our data highlighted that patients report improved physical functionality, which significantly correlates with mental health. However, for accurate measurements, longitudinal studies are necessary to measure the perception of QoL in physical health, mental health, and social relationships.

Potential shortcomings of our study include the risk of selection bias, as the respondents were volunteers. This could limit the applicability of the findings to the entire population of bariatric patients. Without a control group, it could be challenging to determine whether the observed improvements in quality of life can be solely attributed to bariatric surgery. As in all other studies relying on self-reported data from questionnaires, some of the respondents might be subject to recall bias or subjective interpretation. The study has a relatively short follow-up duration. This could restrict the ability to assess the long-term effects and sustainability of improved quality-of-life outcomes.

The study utilized the SF-36 and WHOQOL-BREF questionnaires, which are widely recognized and validated tools for measuring quality of life. This adds credibility to the study's findings and provides a structured and objective approach to evaluating the impact of bariatric surgery on quality of life.

With 76 respondents, the study had a reasonable sample size, which enhances the statistical power and reliability of the results. Assessing patients at different timepoints after the surgical procedure allows for a comprehensive understanding of the overall impact on the quality of life.

5. Conclusions

The current study provides insight into the QoL of patients who underwent different types of bariatric procedures. The findings indicate that following surgery, there was an improvement in the physical and social functioning of patients. The study also points out areas where patients may still encounter difficulties, such as issues related to vitality and limitations associated with mental health. The study can provide valuable insights for medical professionals to develop targeted interventions aimed at improving patient outcomes following bariatric surgery. Additionally, it contributes to the growing body of evidence concerning the impact of bariatric surgery on QoL, thereby guiding future research in this field.

Author Contributions: Conceptualization, R.P.S., D.V.T. and D.A.; methodology, D.A. and D.D.; software, I.C.D. and M.L.C.; validation, R.D., S.T. and R.L.; formal analysis, L.E.C. and A.A.M.; investigation, B.M.C., A.A.M. and L.E.C.; resources, R.D., S.T. and R.L.; data curation, I.C.D. and M.L.C.; writing—original draft preparation, R.P.S.; writing—review and editing, R.P.S. and S.T.; visualization, R.D. and R.L.; supervision, D.V.T., D.A. and D.D.; project administration, B.M.C. and A.A.M. All authors have read and agreed to the published version of the manuscript.

Funding: This research received no external funding.

Institutional Review Board Statement: The study was conducted following the Declaration of Helsinki and approved by the Institutional Ethics Committee of "Grigore T. Popa" University of Medicine and Pharmacy and "St. Spiridon" Clinical Emergency Hospital, Nr. 137/25.01.2022 and Nr.34/17.03.2022, respectively, for studies involving humans.

Informed Consent Statement: Informed consent was obtained from all subjects involved in the study.

Data Availability Statement: The data presented in this study are available on request from the corresponding author.

Acknowledgments: We want to thank Oana Olariu and Ioana Silistraru for their indispensable support and technical assistance throughout this project. We would also like to highlight the efforts of the Romanian Society for Metabolic Surgery (RSMS), a member of IFSO, in implementing a national registry of the obese patient, in an effort for bariatric surgery to be included in national health policies.

Conflicts of Interest: The authors declare no conflict of interest.

References

1. Busutil, R.; Espallardo, O.; Torres, A.; Martínez-Galdeano, L.; Zozaya, N.; Hidalgo-Vega, Á. The Impact of Obesity on Health-Related Quality of Life in Spain. *Health Qual. Life Outcomes* **2017**, *15*, 197. [CrossRef] [PubMed]
2. Rozjabek, H.; Fastenau, J.; LaPrade, A.; Sternbach, N. Adult Obesity and Health-Related Quality of Life, Patient Activation, Work Productivity, and Weight Loss Behaviors in the United States. *Diabetes Metab. Syndr. Obes.* **2020**, *13*, 2049–2055. [CrossRef] [PubMed]
3. World Obesity Atlas 2022. Available online: https://www.worldobesity.org/resources/resource-library/world-obesity-atlas-2022 (accessed on 17 May 2023).
4. Małczak, P.; Mizera, M.; Lee, Y.; Pisarska-Adamczyk, M.; Wysocki, M.; Bała, M.M.; Witowski, J.; Rubinkiewicz, M.; Dudek, A.; Stefura, T.; et al. Quality of Life After Bariatric Surgery-a Systematic Review with Bayesian Network Meta-Analysis. *Obes. Surg.* **2021**, *31*, 5213–5223. [CrossRef] [PubMed]
5. Lins, L.; Carvalho, F.M. SF-36 Total Score as a Single Measure of Health-Related Quality of Life: Scoping Review. *SAGE Open Med.* **2016**, *4*, 2050312116671725. [CrossRef]
6. Buckell, J.; Mei, X.W.; Clarke, P.; Aveyard, P.; Jebb, S.A. Weight Loss Interventions on Health-related Quality of Life in Those with Moderate to Severe Obesity: Findings from an Individual Patient Data Meta-analysis of Randomized Trials. *Obes. Rev.* **2021**, *22*, e13317. [CrossRef]
7. Magallares, A.; Schomerus, G. Mental and Physical Health-Related Quality of Life in Obese Patients before and after Bariatric Surgery: A Meta-Analysis. *Psychol. Health Med.* **2015**, *20*, 165–176. [CrossRef]
8. Dietz, W.H.; Baur, L.A.; Hall, K.; Puhl, R.M.; Taveras, E.M.; Uauy, R.; Kopelman, P. Management of Obesity: Improvement of Health-Care Training and Systems for Prevention and Care. *Lancet* **2015**, *385*, 2521–2533. [CrossRef]
9. Welbourn, R.; Hollyman, M.; Kinsman, R.; Dixon, J.; Liem, R.; Ottosson, J.; Ramos, A.; Våge, V.; Al-Sabah, S.; Brown, W.; et al. Bariatric Surgery Worldwide: Baseline Demographic Description and One-Year Outcomes from the Fourth IFSO Global Registry Report 2018. *Obes. Surg.* **2019**, *29*, 782–795. [CrossRef]

10. Sierżantowicz, R.; Ładny, J.R.; Lewko, J. Quality of Life after Bariatric Surgery-A Systematic Review. *Int. J. Environ. Res. Public Health* **2022**, *19*, 9078. [CrossRef]
11. Arterburn, D.E.; Telem, D.A.; Kushner, R.F.; Courcoulas, A.P. Benefits and Risks of Bariatric Surgery in Adults: A Review. *JAMA* **2020**, *324*, 879–887. [CrossRef]
12. O'Brien, P.E.; Hindle, A.; Brennan, L.; Skinner, S.; Burton, P.; Smith, A.; Crosthwaite, G.; Brown, W. Long-Term Outcomes After Bariatric Surgery: A Systematic Review and Meta-Analysis of Weight Loss at 10 or More Years for All Bariatric Procedures and a Single-Centre Review of 20-Year Outcomes After Adjustable Gastric Banding. *Obes. Surg.* **2019**, *29*, 3–14. [CrossRef] [PubMed]
13. Roth, A.E.; Thornley, C.J.; Blackstone, R.P. Outcomes in Bariatric and Metabolic Surgery: An Updated 5-Year Review. *Curr. Obes. Rep.* **2020**, *9*, 380–389. [CrossRef] [PubMed]
14. Shoar, S.; Saber, A.A. Long-Term and Midterm Outcomes of Laparoscopic Sleeve Gastrectomy versus Roux-En-Y Gastric Bypass: A Systematic Review and Meta-Analysis of Comparative Studies. *Surg. Obes. Relat. Dis.* **2017**, *13*, 170–180. [CrossRef] [PubMed]
15. Shoar, S.; Nguyen, T.; Ona, M.A.; Reddy, M.; Anand, S.; Alkuwari, M.J.; Saber, A.A. Roux-En-Y Gastric Bypass Reversal: A Systematic Review. *Surg. Obes. Relat. Dis.* **2016**, *12*, 1366–1372. [CrossRef] [PubMed]
16. Sánchez-Pernaute, A.; Rubio, M.Á.; Pérez Aguirre, E.; Barabash, A.; Cabrerizo, L.; Torres, A. Single-Anastomosis Duodenoileal Bypass with Sleeve Gastrectomy: Metabolic Improvement and Weight Loss in First 100 Patients. *Surg. Obes. Relat. Dis.* **2013**, *9*, 731–735. [CrossRef]
17. Pantelis, A.G.; Vakis, G.; Kotrotsiou, M.; Lapatsanis, D.P. Status of Body Contouring Following Metabolic Bariatric Surgery in a Tertiary Hospital of Greece—Still a Long Way to Go. *J. Clin. Med.* **2023**, *12*, 3196. [CrossRef]
18. Aitzetmüller-Klietz, M.M.; Raschke, L.; Hirsch, T.; Kückelhaus, M.; Wiebringhaus, P.; Aitzetmüller-Klietz, M.-L.; Harati, K. Factors Influencing Quality of Life after Massive Weight Loss—What Makes the Difference? *Healthcare* **2023**, *11*, 1147. [CrossRef]
19. Hachuła, M.; Kosowski, M.; Zielańska, K.; Basiak, M.; Okopień, B. The Impact of Various Methods of Obesity Treatment on the Quality of Life and Mental Health—A Narrative Review. *Int. J. Environ. Res. Public Health* **2023**, *20*, 2122. [CrossRef]
20. Rego De Figueiredo, I.; Carvalho Vasques, M.; Cunha, N.; Martins, D.; Silva-Nunes, J. Quality of Life in Obese Patients from a Multidisciplinary Bariatric Consultation: A Cross-Sectional Study Comparing to a Non-Bariatric Population and to the General Population. *Int. J. Environ. Res. Public Health* **2022**, *19*, 12029. [CrossRef]
21. Athanasiou, T.; Patel, V.; Darzi, A. *Patient Reported Outcomes and Quality of Life in Surgery*; Springer Nature: Cham, Switzerland, 2023; ISBN 978-3-031-27597-5.
22. Poelemeijer, Y.Q.M.; van der Knaap, E.T.W.; Marang-van de Mheen, P.J.; Demirkiran, A.; Wiezer, M.J.; Hazebroek, E.J.; Greve, J.W.M.; Liem, R.S.L. Measuring Quality of Life in Bariatric Surgery: A Multicentre Study. *Surg. Endosc.* **2020**, *34*, 5522–5532. [CrossRef]
23. De Vries, C.E.E.; Makarawung, D.J.S.; Monpellier, V.M.; Janssen, I.M.C.; De Castro, S.M.M.; Van Veen, R.N. Is the RAND-36 an Adequate Patient-Reported Outcome Measure to Assess Health-Related Quality of Life in Patients Undergoing Bariatric Surgery? *Obes. Surg.* **2022**, *32*, 48–54. [CrossRef]
24. Albarrán-Sánchez, A.; Ramírez-Rentería, C.; Ferreira-Hermosillo, A.; Rodríguez-Pérez, V.; Espinosa-Cárdenas, E.; Molina-Ayala, M.; Boscó-Gárate, I.; Mendoza-Zubieta, V. Quality of life evaluation in Mexican patients with severe obesity before and after bariatric surgery. *Gac. Med. Mex.* **2023**, *157*, 64–69. [CrossRef]
25. Silistraru, I.; Olariu, O.; Ciubara, A.; Roșca, Ș.; Roșca, R. O.; Stanciu, S.; Condratovici, A.P.; Ciureanu, I.-A. Burnout and Online Medical Education: Romanian Students in Lockdown and Their Residency Choices. *Int. J. Environ. Res. Public Health* **2022**, *19*, 5449. [CrossRef] [PubMed]
26. Soroceanu, R.P.; Timofte, D.V.; Maxim, M.; Platon, R.L.; Vlasceanu, V.; Ciuntu, B.M.; Pinzariu, A.C.; Clim, A.; Soroceanu, A.; Silistraru, I.; et al. Twelve-Month Outcomes in Patients with Obesity Following Bariatric Surgery—A Single Centre Experience. *Nutrients* **2023**, *15*, 1134. [CrossRef] [PubMed]
27. Gasmi, A.; Bjørklund, G.; Mujawdiya, P.K.; Semenova, Y.; Peana, M.; Dosa, A.; Piscopo, S.; Gasmi Benahmed, A.; Costea, D.O. Micronutrients Deficiencies in Patients after Bariatric Surgery. *Eur. J. Nutr.* **2022**, *61*, 55–67. [CrossRef] [PubMed]
28. Niroomand, M.; Fotouhi, A.; Irannejad, N.; Hosseinpanah, F. Does High-Dose Vitamin D Supplementation Impact Insulin Resistance and Risk of Development of Diabetes in Patients with Pre-Diabetes? A Double-Blind Randomized Clinical Trial. *Diabetes Res. Clin. Pract.* **2019**, *148*, 1–9. [CrossRef]
29. Pinzariu, A.C.; Pasca, S.A.; Sindilar, A.; Drochioi, C.; Balan, M.; Oboroceanu, T.; Niculescu, S.; Crauciuc, D.V.; Crauciuc, E.G.; Luca, A.; et al. Adipose Tissue Remodeling by Prolonged Administration of High Dose of Vitamin D3 in Rats Treated to Prevent Sarcopenia. *Rev. Chim.* **2017**, *68*, 2139–2143. [CrossRef]
30. Pinzariu, A.C.; Oboroceanu, T.; Eloae, F.Z.; Hristov, I.; Costan, V.V.; Labusca, L.; Cianga, P.; Verestiuc, L.; Hanganu, B.; Crauciuc, D.V.; et al. Vitamin D as a Regulator of Adipocyte Differentiation Effects in Vivo and in Vitro. *Rev. Chim.* **2018**, *69*, 731–734. [CrossRef]
31. Milaneschi, Y.; Simmons, W.K.; Van Rossum, E.F.C.; Penninx, B.W. Depression and Obesity: Evidence of Shared Biological Mechanisms. *Mol. Psychiatry* **2019**, *24*, 18–33. [CrossRef]
32. The LifeLines Cohort Study; Robinson, M.R.; English, G.; Moser, G.; Lloyd-Jones, L.R.; Triplett, M.A.; Zhu, Z.; Nolte, I.M.; Van Vliet-Ostaptchouk, J.V.; Snieder, H.; et al. Genotype–Covariate Interaction Effects and the Heritability of Adult Body Mass Index. *Nat. Genet.* **2017**, *49*, 1174–1181. [CrossRef]

33. Sullivan, P.F.; Neale, M.C.; Kendler, K.S. Genetic Epidemiology of Major Depression: Review and Meta-Analysis. *Am. J. Psychiatry* **2000**, *157*, 1552–1562. [CrossRef] [PubMed]
34. Pigeyre, M.; Yazdi, F.T.; Kaur, Y.; Meyre, D. Recent Progress in Genetics, Epigenetics and Metagenomics Unveils the Pathophysiology of Human Obesity. *Clin. Sci.* **2016**, *130*, 943–986. [CrossRef]
35. ReproGen Consortium; Schizophrenia Working Group of the Psychiatric Genomics Consortium; The RACI Consortium; Finucane, H.K.; Bulik-Sullivan, B.; Gusev, A.; Trynka, G.; Reshef, Y.; Loh, P.-R.; Anttila, V.; et al. Partitioning Heritability by Functional Annotation Using Genome-Wide Association Summary Statistics. *Nat. Genet.* **2015**, *47*, 1228–1235. [CrossRef] [PubMed]
36. Wheeler, E.; Huang, N.; Bochukova, E.G.; Keogh, J.M.; Lindsay, S.; Garg, S.; Henning, E.; Blackburn, H.; Loos, R.J.F.; Wareham, N.J.; et al. Genome-Wide SNP and CNV Analysis Identifies Common and Low-Frequency Variants Associated with Severe Early-Onset Obesity. *Nat. Genet.* **2013**, *45*, 513–517. [CrossRef] [PubMed]
37. O'Brien, P.E.; Sawyer, S.M.; Laurie, C.; Brown, W.A.; Skinner, S.; Veit, F.; Paul, E.; Burton, P.R.; McGrice, M.; Anderson, M.; et al. Laparoscopic Adjustable Gastric Banding in Severely Obese Adolescents: A Randomized Trial. *JAMA* **2010**, *303*, 519. [CrossRef]
38. Fontaine, K.R.; Barofsky, I. Obesity and Health-Related Quality of Life. *Obes. Rev.* **2001**, *2*, 173–182. [CrossRef]
39. Ramada Faria, G.F.; Nunes Santos, J.M.; Simonson, D.C. Quality of Life after Gastric Sleeve and Gastric Bypass for Morbid Obesity. *Porto Biomed. J.* **2017**, *2*, 40–46. [CrossRef]
40. Callegari, A.; Michelini, I.; Sguazzin, C.; Catona, A.; Klersy, C. Efficacy of the SF-36 Questionnaire in Identifying Obese Patients with Psychological Discomfort. *Obes. Surg.* **2005**, *15*, 254–260. [CrossRef]

Disclaimer/Publisher's Note: The statements, opinions and data contained in all publications are solely those of the individual author(s) and contributor(s) and not of MDPI and/or the editor(s). MDPI and/or the editor(s) disclaim responsibility for any injury to people or property resulting from any ideas, methods, instructions or products referred to in the content.

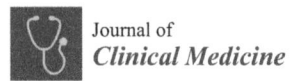

Article

Larissa Heart Failure Risk Score and Mode of Death in Acute Heart Failure: Insights from REALITY-AHF

Andrew Xanthopoulos [1], Angeliki Bourazana [1], Yuya Matsue [2], Yudai Fujimoto [2], Shogo Oishi [3], Eiichi Akiyama [4], Satoshi Suzuki [5], Masayoshi Yamamoto [6], Keisuke Kida [7], Takahiro Okumura [8], Grigorios Giamouzis [1], John Skoularigis [1], Filippos Triposkiadis [1,*] and Takeshi Kitai [9,10,*]

1. Department of Cardiology, University Hospital of Larissa, 41110 Larissa, Greece
2. Department of Cardiovascular Medicine, Juntendo University Graduate School of Medicine, Tokyo 113-0033, Japan
3. Department of Cardiology, Himeji Cardiovascular Center, Himeji 670-8560, Japan
4. Division of Cardiology, Yokohama City University Medical Center, Yokohama 232-0024, Japan
5. Department of Cardiovascular Medicine, Fukushima Medical University, Fukushima 960-1295, Japan
6. Cardiovascular Division, Faculty of Medicine, University of Tsukuba, Tsukuba 305-8577, Japan
7. Department of Pharmacology, St. Marianna University School of Medicine, Kawasaki 216-8511, Japan
8. Department of Cardiology, Nagoya University Graduate School of Medicine, Nagoya 466-8550, Japan
9. Department of Cardiovascular Medicine, Kobe City Medical Center General Hospital, Kobe 650-0047, Japan
10. Department of Cardiovascular Medicine, National Cerebral and Cardiovascular Center, Osaka 564-8565, Japan
* Correspondence: ftriposkiadis@gmail.com (F.T.); t-kitai@kcho.jp (T.K.); Tel.: +30-2413502019 (F.T.); +81-661-701-070 (T.K.); Fax: +81-661-701 346 (T.K.)

Abstract: Patients with heart failure (HF) patients may die either suddenly (sudden cardiac death/SCD) or progressively from pump failure. The heightened risk of SCD in patients with HF may expedite important decisions about medications or devices. We used the Larissa Heart Failure Risk Score (LHFRS), a validated risk model for all-cause mortality and HF rehospitalization, to investigate the mode of death in 1363 patients enrolled in the Registry Focused on Very Early Presentation and Treatment in Emergency Department of Acute Heart Failure (REALITY-AHF). Cumulative incidence curves were generated using a Fine–Gray competing risk regression, with deaths that were not due to the cause of death of interest as a competing risk. Likewise, the Fine–Gray competing risk regression analysis was used to evaluate the association between each variable and the incidence of each cause of death. The AHEAD score, a well-validated HF risk score ranging from 0 to 5 (atrial fibrillation, anemia, age, renal dysfunction, and diabetes mellitus), was used for the risk adjustment. Patients with LHFRS 2–4 exhibited a significantly higher risk of SCD (HR hazard ratio adjusted for AHEAD score 3.15, 95% confidence interval (CI) (1.30–7.65), $p = 0.011$) and HF death (adjusted HR for AHEAD score 1.48, 95% CI (1.04–2.09), $p = 0.03$), compared to those with LHFRS 0,1. Regarding cardiovascular death, patients with higher LHFRS had significantly increased risk compared to those with lower LHFRS (HR 1.44 adjusted for AHEAD score, 95% CI (1.09–1.91), $p = 0.01$). Lastly, patients with higher LHFRS exhibited a similar risk of non-cardiovascular death compared to those with lower LHFRS (HR 1.44 adjusted for AHEAD score, 95% CI (0.95–2.19), $p = 0.087$). In conclusion, LHFRS was associated independently with the mode of death in a prospective cohort of hospitalized HF patients.

Keywords: Larissa heart failure risk score; mode of death; sudden cardiac death; mortality

Citation: Xanthopoulos, A.; Bourazana, A.; Matsue, Y.; Fujimoto, Y.; Oishi, S.; Akiyama, E.; Suzuki, S.; Yamamoto, M.; Kida, K.; Okumura, T.; et al. Larissa Heart Failure Risk Score and Mode of Death in Acute Heart Failure: Insights from REALITY-AHF. *J. Clin. Med.* 2023, 12, 3722. https://doi.org/10.3390/jcm12113722

Academic Editor: Daniele Masarone

Received: 22 February 2023
Revised: 24 May 2023
Accepted: 25 May 2023
Published: 28 May 2023

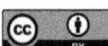

Copyright: © 2023 by the authors. Licensee MDPI, Basel, Switzerland. This article is an open access article distributed under the terms and conditions of the Creative Commons Attribution (CC BY) license (https://creativecommons.org/licenses/by/4.0/).

1. Introduction

Heart failure (HF) is a lethal syndrome affecting 38 million adults globally [1]. Due to the senescence and expansion of the global population, its prevalence continues to rise [2]. Patients with HF suffer a progressive decline in their functional and intellectual capacity, while the risk of sudden cardiac death (SCD) is low. Since its designation as an emerging pandemic in 1997, HF has attracted a host of studies with the purpose of corroborating our mechanistic understanding of the syndrome. Nevertheless, the burden of mortality and hospitalizations varies significantly among the different HF groups [3]. Disparate is also a mode of death where some patients die suddenly while others die from disease progression, such as pump failure or non-cardiovascular death [4]. The evident heterogeneity in the clinical profiles of HF necessitates a profound understanding of the factors associated with the mode of death in HF.

The Larissa Heart Failure Risk Score (LHFRS) is a practical risk stratification model derived from three factors (history of hypertension (yes = 0, no = 2); history of coronary artery disease/myocardial infarction (yes = 1, no = 0); and red blood cell distribution width [RDW] $\geq$ 15% (yes = 1, no = 0); best = 0, worst = 4) [5,6]. It was validated in the external cohort REALITY-AHF [7], which can reliably correlate time to treatment and clinical outcomes among the divergent group of HF patients admitted to the emergency department (ED) [8,9]. In the current study, we assessed the potential associations between the mode of death in HF and the LHFRS in the population of patients enrolled in the REALITY-AHF study.

2. Methods

2.1. Study Population

The REALITY-AHF (Registry Focused on Very Early Presentation and Treatment in Emergency Department of Acute Heart Failure) was a prospective, multicenter, observational cohort study that primarily aimed to assess the association between time to treatment and clinical outcomes in patients with acute HF (AHF) admitted through the emergency department (ED). Enrollment started in August 2014 and was completed in December 2015. Among the 20 participating hospitals, 9 were university hospitals and 11 were non-university teaching hospitals.

The study design and results have been reported elsewhere in detail [8–10]. In brief, patients were included if they were aged $\geq$20 years and diagnosed with AHF in the ED within 3 h of their first evaluation by caregivers. Only the first hospitalization during the study period was registered, and the AHF diagnosis was made based on the Framingham criteria. Exclusion criteria were as follows: (1) treatment with an intravenous (IV) drug before ED arrival; (2) previous heart transplantation; (3) chronic peritoneal dialysis or hemodialysis; (4) acute myocarditis; and (5) acute coronary syndrome requiring emergent or urgent revascularization. The study complied with the 1975 Declaration of Helsinki, and the Institutional Review Board (IRB) approval was obtained from each participating center.

In this study, we enrolled 1363 patients for whom LHFRS data were available.

2.2. Definitions

The red blood cell distribution width (RDW) was calculated as follows: (standard deviation of mean corpuscular volume divided by mean corpuscular volume) $\times$ 100. For an event causing death, the event and death were considered separate events only if the interval that separated the event and the death was 24 h or greater. In cases where the event and death were separated by less than 24 h, death was the only adjudicated event. All deaths were considered cardiovascular unless a non-cardiovascular cause of death was established. Cardiovascular deaths included death due to HF, myocardial infarction, SCD, other cardiovascular causes (e.g., stroke and cardiovascular intervention), and presumed cardiovascular causes [10]. Death due to HF is defined as death occurring in the context of clinically worsening symptoms and/or signs of HF without the evidence of another cause of death: (1) New or increasing symptoms and/or signs of HF requiring the initiation of, or an increase in, treatment directed at HF or occurring in a subject already receiving treatment; (2) HF symptoms or signs requiring continuous i.v. therapy or oxygen administration; (3) confinement to bed entirely due to HF symptoms; (4) pulmonary edema is sufficient to cause tachypnea and distress not occurring in the context of myocardial infarction or as a consequence of an arrhythmia occurring in the absence of worsening HF; (5) cardiogenic shock not occurring in the context of myocardial infarction or as a consequence of an arrhythmia occurring in the absence of worsening HF. In the current analysis, all-cause death was divided into cardiovascular and non-cardiovascular diseases. Cardiovascular death was divided into HF death, SCD, and other cardiovascular deaths.

2.3. Outcomes

The outcomes of interest were as follows: (a) SCD (primary endpoint); (b) death due to HF (secondary endpoint); (c) cardiovascular death (secondary endpoint); and (d) non-cardiovascular death (secondary endpoint), within 1-year after discharge.

2.4. Statistical Analysis

Categorical variables are shown as numbers and percentages and were compared using the Chi-squared test or Fisher's exact test, as appropriate. Continuous variables were expressed as mean and standard deviation or median and interquartile range (IQR). Depending on their distribution (qualitatively judged via histogram and Q-Q plot), continuous variables were compared using Student's *t*-test or Wilcoxon rank-sum test, as appropriate. Two-sided p values < 0.05 were considered statistically significant. Cumulative incidence curves were generated using a Fine–Gray competing risk regression, with deaths that were not due to the cause of death of interest as a competing risk. Likewise, the Fine–Gray competing risk regression analysis was used to evaluate the association between each variable and the incidence of each cause of death. Clinical follow-up data were obtained from medical records or directly from patients either in person or during telephone interviews. We used the AHEAD score for risk adjustment, which is a well-validated HF risk score ranging from 0 to 5 and includes the following variables: atrial fibrillation, anemia (haemoglobin <130 g/l for men and 120 g/l for women), age >70 years), renal dysfunction (creatinine >130 μmol/l), and diabetes mellitus [11,12]. Proportional hazard assumption violations were estimated using generalized linear regression of scaled Schoenfeld residuals over time. Statistical analyses were performed using the statistical software program R version 4.1.3 (R Foundation for Statistical Computing, Vienna, Austria).

3. Results

3.1. Baseline Characteristics

The baseline characteristics of the study population (1363 HF patients) stratified by the LHFRS score are presented in Table 1. Patients with higher LHFRS scores (i.e., 2–4) were younger and had lower admission systolic or diastolic blood pressure compared to patients with lower LHFRS (i.e., 0–1) scores. Additionally, they had a lesser history of hypertension and lower values of hemoglobin, white blood cells, glucose, and sodium. In contrast, patients with LHFRS 0 or 1 had a lesser history of coronary artery disease and lower values of RDW than those with LHFRS 2–4. Regarding medical therapy at admission, beta-blockers, mineralocorticoid receptor antagonists (MRAs), and loop diuretics were more frequently noted in the higher LHFRS categories, whereas angiotensin-receptor blockers (ARBs) were noted in the lower LHFRS categories.

Table 1. Baseline characteristics of the study population.

Variables	LHFRS = 0, 1 n = 789	LHFRS = 2–4 n = 574	p Value
Age (mean (SD))	78.47 (12.10)	75.56 (12.90)	<0.001
Males, n (%)	430 (54.5)	339 (59.1)	0.105
Systolic Blood Pressure (mean (SD))	154.90 (35.67)	135.47 (33.20)	<0.001
Diastolic Blood Pressure (mean (SD))	85.74 (25.67)	78.86 (22.63)	<0.001

Table 1. *Cont.*

Variables	LHFRS = 0, 1 n = 789	LHFRS = 2–4 n = 574	p Value
Heart Rate (mean (SD))	96.98 (27.80)	96.56 (28.48)	0.784
Ambulance, n (%)	452 (57.3)	306 (53.3)	0.16
De novo HF, n (%)	400 (50.7)	247 (43.0)	0.006
Symptom onset (%)			0.013
6 h	188 (23.8)	108 (18.8)	
≤2 days	190 (24.1)	122 (21.3)	
>2 days	411 (52.1)	344 (59.9)	
ECG rhythm (%)			0.001
Sinus rhythm	446 (56.5)	268 (46.7)	
Atrial fibrillation	262 (33.2)	239 (41.6)	
Other	81 (10.3)	67 (11.7)	
Echo visual estimation of LVEF (%)			<0.001
<35	243 (32.3)	256 (46.7)	
35–50	228 (30.3)	141 (25.7)	
>50	281 (37.4)	151 (27.6)	
Heart Failure Symptoms/Signs			
Jugular Venous Distension, n (%)	428 (54.7)	319 (56.2)	0.623
Orthopnea, n (%)	471 (59.8)	290 (50.5)	0.001
Rales, n (%)	512 (64.9)	355 (62.0)	0.291
Peripheral edema, n (%)	531 (67.3)	393 (68.6)	0.658
Pulmonary edema, n (%)	594 (75.3)	378 (65.9)	<0.001
Comorbidities/Risk factors			
Hypertension, n (%)	789 (100.0)	131 (22.8)	<0.001
Diabetes Mellitus, n (%)	305 (38.7)	193 (33.6)	0.065
Coronary Artery Disease, n (%)	213 (27.0)	224 (39.0)	<0.001
Peripheral Arterial Disease, n (%)	64 (8.1)	39 (6.8)	0.421
Chronic Obstructive Pulmonary Disease, n (%)	78 (9.9)	53 (9.2)	0.756
Smoker, n (%)	287 (36.4)	212 (37.0)	0.858
Laboratory Variables			
Hemoglobin (mean (SD))	11.83 (2.23)	11.56 (2.36)	0.033
RDW-CV (mean (SD))	14.56 (1.64)	15.56 (2.30)	<0.001
White Blood Cells (median [IQR])	7800 [5900, 10,400]	7000 [5500, 9300]	<0.001
Glucose (mean (SD))	166.65 (75.96)	157.20 (76.26)	0.026
Blood Urine Nitrogen (median [IQR])	24.50 [17.80, 34.60]	25 [18.42, 36]	0.288
Creatinine (median [IQR])	1.13 [0.86, 1.64]	1.12 [0.85, 1.58]	0.585
Estimated Glomerular Filtration Rate (mean (SD))	55.17 (25.14)	58.00 (26.22)	0.044
Aspartate Aminotransferase (median [IQR])	30 [23, 44]	33 [23, 49]	0.068
Alanine Aminotransferase (median [IQR])	21 [14, 34]	22 [14, 37]	0.286
Na^+ (mean (SD))	139.20 (4.61)	138.28 (4.44)	<0.001

Table 1. Cont.

Variables	LHFRS = 0, 1 n = 789	LHFRS = 2–4 n = 574	p Value
CRP (median [IQR])	0.58 [0.19, 2.26]	0.75 [0.22, 2.04]	0.175
Medications at admission			
ACE-inhibitors, n (%)	135 (17.1)	99 (17.2)	1
Angiotensin Receptor Blockers, n (%)	296 (37.5)	121 (21.1)	<0.001
Beta Blockers, n (%)	330 (42.0)	280 (49.0)	0.013
Mineralocorticoid Antagonists, n (%)	131 (16.6)	171 (29.8)	<0.001
Loop diuretics, n (%)	376 (48.1)	332 (57.9)	<0.001
Medications at discharge			
ACE-inhibitors, n (%)	246 (32.8)	193 (36.2)	0.220
Angiotensin Receptor Blockers, n (%)	284 (37.8)	119 (22.3)	<0.001
Beta Blockers, n (%)	546 (72.4)	395 (73.8)	0.616
Mineralocorticoid Antagonists, n (%)	318 (42.1)	264 (49.3)	0.012
Loop diuretics, n (%)	640 (84.7)	460 (85.7)	0.674

LVEF, left ventricular ejection fraction; RDW, red blood cell distribution width; CRP, C-reactive protein. ECG: electrocardiogram, LVEF: left ventricular ejection fraction, RDW: red blood cell distribution width, Na$^+$: sodium, CRP: C-reactive protein, ACE-inhibitors: angiotensin converting enzyme inhibitors.

3.2. Study Outcomes

During a median follow-up of 1 year, 284 deaths were observed: SCD (n = 23), heart failure deaths (n = 125), other cardiovascular deaths (n = 48), and non-cardiovascular deaths (n = 88). Patients with LHFRS 2–4 exhibited a significantly higher risk of SCD compared to those with LHFRS 0,1 (HR hazard ratio adjusted for AHEAD score 3.15, 95% confidence interval (CI) (1.30–7.65), p = 0.011) (Figure 1A, Table 2). The results were similar when medical treatment at discharge and estimated glomerular filtration rate (eGFR) were used also for risk adjustment (Please see Supplementary Table S1). Patients with LHFRS 2–4 demonstrated a significantly higher risk of HF death compared to those with LHFRS 0,1 (adjusted HR for AHEAD score 1.48, 95% CI (1.04–2.09), p = 0.03) (Figure 1B, Table 2).

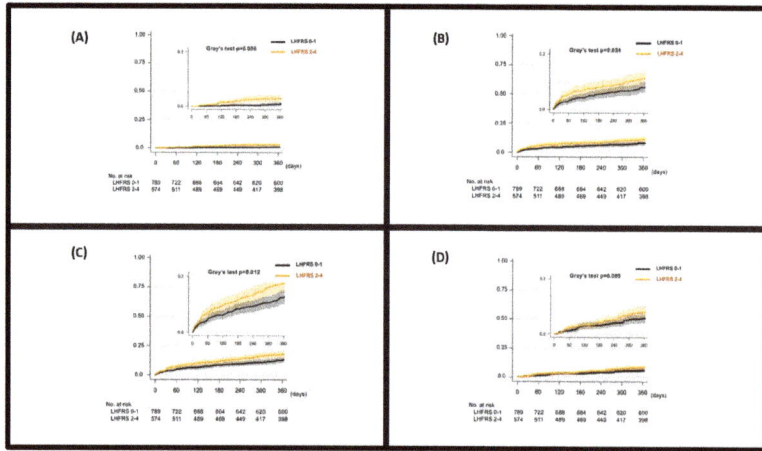

Figure 1. Cumulative incidence curves for (**A**) sudden cardiac death (SCD), (**B**) heart failure (HF) death, (**C**) cardiovascular (CV) death, and (**D**) non-cardiovascular (non-CV) death, based on the Larissa Heart Failure Risk Score (LHFRS).

Table 2. Comparison of risk (unadjusted and adjusted for the AHEAD score) of sudden cardiac death (SCD), heart failure (HF) death, cardiovascular (CV) death, and non-cardiovascular (non-CV) death, in patients with LHFRS 0, 1 vs. LHFRS 2–4.

	Sudden Cardiac Death					
Groups	Unadjusted			Adjusted for AHEAD Score		
	HR	95% CI	p Value	HR	95% CI	p Value
AHEAD score	1.33	1.02–1.72	0.033	1.23	0.93–1.63	0.15
LARISSA Score 0,1		1 (Reference)			1 (Reference)	
LARISSA Score 2–4	3.14	1.29–7.61	0.008	3.15	1.30–7.65	0.011
	Heart Failure Death					
Groups	Unadjusted			Adjusted for AHEAD score		
	HR	95% CI	p value	HR	95% CI	p value
AHEAD score	1.43	1.24–1.64	<0.001	1.38	1.18–1.60	<0.001
LARISSA Score 0,1		1 (Reference)			1 (Reference)	
LARISSA Score 2–4	1.46	1.03–2.07	0.034	1.48	1.04–2.09	0.03
	Cardiovascular Death					
Groups	Unadjusted			Adjusted for AHEAD score		
	HR	95% CI	p value	HR	95% CI	p value
AHEAD score	1.38	1.23–1.54	<0.001	1.32	1.17–1.49	<0.001
LARISSA Score 0,1		1 (Reference)			1 (Reference)	
LARISSA Score 2–4	1.43	1.08–1.89	0.012	1.44	1.09–1.91	0.01
	Non-cardiovascular Death					
Groups	Unadjusted			Adjusted for AHEAD score		
	HR	95% CI	p value	HR	95% CI	p value
AHEAD score	1.26	1.09–1.47	0.002	1.28	1.13–1.42	0.003
LARISSA Score 0,1		1 (Reference)			1 (Reference)	
LARISSA Score 2–4	1.44	0.95–2.18	0.089	1.44	0.95–2.19	0.087

Regarding cardiovascular death, patients with higher LHFRS had a significantly increased risk compared to those with lower LHFRS (HR 1.44 adjusted for AHEAD score, 95% CI (1.09–1.91), p = 0.01) (Figure 1C, Table 2). Lastly, patients with higher LHFRS exhibited a numerically higher risk of non-cardiovascular death compared to those with lower LHFRS, but it did not reach a statistically significant threshold (HR 1.44 adjusted for AHEAD score, 95% CI (0.95–2.19), p = 0.087) (Figure 1D, Table 2). LVEF did not modify the association between high/low LHFRS scores and the study outcomes (all p values for interaction were >0.05).

4. Discussion

In the REALITY-AHF trial, patients with AHF admitted to the ED were studied concerning the time of the first administration of IV diuretics and its clinical implication. A time-to-treatment benefit was observed, as patients with early diuretic administration (<60 min) demonstrated significantly lower in-hospital mortality [8,10]. The LHFRS was validated in the REALITY-AHF as an independent predictor of the primary and secondary outcomes of all-cause mortality and HF readmission [7]. In the present study, the cause of death was adjudicated according to the score's three very specific variables: history of hypertension, history of coronary artery disease/myocardial infarction, and RDW value. A higher risk of SCD, HF death, and a significantly increased risk of cardiovascular death in the groups with higher LHFRS (2–4) highlighted those in greater hazard.

In the present analysis, we noticed that in the higher (2–4) group, a significant proportion of patients (27.6%) had preserved left ventricular ejection fraction (LVEF), whereas 32.3% of patients had LVEF <35%. This study population, which also encompasses patients with lower mean age, is a significant peril of SCD [13]. Since previous trials and risk scores using LVEF as a discriminator failed to demonstrate a significant benefit in patients with preserved LVEF, a notable proportion of HF patients forfeit treatment for SCD prevention, such as sacubitril-valsartan [14]. In the present work, we observed an independent association between the LHFRS and the mode of death, without considering LVEF, and provided a larger group of patients with prompt and appropriate medical care [15,16]. Since arrhythmic death is the cause in the majority of cases with SCD, patients in the aforementioned group would benefit from SCD reduction approaches, such as ventricular ectopy invigilation during their hospitalization and outpatients. A recent meta-analysis of seven randomized clinical trials, including patients with HF and reduced or preserved LVEF, revealed an association between the use of sodium-glucose transport protein 2 (SGLT2) inhibitors and reduced risk of SCD (risk ratios: 0.68; 95% [CI]: 0.48–0.95; $p = 0.03$; $I^2 = 0\%$) [17].

Another differentiating characteristic between LHFRS and the majority of the rest risk scores in HF is the ability of the first to reveal "high risk" AHF patients at the time of initial hospitalization, whereas most other models were applied to patients with chronic HF. The Seattle Heart Failure Model (SHFM) provides information about the likely mode of death among ambulatory HF patients, and the prognostication of the mode of death in PARAGON was evaluated in a group of patients with chronic HF [18,19]. Likewise, the evaluation of the mode of death in the PARADIGM-HF patients was achieved not on a single time point but integrated baseline characteristics as well as covariates that were collected from outpatient visits [20]. Similarly, CHARM, GISSI-HF, and MAGGIC prediction scores were performed in ambulatory HF patients [21]. The Metabolic Exercise test data combined with Cardiac and Kidney Indexes (MECKI) score is an established risk model in patients with systolic HF (i.e., LVEF < 40%) consisting of six variables: hemoglobin, serum sodium, kidney function by means of modification of diet in renal disease (MDRD), echocardiographic left ventricle ejection fraction, peak oxygen consumption (% predicted) and VE/VCO2 slope [22]. It was developed 10 years ago based on 2715 HF patients recruited and prospectively followed in 13 Italian HF centers and demonstrated excellent predictive value for the combined endpoint of death or heart transplantation with an area under the curve (AUC) ranging from 0.80 for events occurring within one year to 0.76 for events occurring within four years [23]. The MECKI score has been validated in different populations and has been proven to be a simple, practical tool for risk stratification in HF patients.

The contribution of risk stratification models in clinical practice is principal since they can change the trajectory of the disease by providing the option of timely therapy. However, their applicability in daily clinical practice has not been established, as most physicians find their use challenging [24,25]. The LHFRS is an easily obtainable risk stratification model since it consists of only three variables, which are typically obtained early at every admission in the ED. Other prognostic risk models have also been established in AHF, such as the Organized Program to Initiate Lifesaving Treatment in Hospitalized Patients with Heart Failure (OPTIMIZE-HF) scoring system [26], the Acute Decompensated Heart failure/N-Terminal proB-type Natriuretic Peptide (ADHF/NT-proBNP) risk score [27,28], the Acute Physiology and Chronic Health Evaluation-Heart Failure (APACHE-HF) scoring system [29] and the Evaluation Study of Congestive Heart Failure and Pulmonary Artery Catheterization Effectiveness (ESCAPE) discharge model [30]. The OPTIMIZE-HF scoring system is a useful bedside tool that includes the following eight variables: age, weight, systolic blood pressure, sodium, creatinine, history of liver disease, history of depression, and history of reactive airway disease. The scoring system has been utilized for the prediction of mortality risk (C-index of 0.72) in hospitalized HF patients within 60 days after their discharge [26]. The ADHF/NT-proBNP risk score contains a total of eight variables (chronic obstructive pulmonary disease, systolic blood pressure, eGFR, serum sodium, hemoglobin, NT-proBNP, LVEF, and tricuspid regurgitation moderate to severe), and the possible total score ranges from 0 to 22 [27]. The ADHF/NT-proBNP score exhibited an excellent discriminative ability for the endpoint of 1-year mortality (C index of 0.839) in a cohort of 453 ADHF patients (derivation cohort) and was successfully validated (C index of 0.768) in a cohort of 371 ADHF patients (validation cohort) [27]. The ADHF/NT-proBNP score has also been reported to predict 1-year mortality in 445 hospitalized advanced HF patients [28]. The APACHE- HF scoring system (mean arterial pressure, pulse, serum sodium, serum potassium, hematocrit, serum creatinine, age, and Glasgow Coma Scale) was found to be reliable in predicting adverse outcomes in 824 AHF patients and outperformed the more complex APACHE II (body temperature, mean blood pressure, pulse, respiratory rate, A-a DO2 (FiO2 $\geq$ 0.5), PaO2 (FiO2 < 0.5), arterial blood, serum sodium, serum potassium, hematocrit, creatinine, white blood cells, and Glasgow Coma Scale), as well as the modified APACHE II scoring system (age, mean blood pressure, pulse, serum sodium, serum potassium, serum creatinine, and Glasgow Coma Scale) [29]. The ESCAPE discharge risk model (age, blood urine nitrogen, 6 min walking test, sodium, cardiopulmonary resuscitation/mechanical ventilation, diuretic dose, no beta-blocker at discharge, discharge brain natriuretic peptide (BNP)) has been shown to predict the risk of death at 6 months (C-index of 0.739) in a cohort of 423 patients with advanced decompensated systolic HF [30]. However, the majority of these risk models are either complicated, using many variables, or limited to systolic HF groups.

Among the comparison of major HF risk models, including CHARM, MAGGIC, GISSI-HF, and SHFM, MAGGIC showed the best overall accuracy in predicting one-year mortality, using 11 variables, whereas SHFM, being the most sophisticated, using 24 variables, demonstrated a lower overestimation of mortality [18,21,31]. On the other hand, the use of oversimplified risk scores may be of doubtful clinical value. Thus, the use of bilirubin level as a discriminator in PRAISE (The Prospective Randomized Amlodipine Evaluation Study) cohort patients signified an increased risk of pump failure death but failed to detect those in danger of SCD [32].

5. Strengths and Limitations

The LHFRS was validated in the REALITY-HF patient population and applied to hospitalized patients only. Certainly, in the trajectory of HF, emerging biomarkers, such as electrolyte disturbances, hypoalbuminemia, and hyperuricemia, can significantly influence the disease outcome and should be monitored in an extended timeline. However, previous analyses have been mainly limited to chronic HF patients. Another substantial limitation is that, due to the disunity of HF pathophysiology, at present LHFRS cannot be used to guide treatment in AHF. Lastly, patients participating in the REALITY-AHF were not on the more recently approved life-prolonging HF drugs (endorsed by international guidelines), such as angiotensin receptor neprilysin inhibitor (ARNI) or SGLT2 inhibitors [33,34], since enrollment of these patients took place earlier (2014–2015); therefore, these drugs were not available. Despite these limitations, the present work demonstrates, for the first time, the independent association of simple LHFRS with SCD and death from heart (pump) failure in a "real world" cohort of hospitalized patients with AHF. In this regard, a high LHFRS score may identify patients at a greater risk of SCD, HF, or cardiovascular death and orientate them to close monitoring in established HF centers.

6. Conclusions

Increased LHFRS was independently associated with SCD and HF death in a prospective cohort of AHF patients.

Supplementary Materials: The following supporting information can be downloaded at: https://www.mdpi.com/article/10.3390/jcm12113722/s1, Table S1. Comparison of risk of sudden cardiac death (SCD) in patients with LHFRS 0,1 vs. LHFRS 2–4.

Author Contributions: Conceptualization, A.X. and T.K.; methodology, A.X., T.K., Y.M., G.G., J.S. and F.T.; validation, A.B., Y.F. and S.O.; formal analysis, T.K.; investigation, Y.F., S.O., E.A., S.S., M.Y., K.K. and T.O.; data curation, Y.F., S.O., E.A., S.S., M.Y., K.K. and T.O.; writing—original draft preparation, A.X., A.B. and T.K.; writing—review and editing, Y.M., G.G., J.S. and F.T.; visualization, A.X., A.B., T.K. and Y.M.; supervision, A.X., T.K., Y.M., F.T. and J.S. All authors have read and agreed to the published version of the manuscript.

Funding: This research received no external funding.

Institutional Review Board Statement: The study was conducted in accordance with the Declaration of Helsinki, and approved by the Institutional Review Board (or Ethics Committee) of each participating center (UMIN000014105).

Informed Consent Statement: As obtaining written informed consent at the ED may cause a delay in the ED management timeline and subsequently bias the results, we used an opt-out method for participant recruitment. All participants were notified of their participation in the study and it was explained that they were free to opt out of the participation at any time.

Data Availability Statement: The registry focused on very early presentation and treatment in the emergency department of acute heart failure syndrome (REALITY-AHF) (UMIN000014105).

Conflicts of Interest: The authors declare no conflict of interest.

References

1. Ziaeian, B.; Fonarow, G.C. Epidemiology and aetiology of heart failure. *Nat. Rev. Cardiol.* **2016**, *13*, 368–378. [CrossRef] [PubMed]
2. Groenewegen, A.; Rutten, F.H.; Mosterd, A.; Hoes, A.W. Epidemiology of heart failure. *Eur. J. Heart Fail.* **2020**, *22*, 1342–1356. [CrossRef] [PubMed]
3. Roger, V.L. Epidemiology of Heart Failure: A Contemporary Perspective. *Circ. Res.* **2021**, *128*, 1421–1434. [CrossRef]
4. Loungani, R.S.; Teerlink, J.R.; Metra, M.; Allen, L.A.; Butler, J.; Carson, P.E.; Chen, C.W.; Cotter, G.; Davison, B.A.; Eapen, Z.J.; et al. Cause of Death in Patients with Acute Heart Failure: Insights From RELAX-AHF-2. *JACC Heart Fail.* **2020**, *8*, 999–1008. [CrossRef]
5. Xanthopoulos, A.; Giamouzis, G.; Tryposkiadis, K.; Paraskevopoulou, E.; Karagiannis, G.; Patsilinakos, S.; Parissis, J.; Farmakis, D.; Butler, J.; Skoularigis, J.; et al. A simple score for early risk stratification in acute heart failure. *Int. J. Cardiol.* **2016**, *230*, 248–254. [CrossRef] [PubMed]
6. Xanthopoulos, A.; Tryposkiadis, K.; Giamouzis, G.; Konstantinou, D.; Giannakoulas, G.; Karvounis, H.; Kattan, M.W.; Skoularigis, J.; Parissis, J.; Starling, R.C.; et al. Larissa Heart Failure Risk Score: A proposed simple score for risk stratification in chronic heart failure. *Eur. J. Heart Fail.* **2017**, *20*, 614–616. [CrossRef]
7. Kitai, T.; Xanthopoulos, A.; Tang, W.W.; Kaji, S.; Furukawa, Y.; Oishi, S.; Akiyama, E.; Suzuki, S.; Yamamoto, M.; Kida, K.; et al. Validation of the Larissa Heart Failure Risk Score for risk stratification in acute heart failure. *Int. J. Cardiol.* **2019**, *307*, 119–124. [CrossRef]
8. Matsue, Y.; Damman, K.; Voors, A.A.; Kagiyama, N.; Yamaguchi, T.; Kuroda, S.; Okumura, T.; Kida, K.; Mizuno, A.; Oishi, S.; et al. Time-to-Furosemide Treatment and Mortality in Patients Hospitalized with Acute Heart Failure. *J. Am. Coll. Cardiol.* **2017**, *69*, 3042–3051. [CrossRef]
9. Kitai, T.; Tang, W.H.W.; Xanthopoulos, A.; Murai, R.; Yamane, T.; Kim, K.; Oishi, S.; Akiyama, E.; Suzuki, S.; Yamamoto, M.; et al. Impact of early treatment with intravenous vasodilators and blood pressure reduction in acute heart failure. *Open Heart* **2018**, *5*, e000845. [CrossRef]
10. Kagiyama, N.; Matsue, Y. The time-to-treatment concept in acute heart failure: Lessons and implications from REALITY-AHF. *Anatol. J. Cardiol.* **2018**, *20*, 125–129. [CrossRef]
11. Spinar, J.; Jarkovsky, J.; Spinarova, L.; Mebazaa, A.; Gayat, E.; Vitovec, J.; Linhart, A.; Widimsky, P.; Miklik, R.; Zeman, K.; et al. AHEAD score—Long-term risk classification in acute heart failure. *Int. J. Cardiol.* **2015**, *202*, 21–26. [CrossRef]
12. Chen, Y.J.; Sung, S.H.; Cheng, H.M.; Huang, W.M.; Wu, C.L.; Huang, C.J.; Hsu, P.F.; Yeh, J.S.; Guo, C.Y.; Yu, W.C.; et al. Performance of AHEAD Score in an Asian Cohort of Acute Heart Failure with Either Preserved or Reduced Left Ventricular Systolic Function. *J. Am. Heart Assoc.* **2017**, *6*, e004297. [CrossRef] [PubMed]
13. Vaduganathan, M.; Patel, R.B.; Shah, S.J.; Butler, J. Sudden cardiac death in heart failure with preserved ejection fraction: A target for therapy? *Heart Fail. Rev.* **2016**, *21*, 455–462. [CrossRef] [PubMed]
14. Rohde, L.E.; Chatterjee, N.A.; Vaduganathan, M.; Claggett, B.; Packer, M.; Desai, A.S.; Zile, M.; Rouleau, J.; Swedberg, K.; Lefkowitz, M.; et al. Sacubitril/Valsartan and Sudden Cardiac Death According to Implantable Cardioverter-Defibrillator Use and Heart Failure Cause: A PARADIGM-HF Analysis. *JACC Heart Fail.* **2020**, *8*, 844–855. [CrossRef]
15. Odajima, S.; Tanaka, H.; Fujimoto, W.; Kuroda, K.; Yamashita, S.; Imanishi, J.; Iwasaki, M.; Todoroki, T.; Okuda, M.; Hayashi, T.; et al. Efficacy of Renin-angiotensin-aldosterone-system inhibitors for heart failure with preserved ejection fraction and left ventricular hypertrophy -from the KUNIUMI Registry Acute Cohort. *J. Cardiol.* **2022**, *79*, 703–710. [CrossRef]

16. Saku, K.; Yokota, S.; Nishikawa, T.; Kinugawa, K. Interventional heart failure therapy: A new concept fighting against heart failure. *J. Cardiol.* **2021**, *80*, 101–109. [CrossRef]
17. Oates, C.P.; Santos-Gallego, C.G.; Smith, A.; Basyal, B.; Moss, N.; Kawamura, I.; Musikantow, D.R.; Turagam, M.K.; Miller, M.A.; Whang, W.; et al. SGLT2 inhibitors reduce sudden cardiac death risk in heart failure: Meta-analysis of randomized clinical trials. *J. Cardiovasc. Electrophysiol.* **2023**, *34*, 1277–1285. [CrossRef] [PubMed]
18. Mozaffarian, D.; Anker, S.D.; Anand, I.; Linker, D.T.; Sullivan, M.D.; Cleland, J.G.; Carson, P.E.; Maggioni, A.P.; Mann, D.L.; Pitt, B.; et al. Prediction of mode of death in heart failure: The Seattle Heart Failure Model. *Circulation* **2007**, *116*, 392–398. [CrossRef] [PubMed]
19. Desai, A.S.; Vaduganathan, M.; Cleland, J.G.; Claggett, B.L.; Barkoudah, E.; Finn, P.; McCausland, F.R.; Yilmaz, M.B.; Lefkowitz, M.; Shi, V.; et al. Mode of Death in Patients with Heart Failure and Preserved Ejection Fraction: Insights From PARAGON-HF Trial. *Circ. Heart Fail.* **2021**, *14*, e008597. [CrossRef]
20. Rohde, L.E.; Vaduganathan, M.; Claggett, B.L.; Polanczyk, C.A.; Dorbala, P.; Packer, M.; Desai, A.S.; Zile, M.; Rouleau, J.; Swedberg, K.; et al. Dynamic changes in cardiovascular and systemic parameters prior to sudden cardiac death in heart failure with reduced ejection fraction: A PARADIGM-HF analysis. *Eur. J. Heart Fail.* **2021**, *23*, 1346–1356. [CrossRef]
21. Canepa, M.; Fonseca, C.; Chioncel, O.; Laroche, C.; Crespo-Leiro, M.G.; Coats, A.J.; Mebazaa, A.; Piepoli, M.F.; Tavazzi, L.; Maggioni, A.P.; et al. Performance of Prognostic Risk Scores in Chronic Heart Failure Patients Enrolled in the European Society of Cardiology Heart Failure Long-Term Registry. *JACC: Heart Fail.* **2018**, *6*, 452–462. [CrossRef] [PubMed]
22. Agostoni, P.; Corrà, U.; Cattadori, G.; Veglia, F.; La Gioia, R.; Scardovi, A.B.; Emdin, M.; Metra, M.; Sinagra, G.; Limongelli, G.; et al. Metabolic exercise test data combined with cardiac and kidney indexes, the MECKI score: A multiparametric approach to heart failure prognosis. *Int. J. Cardiol.* **2013**, *167*, 2710–2718. [CrossRef] [PubMed]
23. Salvioni, E.; Bonomi, A.; Re, F.; Mapelli, M.; Mattavelli, I.; Vitale, G.; Sarullo, F.M.; Palermo, P.; Veglia, F.; Agostoni, P. The MECKI score initiative: Development and state of the art. *Eur. J. Prev. Cardiol.* **2020**, *27*, 5–11. [CrossRef] [PubMed]
24. Tung, Y.-C.; Chang, G.-M.; Chang, H.-Y.; Yu, T.-H. Relationship between Early Physician Follow-Up and 30-Day Readmission after Acute Myocardial Infarction and Heart Failure. *PLoS ONE* **2017**, *12*, e0170061. [CrossRef] [PubMed]
25. Miró, Ò.; Rossello, X.; Platz, E.; Masip, J.; Gualandro, D.M.; Peacock, W.F.; Price, S.; Cullen, L.; DiSomma, S.; de Oliveira, M.T., Jr.; et al. Risk stratification scores for patients with acute heart failure in the Emergency Department: A systematic review. *Eur. Heart J. Acute Cardiovasc. Care* **2020**, *9*, 375–398. [CrossRef]
26. O'Connor, C.M.; Abraham, W.T.; Albert, N.M.; Clare, R.; Stough, W.G.; Gheorghiade, M.; Greenberg, B.H.; Yancy, C.W.; Young, J.B.; Fonarow, G.C. Predictors of mortality after discharge in patients hospitalized with heart failure: An analysis from the Organized Program to Initiate Lifesaving Treatment in Hospitalized Patients with Heart Failure (OPTIMIZE-HF). *Am. Heart J.* **2008**, *156*, 662–673. [CrossRef]
27. Scrutinio, D.; Ammirati, E.; Guida, P.; Passantino, A.; Raimondo, R.; Guida, V.; Braga, S.S.; Pedretti, R.; Lagioia, R.; Frigerio, M.; et al. Clinical utility of N-terminal pro-B-type natriuretic peptide for risk stratification of patients with acute decompensated heart failure. Derivation and validation of the ADHF/NT-proBNP risk score. *Int. J. Cardiol.* **2013**, *168*, 2120–2126. [CrossRef]
28. Scrutinio, D.; Ammirati, E.; Guida, P.; Passantino, A.; Raimondo, R.; Guida, V.; Sarzi Braga, S.; Canova, P.; Mastropasqua, F.; Frigerio, M.; et al. The ADHF/NT-proBNP risk score to predict 1-year mortality in hospitalized patients with advanced decompensated heart failure. *J. Heart Lung Transpl.* **2014**, *33*, 404–411. [CrossRef]
29. Okazaki, H.; Shirakabe, A.; Hata, N.; Yamamoto, M.; Kobayashi, N.; Shinada, T.; Tomita, K.; Tsurumi, M.; Matsushita, M.; Yamamoto, Y.; et al. New scoring system (APACHE-HF) for predicting adverse outcomes in patients with acute heart failure: Evaluation of the APACHE II and Modified APACHE II scoring systems. *J. Cardiol.* **2014**, *64*, 441–449. [CrossRef]
30. O'Connor, C.M.; Hasselblad, V.; Mehta, R.H.; Tasissa, G.; Califf, R.M.; Fiuzat, M.; Rogers, J.G.; Leier, C.V.; Stevenson, L.W. Triage After Hospitalization with Advanced Heart Failure: The ESCAPE (Evaluation Study of Congestive Heart Failure and Pulmonary Artery Catheterization Effectiveness) Risk Model and Discharge Score. *J. Am. Coll. Cardiol.* **2010**, *55*, 872–878. [CrossRef]
31. Rogers, J.K.; Pocock, S.J.; McMurray, J.J.; Granger, C.B.; Michelson, E.L.; Östergren, J.; Pfeffer, M.A.; Solomon, S.D.; Swedberg, K.; Yusuf, S. Analysing recurrent hospitalizations in heart failure: A review of statistical methodology, with application to CHARM-Preserved. *Eur. J. Heart Fail.* **2013**, *16*, 33–40. [CrossRef] [PubMed]
32. Wu, A.H.; Levy, W.; Welch, K.B.; Neuberg, G.W.; O'Connor, C.M.; Carson, P.E.; Miller, A.B.; Ghali, J.K. Association Between Bilirubin and Mode of Death in Severe Systolic Heart Failure. *Am. J. Cardiol.* **2013**, *111*, 1192–1197. [CrossRef] [PubMed]
33. McDonagh, T.A.; Metra, M.; Adamo, M.; Gardner, R.S.; Baumbach, A.; Böhm, M.; Burri, H.; Butler, J.; Čelutkienė, J.; Chioncel, O.; et al. 2021 ESC Guidelines for the diagnosis and treatment of acute and chronic heart failure. *Eur. Heart J.* **2021**, *42*, 3599–3726. [CrossRef] [PubMed]
34. Heidenreich, P.A.; Bozkurt, B.; Aguilar, D.; Allen, L.A.; Byun, J.J.; Colvin, M.M.; Deswal, A.; Drazner, M.H.; Dunlay, S.M.; Evers, L.R.; et al. 2022 AHA/ACC/HFSA Guideline for the Management of Heart Failure: Executive Summary: A Report of the American College of Cardiology/American Heart Association Joint Committee on Clinical Practice Guidelines. *Circulation* **2022**, *145*, e876–e894. [CrossRef] [PubMed]

Disclaimer/Publisher's Note: The statements, opinions and data contained in all publications are solely those of the individual author(s) and contributor(s) and not of MDPI and/or the editor(s). MDPI and/or the editor(s) disclaim responsibility for any injury to people or property resulting from any ideas, methods, instructions or products referred to in the content.

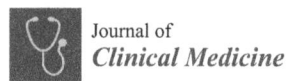

Article

Validation of the Surgical Outcome Risk Tool (SORT) and SORT v2 for Predicting Postoperative Mortality in Patients with Pancreatic Cancer Undergoing Surgery

Anna P. Karamolegkou [1,*], Maria P. Fergadi [2], Dimitrios E. Magouliotis [3,4], Athina A. Samara [4], Evangelos Tatsios [4], Andrew Xanthopoulos [5], Chryssa Pourzitaki [6], David Walker [3] and Dimitris Zacharoulis [4]

1 Department of Anesthesiology, Hippocration General Hospital of Athens, 11527 Athens, Greece
2 Department of Radiology, University of Thessaly, Biopolis, 38221 Larissa, Greece
3 Division of Surgery and Interventional Science, Faculty of Medical Sciences, University College London, London WC1E 6AU, UK
4 Department of Surgery, University of Thessaly, Biopolis, 41110 Larissa, Greece
5 Department of Cardiology, University of Thessaly, 38221 Larissa, Greece
6 Department of Clinical Pharmacology, Faculty of Medicine, School of Health Sciences, Aristotle University of Thessaloniki, 54124 Thessaloniki, Greece
* Correspondence: annamad97@gmail.com

Abstract: Background: Pancreatic cancer surgery is related to significant mortality, thus necessitating the accurate assessment of perioperative risk to enhance treatment decision making. A Surgical Outcome Risk Tool (SORT) and SORT v2 have been developed to provide enhanced risk stratification. Our aim was to validate the accuracy of SORT and SORT v2 in pancreatic cancer surgery. Method: Two hundred and twelve patients were included and underwent pancreatic surgery for cancer. The surgeries were performed by a single surgical team in a single tertiary hospital (2016–2022). We assessed a total of four risk models: SORT, SORT v2, POSSUM (Physiology and Operative Severity Score for the enumeration of Mortality and Morbidity), and P-POSSUM (Portsmouth-POSSUM). The accuracy of the model was evaluated using an observed-to-expected (O:E) ratio and the area under the curve (AUC). Results: The 30-day mortality rate was 3.3% (7 patients). Both SORT and SORT v2 demonstrated excellent discrimination traits (AUC: 0.98 and AUC: 0.98, respectively) and provided the best-performing calibration in the total analysis. However, both tools underestimated the 30-day mortality. Furthermore, both reported a high level of calibration and discrimination in the subgroup of patients undergoing pancreaticoduodenectomy, with previous ERCP, and CA19-9 $\geq$ 500 U/mL. Conclusions: SORT and SORT v2 are efficient risk-assessment tools that should be adopted in the perioperative pathway, shared decision-making (SDM) process, and counseling of patients with pancreatic cancer undergoing surgery.

Keywords: risk assessment; risk tool; sort; surgical outcome risk tool; pancreatic cancer

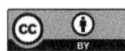

1. Introduction

Pancreatic cancer (PC) represents a major cancer-related cause of death and is currently the fourth most common cause of cancer-related mortality in the USA [1,2]. Most of the cases diagnosed with PC are adenocarcinomas (PDAC) and are commonly located in the pancreatic head or neck [3,4]. In spite of the important advances in anticancer research, PC-associated mortality continues to rise and the prognosis continues to be poor. Thus, it is projected that by 2030, PC will represent the second-highest cancer-related cause of mortality [5,6], with most patients undergoing potentially curative surgery. The treatment strategy for pancreatic cancer should be multidisciplinary, including regimens of chemo- and radiotherapy in conjunction with surgery [7]. On this basis, there is an urgent need for an accurate assessment of the patient's perioperative risk to facilitate shared decision-making (SDM) and the informed consent process while raising the standards of clinical practice quality on the perioperative pathway. In addition, the adoption of a specific and sensitive risk-stratification tool allows for the accurate comparative evaluation of surgical results among institutions, departments, and surgeons for either service evaluation or clinical audit. Several such tools have been implemented into clinical practice [8]. Despite the increasing interest in more advanced risk-stratification tools, risk prediction models remain the most easily accessible choice for this purpose. Nonetheless, they are not frequently employed in everyday practice, potentially due to poor awareness amongst clinicians and with concerns about their accuracy and complexity [9].

The Surgical Outcome Risk Tool (SORT) was proposed following the 2011 National Confidential Enquiry into Patient Outcome and Death (NCEPOD) report [9]. It was developed with the goal of providing a tool that could easily provide an enhanced level of risk stratification for surgical patients in a user-friendly manner [9]. In order to be user-friendly, SORT utilizes only six clinical data variables [9]. Currently, it has been compared favorably with other previously validated risk-stratification tools, such as the ASA physical status (ASA PS) grade, and has been externally validated in groups of patients undergoing hip fracture surgery [10] and colorectal surgery [11]. In both groups [10,11], SORT was associated with acceptable discrimination and calibration levels.

Our previous study implementing preliminary outcomes [12] was the first to validate SORT in patients undergoing surgery for pancreatic cancer, but we did not perform a comparison with other traditional risk-stratification tools. Furthermore, in that study [12], the number of included patients was limited. In addition, an updated version of SORT (SORT v2) has been developed that takes into consideration the physician's risk estimation of the surgery [13]. In this context, the present study aimed to validate the SORT and SORT v2 models in adult patients undergoing surgery for pancreatic cancer and compare them with other traditional risk prediction models.

2. Methods
2.1. Data Extraction Strategy

The current study was performed according to a protocol designed and agreed upon by all authors. Data were extracted from a prospectively maintained database of consecutive patients with pancreatic cancer who underwent surgery between 1 January 2015, and 31 August 2022. All procedures were performed by a single surgical team led by the senior author (D.Z.) at the Department of Surgery, University Hospital of Larissa, Greece. Ethical approval was obtained by the Scientific Committee of the hospital (Protocol number: 50271/30-10-19). Informed consent was waived based on the retrospective nature of the present study. No imputation methods were employed for missing data.

We extracted and included data regarding age, gender, body mass index (BMI), ASA (American Society of Anesthesiology) grade, history of previous operations, operative priority, surgical severity, malignancy status, staging, and type of procedure. We defined mortality as any patient death that occurred during the first 30 days or during the hospital stay if longer than 30 days. The predicted risk of mortality was determined using the SORT and SORT v2 models. Moreover, the predicted mortality was calculated by employing POSSUM and P-POSSUM for all patients. In all cases where the patients' data were incomplete, they were excluded from the analysis.

In order to identify the accuracy of each model, we performed separate sensitivity analyses. These additional analyses were performed to evaluate the discrimination and calibration traits of each model relevant to predicting the perioperative mortality risk based on (1) a procedure-related variable: surgical operation (pancreaticoduodenectomy or total pancreatectomy or distal pancreatectomy); (2) cancer-related variables: CA19-9 levels ($\geq$500 mU/L vs. <500 mU/L), neoadjuvant treatment (received or not); and (3) patient-related variables: age ($\geq$70 vs. <70), pre-operative ERCP (yes or no), and postoperative pancreatic fistula (POPF) (yes or no). The risk for POPF was assessed using the formula described by Weng et al. [14]. We employed these variables given that they might affect postoperative mortality.

2.2. Primary and Secondary Endpoints

The validation of the SORT and SORT v2 models in adult patients with PC undergoing surgery was set as the primary endpoint of the present study. Secondary endpoints included (1) the comparison of SORT and SORT v2 with the POSSUM and P-POSSUM models regarding their discrimination and calibration traits in predicting perioperative mortality and (2) a subgroup sensitivity analysis.

2.3. Statistical Analysis

The SORT score was calculated using the method and web platform developed and proposed by Protopappa et al. [9], in addition with the updated version incorporating subjective information to calculate the SORT v2 score [13]. The SORT and SORT v2 models implement five variables: ASA physical status, operative priority level (elective, urgent, immediate), surgical specialties (gastrointestinal, thoracic, or vascular surgery), surgical severity (major/complex), and malignancy status, age (65–79 or ≥80 years). Surgical severity is calculated automatically upon the entry of procedure details. According to the developers' guidelines, if the procedure performed is not listed, the nearest available procedure is used for calculation [13]. The procedures from the list we used were "total pancreatectomy" and "distal pancreatectomy", both associated with major severity. SORT v2 also implements the physician's perceived mortality risk [13]. The POSSUM and P-POSSUM scores were calculated by employing the method proposed by Copland [15] and Prytherch [16], respectively.

Discrimination (the ability to distinguish patients who died from patients who did not die) and calibration (the ability to successfully predict the mortality rate) traits of the SORT and SORT v2 models were assessed. Discrimination was assessed by producing receiver-operating characteristic (ROC) curves and calculating the area under the ROC curve (AUC). The AUC was determined by calculating the 95% confidence intervals and was compared by employing nonparametric paired tests, as described by DeLong [17]. The model discrimination was defined as poor, fair, or excellent when the AUC was of <0.70, 0.70–0.79, and 0.80–1.00, respectively [17].

The calibration was calculated for each included model by measuring the expected mortality and then comparing it with the observed mortality. An observed-to-expected ratio of 1 represented perfect accuracy, a ratio < 1 represented an overestimation of mortality rate, and a ratio of >1 demonstrated an underprediction. Furthermore, calibration was also assessed by employing the Hosmer–Lemeshow (H-L) goodness of fit test, with a lack of fit defined as a p-value ≤ 0.05 [18]. In cases where the outcome variable separated the predictor variable completely, a perfect separation was described.

All extracted data were tabulated using Microsoft® Excel 16.61 (Microsoft, Redmond, WA, USA) and were analyzed by employing Prism® Graphpad 9.3.1 for Mac (GraphPad Software, San Diego, CA, USA).

3. Results

3.1. Baseline Patient Characteristics

The findings of the current study are presented in accordance with the STROBE (Strengthening the Reporting of Observational Studies in Epidemiology) guidelines [19]. The trial flowchart for the study, which demonstrates the data extraction strategy, is reported in Figure 1. In total, 252 patients were screened, and 212 patients were finally incorporated. The patients' baseline characteristics are presented in Table 1. Of the total group, 78 (36.8%) female patients were included, with a mean age of 67.2 (standard deviation (SD)—10.5) years. Most of the cases presented with a re-sectable tumor (71.7%) and underwent an elective procedure (91.5%). The tumor was located primarily in the head (180 patients—84.9%) of patients. Most of the cases were PDAC 190 (89.6%), with a mean CA19-9 of 502.9 (SD: 1136) U/mL. A total of 178 (84%) patients underwent pancreaticoduodenectomy, sixteen (7.5%) a total pancreatectomy, and eighteen (8.5%) a distal pancreatectomy. Finally, the overall 30-day mortality rate was 3.3%.

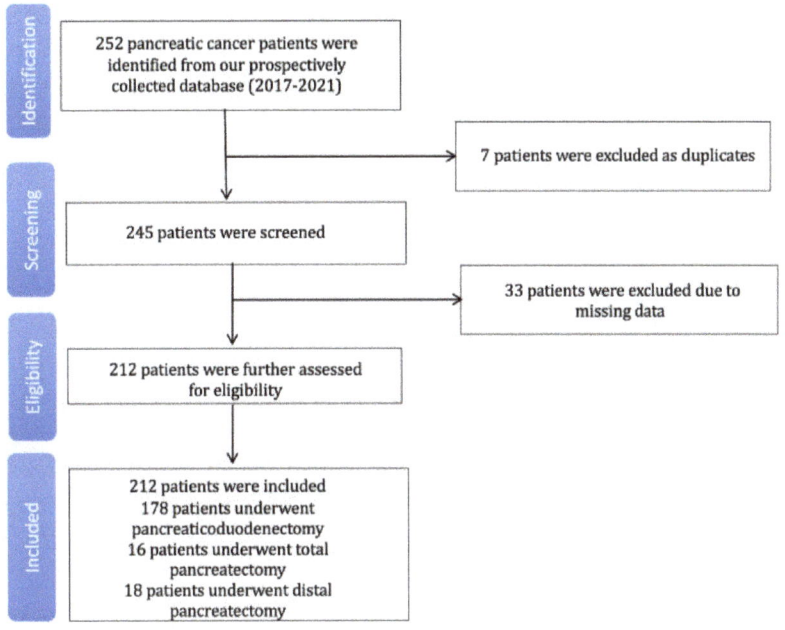

Figure 1. Trial flow.

3.2. Performance of SORT and SORT v2 Models in the Total Dataset

The performance of SORT is presented in Table 2 and Figure 2. In fact, SORT was associated with an excellent discrimination level in the total analysis (AUC: 0.98 (95% CI: 0.95–1.00); $p = 0.001$). SORT v2 presented similar discrimination (AUC: 0.98 (95% CI: 0.97–1.00); $p = 0.001$). Furthermore, SORT demonstrated the lowest Hosmer–Lemeshow value (H-L: 2.97; $p = 0.71$), thus showing the best-performing calibration for all models in the total analysis. SORT v2 demonstrated the second-lowest H–L value (H-L: 5.46; $p = 0.49$). Nonetheless, both SORT and SORT v2 underestimated the mortality determined by observed/expected ratios of >1.

3.3. Comparison of SORT and SORT v2 with Other Mortality Prediction Models in the Entire Dataset

The POSSUM (AUC: 0.72 (95% CI: 0.57–0.88); $p = 0.045$) and P-POSSUM (AUC: 0.75 (95% CI: 0.64–0.86); $p = 0.025$) were associated with a fair discrimination level (Table 2), though both underestimated mortality (Table 2).

3.4. Performance of Mortality Prediction Models in Subgroups

The outcomes derived from the subgroup analysis are shown in Table 3 and Figure 3. The SORT and SORT v2 models demonstrated an excellent discrimination level in predicting perioperative mortality in all subgroups. In certain subgroups, SORT and SORT v2 models demonstrated a perfect separation, which is translated into a perfect prediction of mortality (Table 3). Furthermore, POSSUM and P-POSSUM were inferior in terms of the discrimination level in most of the subgroups when compared with SORT and SORT v2. In addition, SORT demonstrated a high level of calibration in all subgroups, with the lowest value reported in patients undergoing pancreaticoduodenectomy with high levels of CA19-9 and a previous ERCP. In all subgroup analyses except "ERCP or No ERCP", SORT and SORT v2 underestimated the perioperative mortality.

Table 1. Patient baseline characteristics.

Baseline Characteristics	Number of Patients, n = 212
Female, n (%)	78 (36.8)
Mean age, years (SD)	67.2 (10.5)
Age ≥ 70 (%)	82 (38.7)
BMI, (SD)	26.5 (1.9)
Mean previous Operations, n (SD)	1.9 (1)
Pre-operative ERCP, n (%)	82 (38.7)
ASA Class, n (%)	
I	48 (22.6)
II	112 (52.8)
III	42 (19.8)
IV	10 (4.7)
Stage, n (%)	
Re-sectable	152 (71.7)
Borderline re-sectable	60 (28.3)
Mean CA19-9, U/mL (SD)	502.9 (1138)
CA19-9 ≥ 500 U/mL, n (%)	162 (76.4)
CA19-9 < 500 U/mL, n (%)	50 (23.6)
Neoadjuvant treatment, n (%)	56 (26.4)
Operative priority	
Elective	194 (91.5)
Acute	18 (8.5)
Cancer site, n (%)	
Head/Vater	180 (84.9)
Body	14 (6.6)
Tail	18 (8.5)
Pathology, n (%)	
PDAC	190 (89.6)
NET	14 (6.6)
Other	8 (3.8)
Surgical Operation, n (%)	
Pancreaticoduodenectomy	178 (84)
Total pancreatectomy	16 (7.5)
Distal pancreatectomy	18 (8.5)
30-day mortality	7 (3.3)

Abbreviations: ASA: American Society of Anesthesiologists; BMI: Body Mass Index; PDAC: Pancreatic ductal adenocarcinoma; NET: Neuroendocrine Tumor; CA19-9: Carbohydrate antigen 19-9.

Table 2. Discrimination and calibration traits for each score regarding the prediction of mortality in patients with pancreatic cancer undergoing surgery.

Scoring Systems	O	E	O:E	Discrimination		Calibration	
				AUC (95% CI)	p	H-L	p
POSSUM	7	0	-	0.72 (0.57–0.88)	0.045	17.47	0.03
P-POSSUM	7	0	-	0.75 (0.64–0.86)	0.025	9.47	0.31
SORT	7	4	1.75	0.98 (0.95–1.00)	<0.001	2.97	0.71
SORT v2	7	4	1.75	0.98 (0.97–1.00)	<0.001	5.46	0.49

Abbreviations: O: observed; E: expected; AUC: area under curve; 95% CI: 95% confidence interval; H–L: Hosmer–Lemeshow.

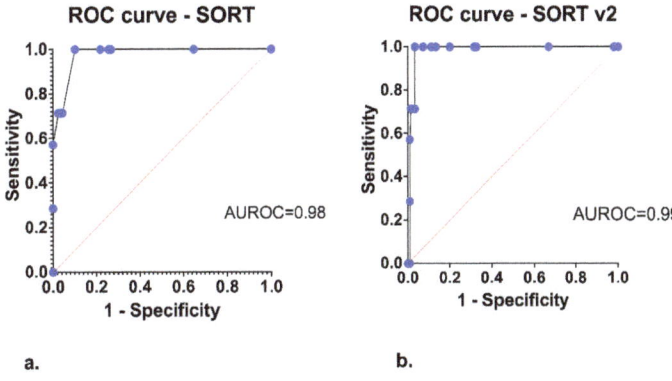

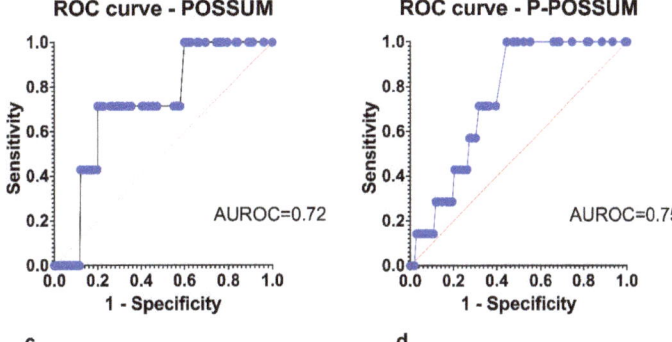

Figure 2. Receiver Operating Characteristic (ROC) curves regarding the discrimination of each model in the total study population. ROC curves regarding. (**a**). Surgical Outcome Risk Tool (SORT), (**b**). SORT v2, (**c**). Physiological and Operative Severity Score (POSSUM), (**d**). Portsmouth-POSSUM (P-POSSUM).

Table 3. Discrimination and calibration traits of each score for predicting mortality in certain subgroups.

Scoring Systems	O	E	O:E	Discrimination		Calibration	
				AUC (95% CI)	p	H-L	p
Pancreaticoduodenectomy (n = 178)							
POSSUM	5	0	-	0.67 (0.50–0.84)	0.193	9.56	0.297
P-POSSUM	5	0	-	0.75 (0.64–0.86)	0.055	11.18	0.192
SORT	5	2	2.5	0.96 (0.92–1.00)	<0.001	2.89	0.822
SORT v2	5	2	2.5	0.98 (0.95–1.00)	<0.001	6.87	0.443
Total pancreatectomy (n = 16)							
POSSUM				perfect seperation			
P-POSSUM				ps			
SORT				ps			
SORT v2				ps			
Distal pancreatectomy (n = 18)							
POSSUM	2	2	1	0.88 (0.71–1.00)	0.092	6.82	0.556
P-POSSUM	2	0	-	0.75 (0.54–0.96)	0.261	17.09	0.017

Table 3. Cont.

Scoring Systems	O	E	O:E	Discrimination		Calibration	
				AUC (95% CI)	p	H-L	p
SORT				ps			
SORT v2				ps			
CA19-9 ≥ 500 mU/L (n = 162)							
POSSUM	5	0	-	0.69 (0.51–0.86)	0.157	9.30	0.318
P-POSSUM	5	0	-	0.76 (0.65–0.87)	0.048	9.88	0.274
SORT	5	2	2.5	0.96 (0.91–1.00)	<0.001	2.82	0.831
SORT v2	5	2	2.5	0.97 (0.95–1.00)	<0.001	6.76	0.562
CA19-9 < 500 mU/L (n = 50)							
POSSUM	2	0	-	0.79 (0.68–0.91)	0.166	18.94	0.015
P-POSSUM	2	0	-	0.71 (0.58–0.84)	0.322	15.29	0.054
SORT				ps			
SORT v2				ps			
Neoadjuvant treatment (n = 56)							
POSSUM	3	2	1.5	0.98 (0.95–1.00)	0.005	0.41	>0.999
P-POSSUM	3	1	3	0.95 (0.88–1.00)	0.009	21.89	0.003
SORT	3	2	1.5	0.91 (0.81–1.00)	0.018	0.83	0.997
SORT v2	3	2	1.5	0.98 (0.95–1.00)	0.005	3.63	0.822
No neoadjuvant treatment (n = 156)							
POSSUM	4	0	-	0.63 (0.42–0.85)	0.370	16.73	0.033
P-POSSUM	4	0	-	0.74 (0.62–0.86)	0.104	12.14	0.145
SORT				ps			
SORT v2	4	2	2	0.99 (0.9671.00)	<0.001	1.29	0.972
≥70 (n = 82)							
POSSUM	2	0	-	0.53 (0.26–0.79)	0.904	8.65	0.373
P-POSSUM	4	0	-	0.65 (0.45–0.84)	0.322	8.52	0.384
SORT	4	2	2	0.94 (0.86–1.00)	0.003	4.50	0.480
SORT v2	4	2	2	0.97 (0.94–1.00)	0.001	0.71	0.994
<70 (n = 130)							
POSSUM	3	0	-	0.92 (0.87–0.97)	0.014	22.27	0.004
P-POSSUM	3	0	-	0.82 (0.75–0.89)	0.059	12.24	0.141
SORT				ps			
SORT v2	3	2	1.5	0.98 (0.96–1.00)	0.004	1.18	0.947
ERCP (n = 82)							
POSSUM	5	4	1.25	0.83 (0.66–1.00)	0.001	16.71	0.033
P-POSSUM	5	2	2.5	0.89 (0.89–1.00)	0.001	6.88	0.550
SORT	5	2	2.5	0.93 (0.85–1.00)	0.001	2.23	0.973
SORT v2	3	2	1.5	0.97 (0.94–1.00)	<0.001	36.27	<0.001
No ERCP (n = 130)							
POSSUM	2	0	-	0.81 (0.75–0.88)	0.130	11.38	0.181
P-POSSUM	2	0	-	0.79 (0.63–0.95)	0.156	7.76	0.458
SORT				ps			
SORT v2	2	2	1	0.98 (0.96–1.00)	0.019	0.52	0.991
High risk for POPF							
POSSUM	4	4	1	0.94 (0.86–1.00)	0.005	6.22	0.622
P-POSSUM	4	2	2	0.91 (0.80–1.00)	0.009	5.64	0.688
SORT	4	3	1.33	0.92 (0.81–1.00)	0.008	0.88	0.997
SORT v2	4	3	1.33	0.98 (0.93–1.00)	0.002	17.81	0.013
Low risk for POPF							
POSSUM	3	0	-	0.59 (0.34–0.84)	0.59	10.60	0.225
P-POSSUM	3	0	-	0.74 (0.67–0.81)	0.15	27.26	0.001
SORT				ps			
SORT v2	3	2	1.5	0.98 (0.97–1.00)	0.004	1.11	0.981

Abbreviations: O: observed; E: expected; AUC: area under curve; 95% CI: 95% confidence interval; H-L: Hosmer–Lemeshow; ps: perfect separation, which is translated into a perfect prediction of mortality; ERCP: endoscopic retrograde cholangiopancreatography; POPF: postoperative pancreatic fistula; Surgical Outcome Risk Tool (SORT); SORT v2; Physiological and Operative Severity Score (POSSUM); Portsmouth-POSSUM (P-POSSUM).

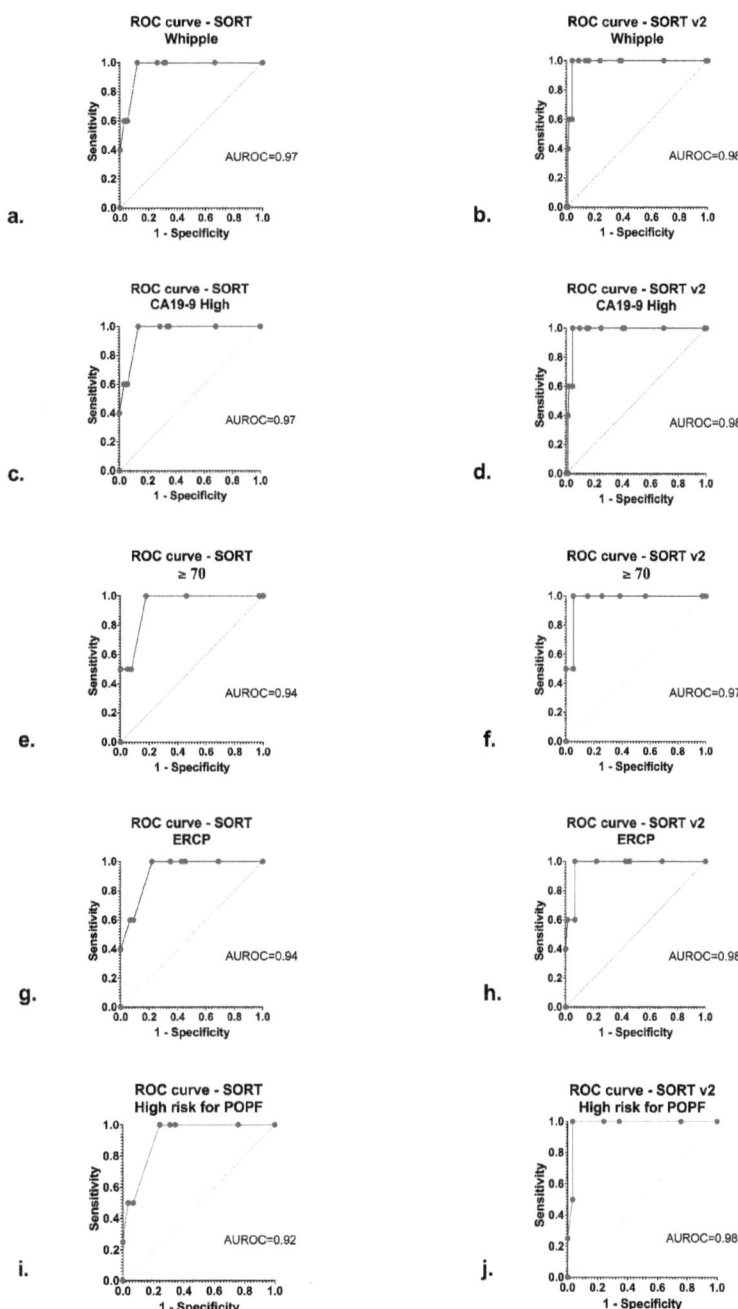

Figure 3. Receiver Operating Characteristic (ROC) curves regarding the discrimination of Surgical Outcome Risk Tool (SORT) and SORT v2 in the following subgroups: (**a**,**b**): pancreaticoduodenectomy procedure; (**c**,**d**): CA19-9 ≥ 500; (**e**,**f**): age ≥ 70; (**g**,**h**): pre-operative endoscopic retrograde cholangiopancreatography (ERCP); (**i**,**j**): High risk for postoperative pancreatic fistula (POPF).

4. Discussion

The current original trial represents the first attempt to validate SORT and SORT v2 models in (1) PC surgery and (2) compare them with additional traditional risk models such as POSSUM and P-POSSUM, and (3) perform a sensitivity subgroup analysis. This study also represents the first external validation of SORT v2 currently provided in the literature and especially in PC surgical patients. The outcomes provided by the present study directly affect daily clinical practice, suggesting the potential value of SORT and SORT v2 in the perioperative pathway and during the counseling and shared decision-making (SDM) processes for patients with PC scheduled for surgery.

SORT remains a useful and probably the most user-friendly risk-stratification tool. It was developed by Protopapa et al. [9], who aimed to accurately predict the 30-day mortality in an objective manner. The present trial demonstrated that six pre-operatively available clinical variables could efficiently predict postoperative mortality with a higher accuracy compared to other traditional risk assessment tools, such as ASA-PS [9]. In the same context, SORT v2 was proposed as an enhanced version of the original SORT as it implements the physician's perception of the perioperative mortality risk [13]. Other risk-stratification tools that have been implemented in clinical practice and were included for comparison in the current study are POSSUM and P-POSSUM. Given that both patients and physicians have implemented these tools in the SDM process, it was important to compare them with SORT and SORT v2. In addition, according to recent evidence [15], traditional risk-stratification tools, such as POSSUM and P-POSSUM, were associated with poor accuracy, while new models are required to provide enhanced calibration and discrimination traits, according to findings derived from prospectively collected data [15]. Our outcomes provide a response to this call for enhanced risk-stratification models in the setting of PC surgery. SORT and SORT v2 demonstrated the best-performing discrimination and calibration characteristics compared with all other risk-stratification models assessed in the present study. Our outcomes not only follow the preliminary outcomes of our previous study [12] but also highlight the superiority of both tools compared with POSSUM and P-POSSUM and validate SORT v2 for the first time. In this context, the outcomes of this study have direct implications for the SDM process of patients with PC regarding their postoperative mortality risk, thus helping patients to co-shape their treatment strategy.

The efficiency of both SORT and SORT v2 was also demonstrated in the sensitivity subgroup analyses. SORT and SORT v2 were associated with excellent discrimination traits and enhanced calibration. However, we should further stress our comparative outcomes regarding patients undergoing pancreaticoduodenectomy with raised levels of CA19-9 and pre-operative ERCP. In this group, SORT and SORT v2 demonstrated excellent calibration and discrimination traits and showed significantly lower H–L values compared to POSSUM and P-POSSUM. Patients with these baseline characteristics represent the most difficult cases faced by our HPB multi-disciplinary teams. These are commonly symptomatic patients, diagnosed through a thorough diagnostic workup after presenting with jaundice. At that stage, they commonly present CA19-9 levels over 500 U/mL, thus demonstrating an aggressive tumor biology, although the tumor is borderline resectable in most of these cases. They also commonly undergo ERCP stenting to alleviate jaundice prior to surgery, especially in cases in which neoadjuvant treatment is chosen. In this context, it is of great importance to have access to such an effective and reliable risk-stratification tool during the MDT meetings when such complex cases are discussed, in addition to during the patients' counseling process.

We have not found a significant difference between SORT and SORT v2, thus proposing that the physicians' estimation of perioperative mortality risk does not significantly affect the original SORT outcomes. Nonetheless, in all analyses, SORT v2 demonstrated slightly better discrimination and calibration compared with SORT. Consequently, it would be interesting to investigate whether there is a discrepancy between SORT and SORT v2 in patients undergoing pancreaticoduodenectomy with vascular reconstruction. Despite our original intention to perform such a subgroup analysis, there were limited available cases that underwent pancreaticoduodenectomy with major vascular reconstruction to perform further analyses. Consequently, this clinically relevant question requires further investigation by a future trial mainly focusing on complex cases. Moreover, the findings of the current study regarding the value of clinical variables employed by SORT remain in accordance with the evidence provided by administrative datasets [20]. Finally, according to our outcomes, SORT and SORT v2 are associated with higher accuracy compared with other pre-operative (BH 2009—Barwon Health 2009) [21] and intraoperative risk-stratification tools (SAS—Surgical Apgar Score) [22], while remaining user-friendly as they implement six clinical variables.

Although POSSUM and P-POSSUM have been extensively validated [2], SORT and SORT v2 have certain advantages. To begin, both tools incorporate only six pre-operative variables, significantly fewer compared with the eighteen perioperative variables of POSSUM and P-POSSUM. They are thus significantly easier to implement in real-life clinical practice. Moreover, POSSUM and P-POSSUM include intra- and postoperative variables that are not available during the pre-operative assessment. Finally, (P-)POSSUM contains certain subjective variables, thus increasing the interobserver variability and heterogeneity and posing a certain bias.

The current study is associated with certain limitations. One limitation is associated with the study design, given that it is a single-institution retrospective trial. Nonetheless, it should be noted that all data was prospectively collected, the patients were consecutive, the surgical team remained the same, and the surgeon's bias regarding patient or surgical approach selection was minimized as this was decided based on MDT suggestions and patients' choices after extensive counseling. In addition, given that one of the most important postoperative complications associated with high morbidity and mortality in pancreatic surgery is POPF, there is a certain limitation related to the lack of this variable in the formulas of all the risk-stratification tools implemented in the present study.

The current outcomes demonstrate that SORT and SORT v2 are feasible, friendly, and efficient risk-stratification tools that should be implemented in the pre-operative counseling and SDM process of patients with PC undergoing surgery, thus enhancing clinical quality in a cost-effective manner. In addition, they are useful instruments to be taken into consideration during multidisciplinary meetings when examining complex cases associated with comorbidities and frailty.

5. Conclusions

In the present study, we validated the SORT and SORT v2 risk-stratification models in adult patients undergoing surgery for pancreatic cancer. Both tools demonstrated the best-performing discrimination and calibration compared with POSSUM and P-POSSUM. The value of SORT and SORT v2 was further confirmed by sensitivity subgroup analyses. Both tools are associated with excellent discrimination and calibration, especially in patients with PC undergoing pancreaticoduodenectomy with pre-operative ERCP and CA19-9 levels over 500 U/mL. SORT represents a feasible and efficient risk stratification tool that can be easily implemented in the perioperative pathway of patients with PC.

Author Contributions: Conceptualization, A.P.K., D.E.M. and D.Z.; Methodology, A.P.K., M.P.F., D.E.M., A.X. and D.Z.; Software, A.P.K., D.E.M. and D.Z.; Validation, M.P.F., D.E.M., A.A.S. and C.P.; Formal analysis, A.P.K., M.P.F., A.A.S., E.T., D.W. and D.Z.; Investigation, A.P.K., M.P.F., D.E.M., A.A.S. and A.X.; Resources, A.A.S., E.T., A.X., C.P. and D.W.; Data curation, A.P.K., E.T., A.X. and D.W.; Writing—original draft, A.P.K., M.P.F., D.E.M., A.A.S., E.T., A.X., C.P., D.W. and D.Z.; Writing—review & editing, A.P.K., M.P.F., D.E.M., A.A.S., E.T., A.X., C.P., D.W. and D.Z.; Visualization, A.P.K., D.E.M., A.A.S. and D.W.; Supervision, C.P., D.W. and D.Z.; Project administration, A.P.K., D.W. and D.Z.; Funding acquisition, E.T. All authors have read and agreed to the published version of the manuscript.

Funding: This research received no external funding.

Institutional Review Board Statement: Ethical approval for the current study was obtained by the Scientific Committee of the University Hospital of Larissa (Protocol number: 50271/30-10-19).

Informed Consent Statement: Not applicable.

Data Availability Statement: All original data is available upon request.

Conflicts of Interest: The authors declare no conflict of interest.

References

1. Ferlay, J.S.; Soerjomataram, I.; Ervik, M.; Dikshit, R.; Eser, S.; Mathers, C.; Rebelo, M.; Parkin, D.M.; Forman, D.; Bray, F. GLOBOCAN 2012 v1.0, Cancer Incidence and Mortality Worldwide: IARC Can-cerBase No. 11 [Internet]. Lyon, France: International Agency for Research on Cancer 2013. Available online: http://globocan.iarc.fr (accessed on 5 June 2019).
2. Siegel, R.L.; Miller, K.D.; Jemal, A. Cancer statistics. *CA Cancer J. Clin.* **2015**, *65*, 5–29. [CrossRef] [PubMed]
3. Wong, H.H.; Chu, P. Immunohistochemical features of the gastrointestinal tract tumors. *J. Gastrointest. Oncol.* **2012**, *3*, 262–284. [CrossRef] [PubMed]
4. Neoptolemos, J.P.; Urrutia, R.; Abbruzzese, J.; Büchler, M.W. (Eds.) *Pancreatic Cancer*; Springer: New York, NY, USA, 2010; Volume LVIII, p. 1390.
5. Yeo, T.P. Demographics, Epidemiology, and Inheritance of Pancreatic Ductal Adenocarcinoma. *Semin. Oncol.* **2015**, *42*, 8–18. [CrossRef] [PubMed]
6. Rahib, L.; Smith, B.D.; Aizenberg, R.; Rosenzweig, A.B.; Fleshman, J.M.; Matrisian, L.M. Projecting cancer incidence and deaths to 2030: The unexpected burden of thyroid, liver, and pancreas cancers in the United States. *Cancer Res.* **2014**, *74*, 2913–2921. [CrossRef] [PubMed]
7. Massani, M.; Stecca, T. Editorial: Neoadjuvant treatment for resectable and borderline resectable pancreatic cancer. *Front. Oncol.* **2023**, *13*, 1138587. [CrossRef] [PubMed]
8. Moonesinghe, S.R.; Mythen, M.G.; Das, P.; Rowan, K.M.; Grocott, M. Risk Stratification Tools for Predicting Morbidity and Mortality in Adult Patients Undergoing Major Surgery: Qualitative systematic review. *Anesthesiology* **2013**, *119*, 959–981. [CrossRef] [PubMed]
9. Protopapa, K.L.; Simpson, J.C.; Smith, N.C.E.; Moonesinghe, S.R. Development and validation of the Surgical Outcome Risk Tool (SORT). *Br. J. Surg.* **2014**, *101*, 1774–1783. [CrossRef] [PubMed]
10. Marufu, T.C.; White, S.M.; Griffiths, R.; Moonesinghe, S.R.; Moppett, I.K. Prediction of 30-day mortality after hip fracture surgery by the Nottingham Hip Fracture Score and the Surgical Outcome Risk Tool. *Anaesthesia* **2016**, *71*, 515–521. [CrossRef] [PubMed]
11. Magouliotis, D.E.; Walker, D.; Baloyiannis, I.; Fergadi, M.P.; Mamaloudis, I.; Chasiotis, G.; Tzovaras, G.A. Validation of the Surgical Outcome Risk Tool (SORT) for Predicting Postoperative Mortality in Colorectal Cancer Patients Undergoing Surgery and Subgroup Analysis. *World J. Surg.* **2021**, *45*, 1940–1948. [CrossRef] [PubMed]
12. Magouliotis, D.E.; Samara, A.; Fergadic, M.P.; Symeonidis, D.; Zacharoulis, D. Validation of the Surgical Outcome Risk Tool (SORT) in patients with pancreatic cancer undergoing surgery. *Braz. J. Anesthesiol.* **2021**, *71*, 304–305. [CrossRef] [PubMed]
13. Wong, D.J.N.; Harris, S.; Sahni, A.; Bedford, J.R.; Cortes, L.; Shawyer, R.; Wilson, A.M.; Lindsay, H.A.; Campbell, D.; Popham, S.; et al. Developing and validating subjective and objective risk-assessment measures for predicting mortality after major surgery: An international prospective cohort study. *PLoS Med.* **2020**, *17*, e1003253. [CrossRef] [PubMed]
14. Weng, H.; Shu, Y.J.; Bao, R.F.; Shu, Y.J.; Weng, M.Z.; Bao, R.F.; Wang, X.F.; Gu, J.; Wang, Z. Preoperative plain CT value of pancreas can predict the risk of pancreatic fistula after pan-creatoduodenectomy. *Chin. J. Gen. Surg.* **2014**, *29*, 21–24.
15. Copeland, G.P.; Jones, D.; Walters, M. POSSUM: A scoring system for surgical audit. *Br. J. Surg.* **1991**, *78*, 355–360. [CrossRef] [PubMed]
16. Prytherch, D.R.; Whiteley, M.S.; Higgins, B.; Weaver, P.C.; Prout, W.G.; Powell, S.J. POSSUM and Portsmouth POSSUM for pre-dicting mortality. Physiological and operative severity score for the enUmeration of mortality and morbidity. *Br. J. Surg.* **1998**, *85*, 1217–1220. [CrossRef] [PubMed]
17. DeLong, E.R.; DeLong, D.M.; Clarke-Pearson, D.L. Comparing the areas under two or more correlated receiver operating charac-teristic curves: A nonparametric approach. *Biometrics* **1988**, *44*, 837–845. [CrossRef] [PubMed]
18. Hosmer, D.W.; Hosmer, T.; Le Cessie, S.; Lemeshow, S. A comparison of goodness-of-fit tests for the logistic regression model. *Statistics Med.* **1997**, *16*, 965–980. [CrossRef]
19. von Elm, E.; Altman, D.G.; Egger, M.; Pocock, S.J.; Gøtzsche, P.C.; Vandenbroucke, J.P.; STROBE Initiative. The Strengthening the Re-porting of Observational Studies in Epidemiology (STROBE) statement: Guidelines for reporting observational studies. *Ann. Intern. Med.* **2007**, *147*, 573–577, Erratum in: *Ann. Intern. Med.* **2008**, *148*, 168. PMID: 17938396. [CrossRef] [PubMed]
20. García-Torrecillas, J.M.; Olvera-Porcel, M.C.; Ferrer-Márquez, M.; Rosa-Garrido, C.; Rodríguez-Barranco, M.; Lea-Pereira, M.C.; Rubio-Gil, F.; Sánchez, M.-J. Predictive Model of the Risk of In-Hospital Mortality in Colorectal Cancer Surgery, Based on the Minimum Basic Data Set. *Int. J. Environ. Res. Public Health* **2020**, *17*, 4216. [CrossRef] [PubMed]

21. Regenbogen, S.E.; Bordeianou, L.; Hutter, M.M.; Gawande, A.A. The intraoperative Surgical Apgar Score predicts postdischarge complications after colon and rectal resection. *Surgery* **2010**, *148*, 559–566. [CrossRef] [PubMed]
22. Kong, C.H.; Guest, G.D.; Stupart, D.A.; Faragher, I.G.; Chan, S.T.F.; Watters, D. Recalibration and Validation of a Preoperative Risk Prediction Model for Mortality in Major Colorectal Surgery. *Dis. Colon Rectum* **2013**, *56*, 844–849. [CrossRef] [PubMed]

Disclaimer/Publisher's Note: The statements, opinions and data contained in all publications are solely those of the individual author(s) and contributor(s) and not of MDPI and/or the editor(s). MDPI and/or the editor(s) disclaim responsibility for any injury to people or property resulting from any ideas, methods, instructions or products referred to in the content.

Review

Perioperative Fluid Management in Colorectal Surgery: Institutional Approach to Standardized Practice

Philip Deslarzes [1], Jonas Jurt [1], David W. Larson [2], Catherine Blanc [3], Martin Hübner [1] and Fabian Grass [1,*]

[1] Department of Visceral Surgery, Lausanne University Hospital CHUV, University of Lausanne (UNIL), 1005 Lausanne, Switzerland; philip.deslarzes@chuv.ch (P.D.); jonas.jurt@chuv.ch (J.J.); martin.hubner@chuv.ch (M.H.)
[2] Division of Colon and Rectal Surgery, Department of Surgery, Mayo Clinic, 200 First Street SW, Rochester, MN 55905, USA; larson.david2@mayo.edu
[3] Department of Anesthesiology, Lausanne University Hospital CHUV, University of Lausanne (UNIL), 1005 Lausanne, Switzerland; catherine.blanc@chuv.ch
* Correspondence: fabian.grass@chuv.ch

Abstract: The present review discusses restrictive perioperative fluid protocols within enhanced recovery after surgery (ERAS) pathways. Standardized definitions of a restrictive or liberal fluid regimen are lacking since they depend on conflicting evidence, institutional protocols, and personal preferences. Challenges related to restrictive fluid protocols are related to proper patient selection within standardized ERAS protocols. On the other hand, invasive goal-directed fluid therapy (GDFT) is reserved for more challenging disease presentations and polymorbid and frail patients. While the perfusion rate (mL/kg/h) appears less predictive for postoperative outcomes, the authors identified critical thresholds related to total intravenous fluids and weight gain. These thresholds are discussed within the available evidence. The authors aim to introduce their institutional approach to standardized practice.

Keywords: perioperative; enhanced recovery; fluid management; guidance

1. Introduction

Over the last 20 years, fluid management has been increasingly recognized as a sensitive and modifiable parameter of perioperative care, directly affecting postoperative outcomes [1–3]. However, the optimal amount of perioperative fluid administration is controversial, and standardized definitions of a restrictive or liberal regimen are lacking due to conflicting evidence, institutional protocols, and personal preferences [4,5]. In line with these findings, a recent meta-analysis revealed various intra- and postoperative fluid volumes [6].

On the one hand, peri- and postoperative fluids are essential to maintain adequate organ perfusion and tissue fluid homeostasis [7]. An overly restrictive approach may lead to hypotension and decreased organ perfusion, ultimately associated with acute kidney injury (AKI) [4]. Furthermore, perioperative organ injury due to both inflammation and ischemia (due to a demand–supply mismatch) represents a potential hazard, thus needing preventive measures and close perioperative monitoring [8]. Enhanced recovery after surgery (ERAS) pathways aim to decrease the physiological surgical stress response represented by a state of insulin resistance [9]. Several measures, including preoperative carbohydrate loading, perioperative feeding strategies, minimally invasive surgery, and early resumption of a normal diet help to modulate the stress response, promote insulin sensitivity, and attenuate the breakdown of protein. Further consequences related to decreased organ perfusion due to an overly restrictive approach may be cardiovascular dysfunction (perioperative myocardial ischemia due to tachycardia, hypotension, hypoxia, or anemia), neurological complications (including confusional states or delirium), and intestinal dysfunction (including splanchnic or anastomotic hypoperfusion), which may be exacerbated by an excessive use of vasopressors [10,11].

On the other hand, fluid overload may result in harmful "third space" weight gain, associated with higher rates of pulmonary complications, postoperative ileus, altered mental status, and edema-related anastomotic complications, thus impeding postoperative recovery [12–16]. Furthermore, an excessive extracellular fluid volume may lead to abdominal compartment syndrome, which by itself may trigger adverse physiologic effects such as respiratory failure and renal failure [17]. In light of these findings, definitions must be set to guide clinical practice.

In the setting of established ERAS pathways, the authors' institutions attempted to identify "safety" fluid thresholds for colorectal resections [13,18,19]. The present review aims to define optimal fluid management, provide an overview of suggested thresholds, and discuss this institutional practice in the light of available evidence.

2. What Is Optimal Fluid Management?

Optimal fluid management implies a normovolemic state during and beyond the surgical procedure without fluid management-related complications due to overly restrictive or generous fluid administration, least possible postoperative weight gain, and prompt functional recovery. Whether a specific patient can be managed by noninvasive monitoring and according to a "zero fluid" approach as suggested by the ERAS guidelines mainly depends on the disease presentation, physiological state at the time of surgery, comorbidities, and patient frailty [2]. A euvolemic, otherwise healthy patient without significant comorbidities warranting close surveillance going into elective, minimally invasive surgery is thus eligible for a standardized, restrictive fluid strategy, considering the physiologic principles of euvolemia [5]. On the other hand, patients at risk presenting with an impaired physical condition and distress due to a more acute or emergent disease presentation should benefit from invasive monitoring techniques and be treated within a more liberal strategy according to their physiologic reactions to surgery in a non-elective, acute setting [6]. This is even more important given the fact that these fragile patients are prone to postoperative morbidity and are not eligible for a simplified restrictive approach. On the contrary, management of these patients implies several critical perioperative assessments, including an evaluation of fluid responsiveness triggering, if appropriate, the administration of fluid boluses to increase stroke volume [20]. Of note, such a protocol does not necessarily need hemodynamic monitoring devices for reliable prediction but can also be carried out using echography after a passive leg raising test or by inferior vena cava evaluation, both in mechanically ventilated and spontaneously breathing patients [21–23]. In line with these basic principles, both authors' institutions aimed to standardize fluid management over the last years to implement preset thresholds related to IV fluids and weight gain as red flags for guidance in clinical practice.

Definition of a Restrictive versus Liberal Approach

To date, there is no standardized definition of restrictive fluid therapy. The Enhanced Recovery After Surgery (ERAS) guidelines recommend aiming for a "zero fluid" balance and euvolemia intraoperatively and during the first postoperative days in patients undergoing elective colorectal resections [24,25]. Pre-operatively, carbohydrate loading and unrestricted access to clear fluids until 2 h before anesthesia induction help maintain fluid homeostasis and initiate surgery in a euvolemic, physiological state. Intraoperatively, a basal rate of crystalloid solution of <4 mL/kg/h is recommended [24,26]. This approach has been considered "restrictive"; however, its interpretation and application in clinical practice remain vague and subjective. Patients requiring goal-directed fluid therapy (GDFT) should receive boluses to maintain the cardiac stroke volume and, hence, central normovolemia [6]. However, recent guidance reserves a GDFT approach for high-risk patients (e.g., frailty and cardiopulmonary dysfunction) and high-risk procedures (e.g., emergent setting and disease-related distress) with large intravascular fluid loss [25,27,28]. Postoperatively, both early IV fluid lock and resumption of liquids and solids allow for adherence to the natural process of fluid homeostasis according to individual needs [29].

In a recent meta-analysis including 18 randomized controlled trials, the median intraoperative fluid administrated in the restrictive group was 1930 mL (interquartile range (IQR): 1480–2470 mL) compared to 3880 mL (IQR: 3000–4400 mL) in the liberal group [30]. On postoperative day 1, the median volume of intravenous fluids was 2340 mL (IQR 1640–3530 mL) versus 4350 mL (3100–5330 mL), respectively. However, important differences were observed among individual trials regarding total fluid volumes in the restrictive and liberal groups [30,31]. Consequently, a liberal approach in a specific trial could be equivalent to a restrictive approach in another trial [30,32]. While the concept of fluid restriction outside high-risk patients and procedures is widely accepted, "safety" thresholds may be valuable adjuncts and serve as red flags for clinical guidance during anesthesia and postoperative surveillance. Several randomized controlled trials compared both approaches (restrictive vs. liberal) and reported on fluid-related thresholds and postoperative complications, as summarized in Table 1.

Table 1 provides an overview of published RCTs comparing restrictive and liberal groups.

Table 1. Randomized controlled trials comparing restrictive and liberal fluid regimens.

Study (Year)	Surgery	N	Total Fluids	IV Fluid Management	mL/kg/h	Weight Day 2 (Δ, kg)	Outcomes Restrictive Group
Lobo 2002 [5]	Elective CS (cancer)	10 (R)	11.6L (IV + oral)	3000 (POD 0)	NA	0	↓ LOS, ↓ gastric emptying
		10 (L)	18L (IV + oral)	5700 (POD 0)		3	↓ time to stool
Brandstrup 2003 [33]	Elective CRS	69 (R)	3.8L (IV + oral POD 0)	2700 (POD 0)	NA	1	↓ cardiopulmonary + tissue-healing complications
		72 (L)	6.2L (IV + oral POD 0)	5400 (POD 0)		3.8	
Nisanevich 2005 [34]	Major abdominal surgery	77 (R)	NA	1400 (IO), 2200 (POD1)	4 RL (IO)	0.5 (POD 1)	↓ LOS, ↓ time to flatus/stool
		75 (L)		3900 (IO), 2000 (POD1)	12 RL (IO)	1.9 (POD 1)	
Kabon 2005 [35]	Elective CS	124 (R)	NA	2500 (IO)	8–10 RL (IO)	NA	→ SSI, nausea
		129 (L)		3900 (IO)	16–18 RL (IO)		
MacKay 2006 [36]	Elective CS	39 (R)	NA	2000 (IO), 2000 (POD1)	NA	NA	→ time to flatus/stool, LOS
		31 (L)		2750 (IO), 2600 (POD1)			
Holte 2007 [37]	Elective CS	16 (R)	1600 (POD 0)	1140 (IO)	5–7 RL	0.8	→ complications, time to stool, LOS
		16 (L)	5100 (POD 0)	3900 (IO)	18 RL	2.9	
Muller 2009 [38]	Elective CS	76 (R)	2700 (POD 0)	1900 (IO)	5 RL (IO)	NA	↓ complications, ↓ LOS
		75 (L)	5200 (POD 0)	3000 (IO)	10 RL (IO)		
Aguilar-Nascimento 2009 [39]	Major abdominal surgery	28 (R)	9.2 L	4400 (IO)	17	NA	↓ LOS, ↓ pulmonary complications
		33 (L)	11.7 L	5400 (IO)	20		

Table 1. Cont.

Study (Year)	Surgery	N	Total Fluids	IV Fluid Management	mL/kg/h	Weight Day 2 (Δ, kg)	Outcomes Restrictive Group
Futier 2010 [40]	Major abdominal surgery	36 (R GDT) 5600 (IO)	NA	3400 (IO) 12.2	7.7 24 (C GDT)	NA	↑ complications (leak, sepsis)
Abraham-Nordling 2012 [41]	Elective CRS	79 (R) 82 (L)	NA	3100 (POD0) 5800 (POD0)	NA	0.8 2.9	↓ overall complications, → LOS, leak, AKI, ↑ cardiac complications
Kaylan 2013 [42]	Elective CRS	121 (R) 119 (L)	NA	1000 (IO), 1900 (POD0) 2000 (IO), 3300 (POD0)	5–7 (L, IO)	−1.4 1.3	→ major complications, LOS, mortality
Hong-Ying 2014 [43]	Elective CRS (cancer)	96 (R) 89 (L)	NA	1600 (IO) 3100 (IO)	NA	0.9 2.8	↓ overall complications, ↑ cardiac complications
Phan 2014 [44]	Elective CRS	50 (R) 50 (L)	NA	1500 (IO) 2100 (IO)	5 (both groups)	NA	→LOS, minor/major complications
Gomez-Izquierdo 2017 [45]	Elective CRS	64 (GDT) 64 (L)	NA	1500 (IO) 2400 (IO)	6 (GDT) 12	0.6 0	→ ileus, LOS, surgical and medical complications
Myles 2018 [4]	Major abdominal surgery	1490 (R) 1493 (L)	NA	1700 (IO), 3700 (24 h) 3000 (IO), 6100 (24 h)	NA	NA	↑ AKI → sepsis, mortality

IV—intravenous, CS—colon surgery, CRS—colorectal surgery, R—restrictive, L—liberal, GDT—goal-directed therapy, NA—not available, LOS—length of stay, POD—postoperative day, IO—intraoperative, AKI—acute kidney injury. Total fluids relate to the total LOS unless specified otherwise. Arrow down: decreased, arrow up: increased, regular arrow: same.

In a former meta-analysis, Varadhan et al. suggested stratifying fluid regimens of the perioperative day into restrictive (<1750 mL/d), balanced (1750–2750 mL/d), and liberal (>2750 mL/d) [32]. The balanced fluid range was calculated to compensate for the daily physiological water loss for an average human in a homeostatic state, estimated between 25–35 mL/kg [46,47]. This volume is supposed to replace the perioperative body water loss to approach a zero fluid balance. Interestingly, this upper cut-off of 2.7 L was independently confirmed by an institutional series of the Mayo Clinic [13].

3. Impact of Fluid Overload on Postoperative Complications

A considerable weight gain of >6 kg after elective colorectal surgery has been observed in several studies, requiring close postoperative surveillance to prevent associated complications, especially in fragile patients prone to pulmonary complications [33]. However, fluid management in these fragile patients represents a particular challenge given that they are at increased risk of experiencing postoperative morbidity. This impedes uncritical assumptions of cause (fluid overload) and effect (complications) patterns. While some of the data suggest a modest correlation between total perioperative IV fluid administration and weight gain [48,49], a dose–response correlation with consequent increased complication rates was observed by others [33,50]. Despite the seemingly easy-to-perform weight measurements in the postoperative period, postoperative weight is reported in only 50% of randomized controlled studies [30], Table 1.

Fluid overload induces prolonged gastric emptying [5], which, together with bowel edema and interstitial third space fluids, causes postoperative ileus (POI). The series of both our institutions confirmed an independent effect of fluid overload and weight gain on POI occurrence [18,51]. These findings were confirmed by others and independently validated [52–54]. Furthermore, similar associations were observed in the setting of ostomy procedures [55,56].

Pulmonary complications after surgery are a major concern, with an occurrence of up to 23% [12,57]. Fluid overload of the interstitial space triggers pulmonary edema, especially in patients with impaired cardiac function [57,58]. A significant decrease in mean blood saturation on the second night after surgery was observed in patients within the liberal fluid administration group; however, there was no increased morbidity in this study [37]. However, the results are conflicting, and cause–effect patterns are hard to establish in fragile patients with cardiopulmonary impairment. Several studies, including an institutional series, revealed that fluid overload and weight gain are associated with an increased risk of pulmonary complications [12,50,59].

Impact of Fluid Management on Renal Function

While perioperative hypotension may impact on several organs, a major concern of overly restrictive perioperative fluid administration is the development of AKI. The evidence is conflicting. A meta-analysis revealed a higher AKI rate in the restrictive group [30]. Further data suggest that even a minor increase in creatinine levels could increase in-hospital mortality in non-cardiac surgical patients [60]. However, no cause–effect patterns could be established due to its retrospective design. Myles et al. published a large multicentric randomized controlled landmark trial comparing restrictive versus liberal fluid administration in major abdominal surgery [4]. In their study, the restrictive approach had no impact on disability-free survival but was associated with a statistically significant AKI increase (8.6% vs. 5% in the restrictive and liberal groups, respectively). Notably, around 50% of patients in this trial were not treated according to the ERAS principles, impeding uncritical extrapolation of the results to the setting of our institutions offering care within longstanding, established, and standardized ERAS pathways [61,62]. A sizeable institutional series of elective patients revealed a low AKI rate of 2.5% according to loss of kidney function and end-stage kidney disease (RIFLE) criteria [63]. In another series of our group, an intraoperative fluid range defined as "balanced" (300 mL–2700 mL) was associated with the lowest rate of POI and a prolonged length of stay but not AKI [13]. Restrictive fluid management during elective colorectal resections appears safe if carried out within standardized pathways and it is supported by respective societies [24,25,64].

4. Fluid Management in the Perioperative Period: Which Indicators

Intraoperative oliguria occurring in isolation should not trigger fluid boluses since the predictive value for postoperative AKI appears low [65]. An institutional series of the Mayo Clinic revealed that a certain degree of postoperative hypotension in up to 10% of patients may persist for less than 20 h without negatively impacting AKI occurrence, which affected <3% [66]. There is a broad consensus that a permissive attitude to physiologic oliguria due to renal vasoconstriction can be adopted in the elective ERAS setting, providing no established cause exists [25]. Based on the available information, intraoperative fluid management should be protocolized to determine an underlying physiologic problem requiring reversal [67]. Standard monitoring integrating clinical data is thus likely sufficient in low-risk procedures, combining maintenance fluids at a low rate of < 4 ml/kg/h in the intraoperative and early postoperative period in the post-anesthesia care unit. Outside this low-risk setting and depending on the surgical risk, GDFT, including advanced hemodynamic monitoring devices, should be used as valuable adjuncts in higher-risk patients or procedures, triggering fluid administration if a decreased cardiac output or surrogates are suspected [68,69].

5. Summary of Institutional Thresholds and Practice Guidance

Based on the above discussed evidence and considering a 7-year experience in ERAS care in both authors' institutions at that time, our groups aimed not only to focus on established, evidence-based perioperative ERAS care but also to standardize fluid management [19]. The need to improve perioperative fluid management standards in our institutions was motivated by the rather low compliance with guidelines, despite growing ERAS experience [19]. Importantly, the aim was not to set inflexible, dogmatic thresholds but to help with guidance in clinical practice. Restrictive fluid management through a zero-balance practice in elective surgery represents one puzzle piece in a comprehensive care pathway aiming to maintain a physiologic state throughout the perioperative period, significantly impacting postoperative recovery [5].

In total, 11 cohort studies of the authors' institutions described fluid management-related thresholds, as summarized in Table 2.

Table 2. Fluid thresholds and related outcomes within the authors' institutions.

Study (Year)	Cohort	N	Critical Fluid-Related Threshold	Outcome Related to Fluid Overload
Abd El Aziz 2022 [13]	Elective CRS	2900	300–2700 mL (IO)	↑ POI, ↑ LOS, ↑ AKI
Grass 2022 [70]	Elective CRS	5′398	3000 mL (IO)	Impeded outpatient strategy in selected patients
Butti 2020 [48]	Major abdominal surgery + IMC stay	111	3 kg (POD 2)	Prolonged IMC stay
Grass 2020 [18]	Elective CRS	4205	3000 mL 2.5 kg (POD 2)	↑ POI
Grass 2020 [71]	Elective CRS	5122	3000 mL (IO)	Prolonged LOS > 48 h
Grass 2020 [72]	Urgent colectomy	224	3000 mL (POD 0), 2.3 kg (POD 2)	↑ overall complications
Grass 2019 [63]	Elective CRS	7103	3800 mL	↑ AKI
Hübner 2019 [50]	Laparoscopic CRS	580	3000 mL (colon) 4000 mL (rectum)	↑ overall, major, respiratory complications
Grass 2019 [56]	Loop ileostomy closure	238	1700 mL (POD 0) 1.2 kg (POD 2)	↑ POI
Pache 2019 [73]	Open CRS	121	3500 kg (POD 0) 3.5 kg (POD 2)	↑ overall, respiratory complications, prolonged LOS
Jurt 2018 [12]	Elective CRS	1298	4 kg (POD 2)	↑ respiratory complications

IV—intravenous, CS—colon surgery, CRS—colorectal surgery, LOS—length of stay, POD—postoperative day, IO—intraoperative, AKI—acute kidney injury, POI—postoperative ileus. Arrow down: decreased, arrow up: increased, regular arrow: same.

The thresholds are displayed with their respective impact on specific outcomes or clinical consequences. Three papers from the Lausanne group tried to identify thresholds through receiver operating characteristics (ROC) curves in different surgical settings: minimally invasive surgery [50], open surgery [73], and lastly, surgery for urgent indications [72]. Interestingly, the thresholds did not differ significantly across the different settings. The Mayo group analyzed an independent large dataset of elective colorectal surgeries with a focus on POI, prolonged LOS, and AKI, which were plotted against the rate of intraoperative Ringer lactate (RL) infusion (mL/kg/h) and total intraoperative volume [13]. Total intraoperative RL ≥ 2.7 L was independently associated with POI and prolonged LOS, but not AKI. Of note, the infusion rate (ml/kg/h) was not retained as a superior predictive tool. Further work focused on patients undergoing major surgery and needing postoperative surveillance in an intermediate care unit [48]. In this particularly vulnerable subgroup of patients, the fluid balance and weight course showed only a modest correlation. Both institutions further focused on POI in their analyses and found comparable results, with a strong correlation of fluid overload and POI in patients undergoing major surgery [18] and in patients undergoing loop ileostomy closure [56]. In the largest dataset of the Mayo group with over 7000 patients, early AKI was very uncommon within the institutional ERP (2.5%), and long-term sequelae were exceptionally low [63]. Interestingly, AKI patients received higher amounts of POD 0 fluids and had increased postoperative weight gain at POD 2. A further study of the Lausanne group revealed a protective effect of high compliance with the ERAS protocol to prevent postoperative pulmonary complications [12]. A threshold of 4 kg at POD 2 appeared to be critical in this setting. Finally, both author groups showed increasing interest in short stay processes in recent years, and excess intraoperative fluids of >3 L turned out to impede early discharge and thus an outpatient strategy [70,71].

Taking the above summarized evidence together, a threshold of 3000 mL intraoperatively serves presently as a red flag in daily clinical practice in both authors' institutions. In addition to the mere focus on IV fluids, weight gain at postoperative day 2 turned out to be a valid surrogate for fluid overload [18].

Besides IV fluid management, several further ERAS care items help to maintain tissue homeostasis and an euvolemic state [24]. Preoperative carbohydrate loading helps to attenuate the catabolic response through a reduction of insulin resistance in response to surgery [74]. Clear fluids can be safely ingested until 2 h before surgery, whereas 6 h fasting for solid food is sufficient [75]. While there is growing evidence in favor of combined mechanical and oral antibiotic bowel preparation, mechanical bowel preparation alone may lead to preoperative dehydration and electrolyte imbalances and should thus be avoided [76]. Postoperatively, early oral nutrition is advocated and has proven its benefits by several meta-analyses and has been endorsed by different nutritional societies [64]. Finally, early mobilization of at least 6 h per day is of utmost importance and helps to prevent muscle loss and to promote functional recovery due to a direct prokinetic effect on the intestines [77]. Figure 1 summarizes the pre, intra, and postoperative measures within the institutions' standardized ERAS protocol.

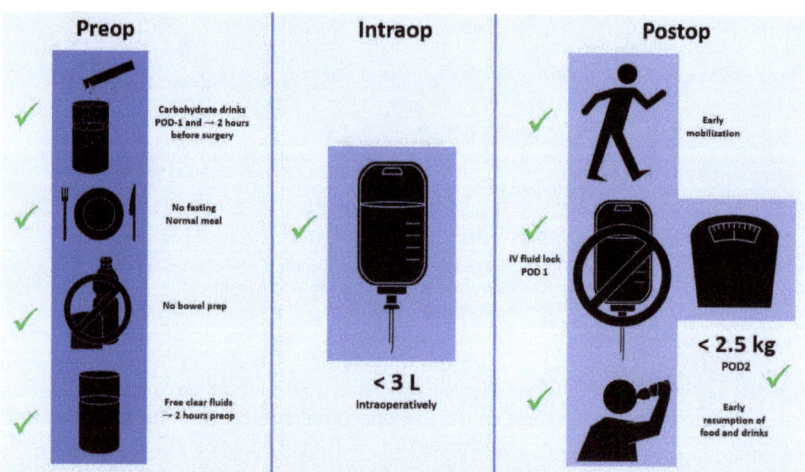

Figure 1. Schematic representation of fluid management-related recommendations within the authors' institutional ERAS pathways.

6. Implications in Daily Clinical Practice

The fast track concept that eventually led to standardized ERAS pathways was introduced 25 years ago by Henrik Kehlet and helped to simplify patient management by targeting the quality and speed of postoperative recovery [78]. Standardization of care is a way to facilitate patient management and improve a multidisciplinary team approach [79]. This holds true for surgical technique, but also intraoperative management and patient care in the ward. Postoperative care protocols with predefined care maps simplify the workflow, especially for frequently performed procedures. Perioperative fluid management represents a key element of ERAS care.

ERAS guidelines suggest aiming for a zero fluid balance for elective colorectal resections, while GDFT should be reserved for high-risk patients and procedures [24,25]. The use of vasopressors is advocated when fluid boluses fail to improve the stroke volume in order to prevent fluid overload [80]. The thresholds described in the present study and used in the authors' institutions cannot replace careful individual risk-stratification in every patient before surgery. However, in the authors' experience, they help with raising awareness among both surgeons and anesthesiologists to discuss fluid management during and after the procedure. Furthermore, a weight gain threshold of 2.5 kg at POD 2 serves as a useful point of reference in the surgical ward. Postoperative body weight is easy to assess and helps to timely launch counterregulatory measures [48,81]. In patients who exceed the threshold, subsequent fluid restriction, diuretics, and the promotion of mobilization can be initiated [50].

7. Conclusions

In conclusion, our practice of restrictive fluid management is based on institutional thresholds to help guide clinical practice, aiming to prevent deleterious fluid overload-related adverse outcomes.

Author Contributions: Conceptualization, P.D., J.J, M.H. and F.G.; methodology, P.D. and F.G.; validation, D.W.L. and C.B.; writing—original draft preparation, P.D., J.J. and F.G.; writing—review and editing, D.W.L., M.H. and C.B. All authors have read and agreed to the published version of the manuscript.

Funding: This research received no external funding.

Informed Consent Statement: Not applicable.

Data Availability Statement: Please contact the authors for specific data.

Conflicts of Interest: The authors declare no conflict of interest.

References

1. Prowle, J.R.; Kirwan, C.J.; Bellomo, R. Fluid management for the prevention and attenuation of acute kidney injury. *Nat. Rev. Nephrol.* **2014**, *10*, 37–47. [CrossRef]
2. Voldby, A.W.; Brandstrup, B. Fluid therapy in the perioperative setting-a clinical review. *J. Intensive Care* **2016**, *4*, 27. [CrossRef]
3. Aga, Z.; Machina, M.; McCluskey, S.A. Greater intravenous fluid volumes are associated with prolonged recovery after colorectal surgery: A retrospective cohort study. *Br. J. Anaesth.* **2016**, *116*, 804–810. [CrossRef]
4. Myles, P.S.; Bellomo, R.; Corcoran, T.; Forbes, A.; Peyton, P.; Story, D.; Christophi, C.; Leslie, K.; McGuinness, S.; Parke, R.; et al. Restrictive versus Liberal Fluid Therapy for Major Abdominal Surgery. *N. Engl. J. Med.* **2018**, *378*, 2263–2274. [CrossRef]
5. Lobo, D.N.; Bostock, K.A.; Neal, K.R.; Perkins, A.C.; Rowlands, B.J.; Allison, S.P. Effect of salt and water balance on recovery of gastrointestinal function after elective colonic resection: A randomised controlled trial. *Lancet* **2002**, *359*, 1812–1818. [CrossRef] [PubMed]
6. Rollins, K.E.; Mathias, N.C.; Lobo, D.N. Meta-analysis of goal-directed fluid therapy using transoesophageal Doppler monitoring in patients undergoing elective colorectal surgery. *BJS Open* **2019**, *3*, 606–616. [CrossRef] [PubMed]
7. Doherty, M.; Buggy, D.J. Intraoperative fluids: How much is too much? *Br. J. Anaesth.* **2012**, *109*, 69–79. [CrossRef]
8. Conrad, C.; Eltzschig, H.K. Disease Mechanisms of Perioperative Organ Injury. *Anesth. Analg.* **2020**, *131*, 1730–1750. [CrossRef]
9. Carli, F. Physiologic considerations of Enhanced Recovery After Surgery (ERAS) programs: Implications of the stress response. *Can. J. Anaesth.* **2015**, *62*, 110–119. [CrossRef] [PubMed]
10. Botto, F.; Alonso-Coello, P.; Chan, M.T.; Villar, J.C.; Xavier, D.; Srinathan, S.; Guyatt, G.; Cruz, P.; Graham, M.; Wang, C.Y.; et al. Myocardial injury after noncardiac surgery: A large, international, prospective cohort study establishing diagnostic criteria, characteristics, predictors, and 30-day outcomes. *Anesthesiology* **2014**, *120*, 564–578. [CrossRef]
11. Klingensmith, N.J.; Coopersmith, C.M. The Gut as the Motor of Multiple Organ Dysfunction in Critical Illness. *Crit. Care Clin.* **2016**, *32*, 203–212. [CrossRef] [PubMed]

12. Jurt, J.; Hubner, M.; Pache, B.; Hahnloser, D.; Demartines, N.; Grass, F. Respiratory Complications After Colorectal Surgery: Avoidable or Fate? *World J. Surg.* **2018**, *42*, 2708–2714. [CrossRef]
13. Abd El Aziz, M.A.; Grass, F.; Calini, G.; Lovely, J.K.; Jacob, A.K.; Behm, K.T.; D'Angelo, A.D.; Shawki, S.F.; Mathis, K.L.; Larson, D.W. Intraoperative Fluid Management a Modifiable Risk Factor for Surgical Quality—Improving Standardized Practice. *Ann. Surg.* **2022**, *275*, 891–896. [CrossRef]
14. Huisman, D.E.; Bootsma, B.T.; Ingwersen, E.W.; Reudink, M.; Slooter, G.D.; Stens, J.; Daams, F.; LekCheck Study, g. Fluid management and vasopressor use during colorectal surgery: The search for the optimal balance. *Surg. Endosc.* **2023**, *37*, 6062–6070. [CrossRef]
15. Ouchi, A.; Sakuramoto, H.; Hoshino, H.; Matsuishi, Y.; Sakaguchi, T.; Enomoto, Y.; Hoshino, T.; Shimojo, N.; Inoue, Y. Association between fluid overload and delirium/coma in mechanically ventilated patients. *Acute Med. Surg.* **2020**, *7*, e508. [CrossRef]
16. Boland, M.R.; Reynolds, I.; McCawley, N.; Galvin, E.; El-Masry, S.; Deasy, J.; McNamara, D.A. Liberal perioperative fluid administration is an independent risk factor for morbidity and is associated with longer hospital stay after rectal cancer surgery. *Ann. R. Coll. Surg. Engl.* **2017**, *99*, 113–116. [CrossRef]
17. Holte, K.; Sharrock, N.E.; Kehlet, H. Pathophysiology and clinical implications of perioperative fluid excess. *Br. J. Anaesth.* **2002**, *89*, 622–632. [CrossRef]
18. Grass, F.; Lovely, J.K.; Crippa, J.; Hubner, M.; Mathis, K.L.; Larson, D.W. Potential Association Between Perioperative Fluid Management and Occurrence of Postoperative Ileus. *Dis. Colon. Rectum* **2020**, *63*, 68–74. [CrossRef]
19. Grass, F.; Hubner, M.; Mathis, K.L.; Hahnloser, D.; Dozois, E.J.; Kelley, S.R.; Demartines, N.; Larson, D.W. Challenges to accomplish stringent fluid management standards 7 years after enhanced recovery after surgery implementation-The surgeon's perspective. *Surgery* **2020**, *168*, 313–319. [CrossRef] [PubMed]
20. Monnet, X.; Malbrain, M.; Pinsky, M.R. The prediction of fluid responsiveness. *Intensive Care Med.* **2023**, *49*, 83–86. [CrossRef] [PubMed]
21. Monnet, X.; Marik, P.; Teboul, J.L. Passive leg raising for predicting fluid responsiveness: A systematic review and meta-analysis. *Intensive Care Med.* **2016**, *42*, 1935–1947. [CrossRef] [PubMed]
22. Sanfilippo, F.; La Via, L.; Dezio, V.; Amelio, P.; Genoese, G.; Franchi, F.; Messina, A.; Robba, C.; Noto, A. Inferior vena cava distensibility from subcostal and trans-hepatic imaging using both M-mode or artificial intelligence: A prospective study on mechanically ventilated patients. *Intensive Care Med. Exp.* **2023**, *11*, 40. [CrossRef] [PubMed]
23. Sanfilippo, F.; La Via, L.; Dezio, V.; Santonocito, C.; Amelio, P.; Genoese, G.; Astuto, M.; Noto, A. Assessment of the inferior vena cava collapsibility from subcostal and trans-hepatic imaging using both M-mode or artificial intelligence: A prospective study on healthy volunteers. *Intensive Care Med. Exp.* **2023**, *11*, 15. [CrossRef]
24. Gustafsson, U.O.; Scott, M.J.; Hubner, M.; Nygren, J.; Demartines, N.; Francis, N.; Rockall, T.A.; Young-Fadok, T.M.; Hill, A.G.; Soop, M.; et al. Guidelines for Perioperative Care in Elective Colorectal Surgery: Enhanced Recovery After Surgery (ERAS®) Society Recommendations: 2018. *World J. Surg.* **2019**, *43*, 659–695. [CrossRef]
25. Thiele, R.H.; Raghunathan, K.; Brudney, C.S.; Lobo, D.N.; Martin, D.; Senagore, A.; Cannesson, M.; Gan, T.J.; Mythen, M.M.; Shaw, A.D.; et al. American Society for Enhanced Recovery (ASER) and Perioperative Quality Initiative (POQI) joint consensus statement on perioperative fluid management within an enhanced recovery pathway for colorectal surgery. *Perioper. Med.* **2016**, *5*, 24. [CrossRef]
26. Feldheiser, A.; Aziz, O.; Baldini, G.; Cox, B.P.; Fearon, K.C.; Feldman, L.S.; Gan, T.J.; Kennedy, R.H.; Ljungqvist, O.; Lobo, D.N.; et al. Enhanced Recovery After Surgery (ERAS) for gastrointestinal surgery, part 2: Consensus statement for anaesthesia practice. *Acta Anaesthesiol. Scand.* **2016**, *60*, 289–334. [CrossRef] [PubMed]
27. Srinivasa, S.; Lemanu, D.P.; Singh, P.P.; Taylor, M.H.; Hill, A.G. Systematic review and meta-analysis of oesophageal Doppler-guided fluid management in colorectal surgery. *Br. J. Surg.* **2013**, *100*, 1701–1708. [CrossRef] [PubMed]
28. Srinivasa, S.; Taylor, M.H.; Singh, P.P.; Yu, T.C.; Soop, M.; Hill, A.G. Randomized clinical trial of goal-directed fluid therapy within an enhanced recovery protocol for elective colectomy. *Br. J. Surg.* **2013**, *100*, 66–74. [CrossRef]
29. Braga, M.; Scatizzi, M.; Borghi, F.; Missana, G.; Radrizzani, D.; Gemma, M.; Perioperative Italian, S. Identification of core items in the enhanced recovery pathway. *Clin. Nutr. ESPEN* **2018**, *25*, 139–144. [CrossRef] [PubMed]
30. Messina, A.; Robba, C.; Calabro, L.; Zambelli, D.; Iannuzzi, F.; Molinari, E.; Scarano, S.; Battaglini, D.; Baggiani, M.; De Mattei, G.; et al. Perioperative liberal versus restrictive fluid strategies and postoperative outcomes: A systematic review and metanalysis on randomised-controlled trials in major abdominal elective surgery. *Crit. Care* **2021**, *25*, 205. [CrossRef]
31. Messina, A.; Robba, C.; Calabro, L.; Zambelli, D.; Iannuzzi, F.; Molinari, E.; Scarano, S.; Battaglini, D.; Baggiani, M.; De Mattei, G.; et al. Association between perioperative fluid administration and postoperative outcomes: A 20-year systematic review and a meta-analysis of randomized goal-directed trials in major visceral/noncardiac surgery. *Crit. Care* **2021**, *25*, 43. [CrossRef] [PubMed]
32. Varadhan, K.K.; Lobo, D.N. A meta-analysis of randomised controlled trials of intravenous fluid therapy in major elective open abdominal surgery: Getting the balance right. *Proc. Nutr. Soc.* **2010**, *69*, 488–498. [CrossRef] [PubMed]
33. Brandstrup, B.; Tonnesen, H.; Beier-Holgersen, R.; Hjortso, E.; Ording, H.; Lindorff-Larsen, K.; Rasmussen, M.S.; Lanng, C.; Wallin, L.; Iversen, L.H.; et al. Effects of intravenous fluid restriction on postoperative complications: Comparison of two perioperative fluid regimens: A randomized assessor-blinded multicenter trial. *Ann. Surg.* **2003**, *238*, 641–648. [CrossRef]

34. Nisanevich, V.; Felsenstein, I.; Almogy, G.; Weissman, C.; Einav, S.; Matot, I. Effect of intraoperative fluid management on outcome after intraabdominal surgery. *Anesthesiology* **2005**, *103*, 25–32. [CrossRef]
35. Kabon, B.; Akca, O.; Taguchi, A.; Nagele, A.; Jebadurai, R.; Arkilic, C.F.; Sharma, N.; Ahluwalia, A.; Galandiuk, S.; Fleshman, J.; et al. Supplemental intravenous crystalloid administration does not reduce the risk of surgical wound infection. *Anesth. Analg.* **2005**, *101*, 1546–1553. [CrossRef] [PubMed]
36. MacKay, G.; Fearon, K.; McConnachie, A.; Serpell, M.G.; Molloy, R.G.; O'Dwyer, P.J. Randomized clinical trial of the effect of postoperative intravenous fluid restriction on recovery after elective colorectal surgery. *Br. J. Surg.* **2006**, *93*, 1469–1474. [CrossRef]
37. Holte, K.; Foss, N.B.; Andersen, J.; Valentiner, L.; Lund, C.; Bie, P.; Kehlet, H. Liberal or restrictive fluid administration in fast-track colonic surgery: A randomized, double-blind study. *Br. J. Anaesth.* **2007**, *99*, 500–508. [CrossRef] [PubMed]
38. Muller, S.; Zalunardo, M.P.; Hubner, M.; Clavien, P.A.; Demartines, N.; Zurich Fast Track Study, G. A fast-track program reduces complications and length of hospital stay after open colonic surgery. *Gastroenterology* **2009**, *136*, 842–847. [CrossRef] [PubMed]
39. de Aguilar-Nascimento, J.E.; Diniz, B.N.; do Carmo, A.V.; Silveira, E.A.; Silva, R.M. Clinical benefits after the implementation of a protocol of restricted perioperative intravenous crystalloid fluids in major abdominal operations. *World J. Surg.* **2009**, *33*, 925–930. [CrossRef] [PubMed]
40. Futier, E.; Constantin, J.M.; Petit, A.; Chanques, G.; Kwiatkowski, F.; Flamein, R.; Slim, K.; Sapin, V.; Jaber, S.; Bazin, J.E. Conservative vs restrictive individualized goal-directed fluid replacement strategy in major abdominal surgery: A prospective randomized trial. *Arch. Surg.* **2010**, *145*, 1193–1200. [CrossRef]
41. Abraham-Nordling, M.; Hjern, F.; Pollack, J.; Prytz, M.; Borg, T.; Kressner, U. Randomized clinical trial of fluid restriction in colorectal surgery. *Br. J. Surg.* **2012**, *99*, 186–191. [CrossRef] [PubMed]
42. Kalyan, J.P.; Rosbergen, M.; Pal, N.; Sargen, K.; Fletcher, S.J.; Nunn, D.L.; Clark, A.; Williams, M.R.; Lewis, M.P. Randomized clinical trial of fluid and salt restriction compared with a controlled liberal regimen in elective gastrointestinal surgery. *Br. J. Surg.* **2013**, *100*, 1739–1746. [CrossRef]
43. Jie, H.Y.; Ye, J.L.; Zhou, H.H.; Li, Y.X. Perioperative restricted fluid therapy preserves immunological function in patients with colorectal cancer. *World J. Gastroenterol.* **2014**, *20*, 15852–15859. [CrossRef] [PubMed]
44. Phan, T.D.; D'Souza, B.; Rattray, M.J.; Johnston, M.J.; Cowie, B.S. A randomised controlled trial of fluid restriction compared to oesophageal Doppler-guided goal-directed fluid therapy in elective major colorectal surgery within an Enhanced Recovery After Surgery program. *Anaesth. Intensive Care* **2014**, *42*, 752–760. [CrossRef]
45. Gomez-Izquierdo, J.C.; Trainito, A.; Mirzakandov, D.; Stein, B.L.; Liberman, S.; Charlebois, P.; Pecorelli, N.; Feldman, L.S.; Carli, F.; Baldini, G. Goal-directed Fluid Therapy Does Not Reduce Primary Postoperative Ileus after Elective Laparoscopic Colorectal Surgery: A Randomized Controlled Trial. *Anesthesiology* **2017**, *127*, 36–49. [CrossRef] [PubMed]
46. Lobo, D.N. Fluid, electrolytes and nutrition: Physiological and clinical aspects. *Proc. Nutr. Soc.* **2004**, *63*, 453–466. [CrossRef] [PubMed]
47. Malbrain, M.; Langer, T.; Annane, D.; Gattinoni, L.; Elbers, P.; Hahn, R.G.; De Laet, I.; Minini, A.; Wong, A.; Ince, C.; et al. Intravenous fluid therapy in the perioperative and critical care setting: Executive summary of the International Fluid Academy (IFA). *Ann. Intensive Care* **2020**, *10*, 64. [CrossRef] [PubMed]
48. Butti, F.; Pache, B.; Winiker, M.; Grass, F.; Demartines, N.; Hubner, M. Correlation of postoperative fluid balance and weight and their impact on outcomes. *Langenbecks Arch. Surg.* **2020**, *405*, 1191–1200. [CrossRef] [PubMed]
49. Tolstrup, J.; Brandstrup, B. Clinical Assessment of Fluid Balance is Incomplete for Colorectal Surgical Patients. *Scand. J. Surg.* **2015**, *104*, 161–168. [CrossRef] [PubMed]
50. Hubner, M.; Pache, B.; Sola, J.; Blanc, C.; Hahnloser, D.; Demartines, N.; Grass, F. Thresholds for optimal fluid administration and weight gain after laparoscopic colorectal surgery. *BJS Open* **2019**, *3*, 532–538. [CrossRef]
51. Grass, F.; Slieker, J.; Jurt, J.; Kummer, A.; Sola, J.; Hahnloser, D.; Demartines, N.; Hubner, M. Postoperative ileus in an enhanced recovery pathway-a retrospective cohort study. *Int. J. Color. Dis.* **2017**, *32*, 675–681. [CrossRef]
52. Lin, Z.; Li, Y.; Wu, J.; Zheng, H.; Yang, C. Nomogram for prediction of prolonged postoperative ileus after colorectal resection. *BMC Cancer* **2022**, *22*, 1273. [CrossRef] [PubMed]
53. Wolthuis, A.M.; Bislenghi, G.; Fieuws, S.; de Buck van Overstraeten, A.; Boeckxstaens, G.; D'Hoore, A. Incidence of prolonged postoperative ileus after colorectal surgery: A systematic review and meta-analysis. *Color. Dis.* **2016**, *18*, O1–O9. [CrossRef]
54. Shereef, A.; Raftery, D.; Sneddon, F.; Emslie, K.; Mair, L.; Mackay, C.; Ramsay, G.; Forget, P. Prolonged Ileus after Colorectal Surgery, a Systematic Review. *J. Clin. Med.* **2023**, *12*, 5769. [CrossRef]
55. Greenberg, A.L.; Kelly, Y.M.; McKay, R.E.; Varma, M.G.; Sarin, A. Risk factors and outcomes associated with postoperative ileus following ileostomy formation: A retrospective study. *Perioper. Med.* **2021**, *10*, 55. [CrossRef] [PubMed]
56. Grass, F.; Pache, B.; Butti, F.; Sola, J.; Hahnloser, D.; Demartines, N.; Hubner, M. Stringent fluid management might help to prevent postoperative ileus after loop ileostomy closure. *Langenbecks Arch. Surg.* **2019**, *404*, 39–43. [CrossRef] [PubMed]
57. Miskovic, A.; Lumb, A.B. Postoperative pulmonary complications. *Br. J. Anaesth.* **2017**, *118*, 317–334. [CrossRef]
58. Danziger, J.; Hoenig, M.P. The Role of the Kidney in Disorders of Volume: Core Curriculum 2016. *Am. J. Kidney Dis.* **2016**, *68*, 808–816. [CrossRef]

59. Brandstrup, B.; Beier-Holgersen, R.; Iversen, L.H.; Starup, C.B.; Wentzel, L.N.; Lindorff-Larsen, K.; Petersen, T.C.; Tonnesen, H. The Influence of Perioperative Fluid Therapy on N-terminal-pro-brain Natriuretic Peptide and the Association With Heart and Lung Complications in Patients Undergoing Colorectal Surgery: Secondary Results of a Clinical Randomized Assessor-blinded Multicenter Trial. *Ann. Surg.* **2020**, *272*, 941–949. [CrossRef] [PubMed]
60. Kork, F.; Balzer, F.; Spies, C.D.; Wernecke, K.D.; Ginde, A.A.; Jankowski, J.; Eltzschig, H.K. Minor Postoperative Increases of Creatinine Are Associated with Higher Mortality and Longer Hospital Length of Stay in Surgical Patients. *Anesthesiology* **2015**, *123*, 1301–1311. [CrossRef]
61. Lovely, J.K.; Maxson, P.M.; Jacob, A.K.; Cima, R.R.; Horlocker, T.T.; Hebl, J.R.; Harmsen, W.S.; Huebner, M.; Larson, D.W. Case-matched series of enhanced versus standard recovery pathway in minimally invasive colorectal surgery. *Br. J. Surg.* **2012**, *99*, 120–126. [CrossRef]
62. Roulin, D.; Donadini, A.; Gander, S.; Griesser, A.C.; Blanc, C.; Hubner, M.; Schafer, M.; Demartines, N. Cost-effectiveness of the implementation of an enhanced recovery protocol for colorectal surgery. *Br. J. Surg.* **2013**, *100*, 1108–1114. [CrossRef]
63. Grass, F.; Lovely, J.K.; Crippa, J.; Mathis, K.L.; Hubner, M.; Larson, D.W. Early Acute Kidney Injury Within an Established Enhanced Recovery Pathway: Uncommon and Transitory. *World J. Surg.* **2019**, *43*, 1207–1215. [CrossRef]
64. Weimann, A.; Braga, M.; Carli, F.; Higashiguchi, T.; Hubner, M.; Klek, S.; Laviano, A.; Ljungqvist, O.; Lobo, D.N.; Martindale, R.G.; et al. ESPEN practical guideline: Clinical nutrition in surgery. *Clin. Nutr.* **2021**, *40*, 4745–4761. [CrossRef] [PubMed]
65. Tallarico, R.T.; McCoy, I.E.; Depret, F.; Legrand, M. Meaning and Management of Perioperative Oliguria. *Anesthesiology* **2023**, *140*, 304–312. [CrossRef] [PubMed]
66. Hubner, M.; Lovely, J.K.; Huebner, M.; Slettedahl, S.W.; Jacob, A.K.; Larson, D.W. Intrathecal analgesia and restrictive perioperative fluid management within enhanced recovery pathway: Hemodynamic implications. *J. Am. Coll. Surg.* **2013**, *216*, 1124–1134. [CrossRef]
67. Romagnoli, S.; Ricci, Z.; Ronco, C. Perioperative Acute Kidney Injury: Prevention, Early Recognition, and Supportive Measures. *Nephron* **2018**, *140*, 105–110. [CrossRef] [PubMed]
68. du Toit, L.; Biccard, B.M. The relationship between intraoperative oliguria and acute kidney injury. *Br. J. Anaesth.* **2019**, *122*, 707–710. [CrossRef] [PubMed]
69. Howitt, S.H.; Oakley, J.; Caiado, C.; Goldstein, M.; Malagon, I.; McCollum, C.; Grant, S.W. A Novel Patient-Specific Model for Predicting Severe Oliguria; Development and Comparison With Kidney Disease: Improving Global Outcomes Acute Kidney Injury Classification. *Crit. Care Med.* **2020**, *48*, e18–e25. [CrossRef] [PubMed]
70. Grass, F.; Hubner, M.; Behm, K.T.; Mathis, K.L.; Hahnloser, D.; Day, C.N.; Harmsen, W.S.; Demartines, N.; Larson, D.W. Development and validation of a prediction score for safe outpatient colorectal resections. *Surgery* **2022**, *171*, 336–341. [CrossRef] [PubMed]
71. Grass, F.; Hubner, M.; Mathis, K.L.; Hahnloser, D.; Dozois, E.J.; Kelley, S.R.; Demartines, N.; Larson, D.W. Identification of patients eligible for discharge within 48 h of colorectal resection. *Br. J. Surg.* **2020**, *107*, 546–551. [CrossRef]
72. Grass, F.; Pache, B.; Butti, F.; Sola, J.; Hahnloser, D.; Demartines, N.; Hubner, M. Fluid management for critical patients undergoing urgent colectomy. *J. Eval. Clin. Pract.* **2020**, *26*, 109–114. [CrossRef] [PubMed]
73. Pache, B.; Hubner, M.; Sola, J.; Hahnloser, D.; Demartines, N.; Grass, F. Receiver operating characteristic analysis to determine optimal fluid management during open colorectal surgery. *Color. Dis.* **2019**, *21*, 234–240. [CrossRef] [PubMed]
74. Gianotti, L.; Biffi, R.; Sandini, M.; Marrelli, D.; Vignali, A.; Caccialanza, R.; Vigano, J.; Sabbatini, A.; Di Mare, G.; Alessiani, M.; et al. Preoperative Oral Carbohydrate Load Versus Placebo in Major Elective Abdominal Surgery (PROCY): A Randomized, Placebo-controlled, Multicenter, Phase III Trial. *Ann. Surg.* **2018**, *267*, 623–630. [CrossRef]
75. Brady, M.; Kinn, S.; Stuart, P. Preoperative fasting for adults to prevent perioperative complications. *Cochrane Database Syst. Rev.* **2003**, *4*, CD004423. [CrossRef]
76. Rollins, K.E.; Javanmard-Emamghissi, H.; Lobo, D.N. Impact of mechanical bowel preparation in elective colorectal surgery: A meta-analysis. *World J. Gastroenterol.* **2018**, *24*, 519–536. [CrossRef] [PubMed]
77. Killewich, L.A. Strategies to minimize postoperative deconditioning in elderly surgical patients. *J. Am. Coll. Surg.* **2006**, *203*, 735–745. [CrossRef]
78. Golder, H.J.; Papalois, V. Enhanced Recovery after Surgery: History, Key Advancements and Developments in Transplant Surgery. *J. Clin. Med.* **2021**, *10*, 1634. [CrossRef]
79. Page, A.J.; Gani, F.; Crowley, K.T.; Lee, K.H.; Grant, M.C.; Zavadsky, T.L.; Hobson, D.; Wu, C.; Wick, E.C.; Pawlik, T.M. Patient outcomes and provider perceptions following implementation of a standardized perioperative care pathway for open liver resection. *Br. J. Surg.* **2016**, *103*, 564–571. [CrossRef] [PubMed]
80. Bijker, J.B.; van Klei, W.A.; Vergouwe, Y.; Eleveld, D.J.; van Wolfswinkel, L.; Moons, K.G.; Kalkman, C.J. Intraoperative hypotension and 1-year mortality after noncardiac surgery. *Anesthesiology* **2009**, *111*, 1217–1226. [CrossRef]
81. Lobo, D.N.; Macafee, D.A.; Allison, S.P. How perioperative fluid balance influences postoperative outcomes. *Best. Pract. Res. Clin. Anaesthesiol.* **2006**, *20*, 439–455. [CrossRef]

Disclaimer/Publisher's Note: The statements, opinions and data contained in all publications are solely those of the individual author(s) and contributor(s) and not of MDPI and/or the editor(s). MDPI and/or the editor(s) disclaim responsibility for any injury to people or property resulting from any ideas, methods, instructions or products referred to in the content.

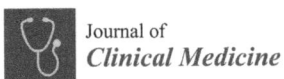

Systematic Review

Accuracy of Artificial Intelligence-Based Technologies for the Diagnosis of Atrial Fibrillation: A Systematic Review and Meta-Analysis

Nikolaos Manetas-Stavrakakis [1,*], Ioanna Myrto Sotiropoulou [1], Themistoklis Paraskevas [2], Stefania Maneta Stavrakaki [3], Dimitrios Bampatsias [4], Andrew Xanthopoulos [5], Nikolaos Papageorgiou [6] and Alexandros Briasoulis [1]

1. Department of Clinical Therapeutics, National and Kapodistrian University of Athens, 157 28 Athens, Greece; mirtosoti@med.uoa.gr (I.M.S.); abriasoulis@med.uoa.gr (A.B.)
2. Department of Internal Medicine, University Hospital of Patras, 265 04 Patras, Greece; themispara@hotmail.com
3. Faculty of Medicine, Imperial College London, London SW7 2BX, UK; s.maneta-stavrakaki17@imperial.ac.uk
4. Division of Cardiology, Columbia University, New York, NY 10027, USA; db3670@cumc.columbia.edu
5. Department of Cardiology, University of Thessaly, 382 21 Larissa, Greece; andrewvxanth@gmail.com
6. Barts Health NHS Trust, St Bartholomew's Hospital, London EC1A 7BE, UK; n.papageorgiou@nhs.net
* Correspondence: nikolaos.manetas-stavrakakis@nhs.net

Abstract: Atrial fibrillation (AF) is the most common arrhythmia with a high burden of morbidity including impaired quality of life and increased risk of thromboembolism. Early detection and management of AF could prevent thromboembolic events. Artificial intelligence (AI)--based methods in healthcare are developing quickly and can be proved as valuable for the detection of atrial fibrillation. In this metanalysis, we aim to review the diagnostic accuracy of AI-based methods for the diagnosis of atrial fibrillation. A predetermined search strategy was applied on four databases, the PubMed on 31 August 2022, the Google Scholar and Cochrane Library on 3 September 2022, and the Embase on 15 October 2022. The identified studies were screened by two independent investigators. Studies assessing the diagnostic accuracy of AI-based devices for the detection of AF in adults against a gold standard were selected. Qualitative and quantitative synthesis to calculate the pooled sensitivity and specificity was performed, and the QUADAS-2 tool was used for the risk of bias and applicability assessment. We screened 14,770 studies, from which 31 were eligible and included. All were diagnostic accuracy studies with case–control or cohort design. The main technologies used were: (a) photoplethysmography (PPG) with pooled sensitivity 95.1% and specificity 96.2%, and (b) single-lead ECG with pooled sensitivity 92.3% and specificity 96.2%. In the PPG group, 0% to 43.2% of the tracings could not be classified using the AI algorithm as AF or not, and in the single-lead ECG group, this figure fluctuated between 0% and 38%. Our analysis showed that AI-based methods for the diagnosis of atrial fibrillation have high sensitivity and specificity for the detection of AF. Further studies should examine whether utilization of these methods could improve clinical outcomes.

Keywords: atrial fibrillation; artificial intelligence; screening

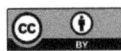

1. Introduction

Atrial fibrillation (AF) is the most common arrhythmia in adults worldwide. AF can be completely asymptomatic, and often its initial presentation includes thromboembolic events, such as strokes. It is estimated that more than 25% of strokes are caused by previously asymptomatic atrial fibrillation. In most of the cases, the stroke could have been prevented if the atrial fibrillation had been detected earlier, and the patients were started on anticoagulation therapy [1].

Given that many of the complications are preventable, many screening strategies have been suggested [2,3]. Currently, the European Society of Cardiology (ESC) guidelines suggest opportunistic screening for people above 65 years old, and systematic screening for people > 75 years old or those with increased risk of stroke [3]. The recommended screening tools include pulse check, single-lead ECG > 30 s. or 12-lead ECG interpreted by a physician [3]. However, since AF is often paroxysmal, these screening methods result in many false negative results, and therefore their use is limited [2].

Over the last few years, mobile heath technology has been developing quickly [4]. So far, various mobile devices and smartwatches with AI algorithms have been developed to detect AF and they demonstrate high diagnostic accuracy against a gold standard (i.e., 12-lead ECG, single-lead ECG, telemetry, Holter monitor, or implantable cardiac monitor) [5–7].

So far, the two main technologies used by AI-based devices to automatically detect AF are the photoplethysmography (PPG) and the single-lead ECG. The former is a photoelectric method that measures changes in blood volume in the peripheral vessels. PPG devices consist of a light source and receptor, and based on the reflected light can detect changes in the blood volume. These changes can be captured in a PPG trace which is then interpreted by an AI algorithm [8,9]. The single-lead ECG methods consist of a portable or wearable device which can record a single-lead ECG trace. To complete this assessment, the individual is asked to keep two parts of their body (e.g., wrist and finger or two fingers, etc.) in touch with the device for a pre-determined time. The recording is then transmitted to an AI application for interpretation [10–12]. These AI methods classify their recordings as "possible AF", "normal" or "no AF", "undiagnosable/unclassified", or "error" [11,12].

Compared to the conventional methods, AI-based devices for the diagnosis of AF are widely available, easy to use, and offer prolonged monitoring times, which increase the chances of detecting paroxysmal episodes of AF [12]. If accurate, they can also accelerate the decision-making process by the physicians, who could use these data without the need to wait for further time-consuming investigations. In addition, single-lead ECG devices can save the ECG tracings, which can then be reviewed by a physician.

On the other hand, the rapid increase in uncertified devices and applications can lead to many false results. This can cause stress to the patients, unnecessary treatments and investigations, and a cost burden for the health care systems [12]. Also, single-lead ECGs are conducted by untrained individuals rather than trained health care professionals, which can result in poor quality tracings and thus unreliable outcomes [12].

The aim of our study is to provide a systematic review and meta-analysis of the diagnostic accuracy of all the available AI-based methods for the diagnosis of atrial fibrillation.

2. Materials and Methods

This systematic review–metanalysis was designed and conducted based on the Preferred Reporting Items for Systematic Reviews and Meta-Analyses (PRISMA) guidelines [13]. PROSPERO registration: https://www.crd.york.ac.uk/prospero/display_record.php?RecordID=357232 accessed on 10 July 2023 [14].

2.1. Inclusion and Exclusion Criteria

We included: (1) diagnostic studies with a cohort or case–control design, (2) studies conducted in adults 18 years old and above, (3) studies which tested AI-based devices to detect AF, (4) studies which used an acceptable reference standard interpreted via a healthcare professional, including 12-lead ECG, 6-lead ECG, single-lead ECG, 3-lead Holter monitor and telemetry, (5) studies that provided true positive, true negative, false positive, and false negative results or provided enough data to calculate them, (6) studies in which unclassified/unreadable results by the devices were reported separately.

Exclusion criteria included: (1) conference abstracts or studies without available full text, (2) studies published in a language other than English, (3) studies that only provided measurement-based instead of individual-based results, (4) studies that validated novel devices without automated interpretation, (5) studies in which the reference standard test was not completed in all the participants.

Unclassified results are the ones that could not be classified by the automated algorithm as AF or not AF. Unreadable results are the ones that could not be interpreted by the automated algorithm, e.g., poor quality or short tracings.

2.2. Data Sources and Search Strategy

To identify all the relevant studies, we searched the databases: (1) PubMed, (2) Embase, (3) Cochrane Library, and (4) Google Scholar. In addition, we conducted a manual search for further eligible studies.

The search in PubMed was undertaken on 31 August 2022, in Cochrane Library and Google Scholar on 3 September 2022 and in the Embase database on 15 October 2022.

The search strategy we used was:

((ai OR artificial intelligence OR machine learning OR ml OR deep learning OR neural network OR wearables OR smartwatches OR wearable OR smartwatch OR applewatch OR alivecor OR iECG) AND (diagnosis OR diagnosing OR detection OR detect OR detecting) AND (af OR atrial fibrillation OR afib OR arrhythmia OR svt OR supraventricular tachycardia OR atrial flutter OR tachycardia)).

The search strategy was created by the first author (NMS), reviewed by a second member of the team (IMS), and approved by the supervising professor (AB).

2.3. Screening

The identified citations were imported in the web application Covidence, which is endorsed by the Cochrane Collaboration for the conduction of systematic reviews [15]. The screening was performed by two independent and blinded researchers (NMS and IMS). Initially, duplicates were removed either automatically by the Covidence web app, or, less frequently, manually by the researchers. Following that, we screened the studies by reading the title and abstract, and then, for the selected studies, we performed a full-text review. Studies that met our inclusion and exclusion criteria were selected. In case of disagreement, the 2 researchers discussed until an agreement was reached.

2.4. Data Extraction

Data extraction was executed in Microsoft Excel, version 16.69. In case of uncertainty, a second researcher was asked to extract the data for the study in question, which was then discussed. In addition, when data calculation was impossible, the authors were contacted. If this was impossible, the study was reviewed by the second researcher before exclusion. For all the included studies, we extracted data including among others: the first author, the year of publication, the setting (inpatient vs. outpatient), the study design, the name of the device, the type of AI algorithm, the duration of the index test, the reference standard, basic demographics, true positive and negative results, false positive and negative results, and unclassified and unreadable results.

2.5. Assessment of Risk of Bias and Applicability

For the assessment of risk of bias and applicability, we used the quality assessment of diagnostic accuracy studies—2 (QUADAS-2) tool, which is recommended by the Cochrane Collaboration and the U.K. National Institute for Health and Care Excellence [16]. We assessed each study in 4 domains (1) selection of participants, (2) index test, (3) reference standard, (4) flow and timing. For each study, we also assessed the first 3 domains regarding its applicability. We used predetermined signaling questions tailored to our review. The assessment of risk of bias and applicability was performed by the main researcher (NMS).

2.6. Statistical Analysis

Data synthesis was conducted separately for the two main types of technology, photoplethysmography (PPG) and single-lead ECG. For the studies that tested technologies other than the above two, we did not perform a quantitative analysis due to lack of sufficient data, however, we describe their results. As effect measures of diagnostic accuracy, we used sensitivity and specificity. For the unclassified/unreadable results, we did not perform a quantitative analysis, however we describe them separately for each group. To present the unclassified/unreadable outcomes, we used their percentages out of total results as the effect measure. Studies that tested more than one device/technology are included as separate studies. We performed subgroup analysis on the PPG (inpatients vs. outpatients) and single-lead ECG groups (inpatients vs. outpatients and duration of index test).

To calculate our summary values and create the graphical interpretations, we used the mada package in R, version 4.2.3 (which uses the bivariate model of Reitsma, which is equivalent with the HSROC of Rutter and Gatsonis when covariates are not used). Also, we used the interactive online application MetaDTA, version 2.0 [17]. For the data synthesis, we used the random effects methodology due to the expected clinical heterogeneity among the studies. Due to the lack of a gold standard for the assessment of heterogeneity in diagnostic accuracy studies, we used the Zhou and Dendukuri approach, which considers the correlation between sensitivity and specificity for the calculation of I^2 [18].

3. Results

3.1. Study Selection

The flowchart (Figure 1) illustrates our study selection process. We identified 14,770 studies from which 43 were selected. From those, 12 studies were excluded in a later stage. Six of them were excluded because they only provided measurement-based, and not patient-based, results [19–23]. The remaining six studies were excluded because they either did not provide enough data or we were unable to communicate with the authors to provide data for analysis [24–29]. In the end, 31 studies were included in our analysis (Figure 1).

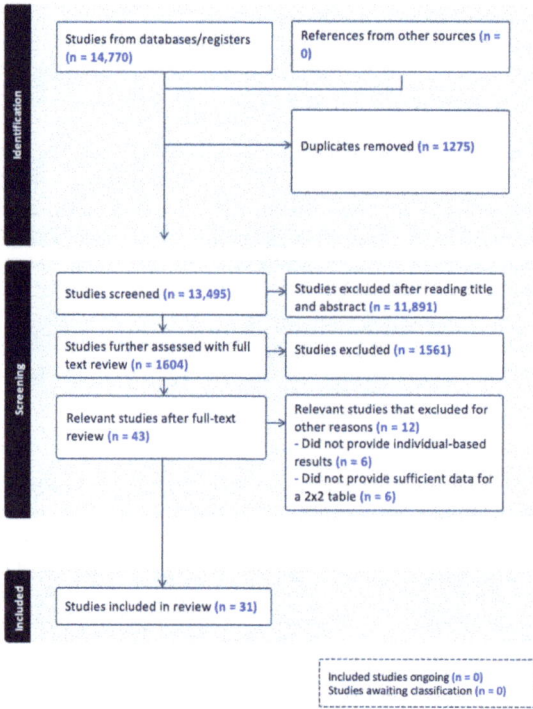

Figure 1. Flow chart (n: number).

3.2. Diagnostic Performance of Photoplethysmography (PPG) Devices

3.2.1. Study Characteristics of PPG Studies

We identified 12 diagnostic accuracy studies that tested PPG devices for the diagnosis of atrial fibrillation. Their characteristics are summarized in Table 1. Nine studies had a case–control design and three had a cohort design. The total number of participants was 4579. The smallest study included 51 patients [30], and the biggest, 1057 [31]. Five studies were conducted in an outpatient setting [11,31–34], five studies in an inpatient setting [30,35–38] and two studies in both settings [39,40]. Eight studies [30,31,33,36–40] used smartwatches, three studies [11,32,35] used mobile phones and one study [34] tested the technology of a remote PPG with the use of industrial camera. Seven studies tested the devices for up to 5 min [11,32,35–37,39,40], and the rest tested the devices from 10 min to up to 1 week [30,31,33,34,38]. Three studies [36–38] tested more than one device/technology, therefore each one was included as a separate study.

3.2.2. Assessment of Risk of Bias and Applicability of PPG Studies

Fourteen studies [11,34–40] were deemed high risk of bias in the participants' domain, and two studies [11,35] in the index test domain. The rest were deemed either low or unclear risk of bias (Figure 2). The studies were low in risk regarding their applicability (Figure 2).

3.2.3. Data Synthesis of the PPG Studies

The total sensitivity for the diagnosis of atrial fibrillation in the PPG group was 95.1% (95% C.I. 92.5–96.8%), the specificity was 96.2% (95%C.I. 94.3–97.5%), the area under the curve (AUC) for the SROC curve was 0.983 and the partial AUC was 0.961. The I^2 was 12.5% (Figures 3 and 4).

Among the studies, the AF prevalence was found to be between 2.5% and 57%, with a median prevalence of 44%. Based on these data, we used the total sensitivity and specificity to calculate the predictive false results in 1000 patients, by using different prevalence values. For prevalence of 5%, PPG devices would have resulted in 47 (95% C.I. 30–71) false positive results and 2 (95% C.I. 1–3) false negative results in 1000 patients. For the median prevalence of our studies, 44%, PPG devices would have resulted in 27 (95% C.I. 18–42) false positive results and 17 (95% C.I. 11–25) false negative results in 1000 patients. For a high prevalence of 60%, PPG devices would have resulted in 20 (95% C.I. 13–30) false positive results and 23 (95% C.I. 15–34) false negative results in 1000 patients.

3.2.4. Subgroup Analysis (Inpatients vs. Outpatients) of the PPG Studies

We did not proceed to a formal subgroup analysis for the PPG studies due to the low number of studies per subgroup, but also because we did not observe clusters in this subgroup's SROC curve (Figure 5).

3.2.5. Unclassified Unreadable Results of the PPG Studies

We found significant heterogeneity among the studies, regarding the unclassified/unreadable results. The reported unclassified/unreadable results ranged from 0% at the lowest [30–33,38] to 43.2% at the highest (Table 1) [37].

Table 1. Study characteristics (PPG, single-lead ECG and miscellaneous).

Author, Year	Setting	Study Design	Device	Algorithm	Time Used	Gold Standard	Age (Mean ± SD)	Sex (Females %)	N	N in AF Group	N in Control Group (Type of Control Group)	Group of AFL	TP	TN	FP	FN	Unclassified/Uninterpretable
Bacevicius et al., 2022 [39]	Inpatients and outpatients	Case-control selected cross-sectional study	Prototype of the wearable device	Automatic PPG-based algorithm (PPG)	2 min.	3-lead Holter	AF: 65.6 ± 11.2, SR: 67.3 ± 14.2	AF: 47.1%, SR: 46.1%	344	121	223 (SR)	Excluded from study	114	216	7	7	Excluded
Chang et al., 2022 [33]	Outpatients	Cohort selected cross-sectional study	Garmin Forerunner 945 smartwatch	Garmin Forerunner 945 smartwatch algorithm (PPG)	24 h	3-lead Holter	All participants: 66.1 ± 12.6 AF: 69.3 ± 11.5 Non-AF: 62.0 ± 12.9	All participants: 36.5% AF: 30.4% Non-AF: 44.3%	200	112	88 (non-AF)	AF group	109	78	10	3	0%
Chen et al., 2020 (A) [40]	Inpatients and outpatients	Case-control selected cross-sectional study	Amazfit Health Band 1S	RealBeats Artificial Intelligence Biological Data Engine (Huami Technology) (PPG)	3 min.	12-lead ECG	AF: 70.4 ± 11.5 Non-AF: 59.3 ± 14.8	AF: females: 43.3% Non-AF: females: 52.6%	401	139	244 (non-AF)	Control group	132	242	2	7	4.5%
Van Haelst et al., 2018 (A) [11]	Outpatients	Case-control selected cross-sectional study	Fibricheck	Fibricheck algorithm (PPG)	3 min.	12-lead ECG	All participants: 77.3 ± 8.0 AF: 78.8 ± 8.0 No AF: 75.9 ± 7.9	All participants: 57.4% AF: 51.1% Non-AF: 63.3%	190	75	93 (non-AF)	AF group	73	83	10	2	11.6%
Mol et al., 2020 [35]	Inpatients	Case-control selected cross-sectional study	Algorithm developed by Happitech (Amsterdam, The Netherlands) (PPG)		90 s	Continuous electrocardiography	All participants: 69 ± 9	All participants: 43%	257	149	108 (SR)	Excluded from study	139	101	2	3	4.7%
Sun et al., 2022 [34]	Outpatients	Case-control selected cross-sectional study	Industrial camera (FLIR BFLY-U3-03S2C-CS)	DCNN model (PPG)	10 min. max or as tolerated	12-lead ECG	69.3 ± 13.0 AF: 74.3 ± 12.5 Non-AF: 67.8 ± 13.0	All participants: 46% AF: 51.4% Non-AF: 44.8%	453	105	348 (no-AF)	Control group	98	342	6	7	Excluded
Tison et al., 2018 [30]	Inpatients	Case-control selected cross-sectional study	Apple Watch	Optimized Cardiogram app (PPG)	20 min prior- and 20 min post-cardioversion	12-lead ECG	All participants: 66.1 ± 10.7	All participants: 16%	51	51	51 (SR)	Excluded from study	50	46	5	1	0%
Väliaho et al., 2019 (A) [36]	Inpatients	Case-control selected cross-sectional study	Empatica E4 wrist band	MATLAB® software version R2017b using AFEvidence or COSEn (PPG)	5 min	3-lead Holter	AF: 72.0 ± 14.3 years SR: 54.5 ± 18.6 years	AF: 42.5% SR: 44.9%	213	106	107 (SR)	Excluded from study	102	105	2	4	Excluded
Väliaho et al., 2019 (B) [36]	Inpatients	Case-control selected cross-sectional study	Empatica E4 wrist band	MATLAB® software version R2017b using AFEvidence or COSEn (PPG)	5 min	3-lead Holter	AF: 72.0 ± 14.3 years SR: 54.5 ± 18.6 years	AF: 42.5% SR: 44.9%	213	106	107 (SR)	Excluded from study	101	105	2	5	Excluded
Väliaho et al., 2021 (A) [41]	Inpatients	Case-control selected cross-sectional study	Empatica E4 wrist band	MATLAB® software version R2017b) with a novel autocorrelation (AC) feature (PPG)	1 min every 10 min, 20 min, 30 min, 60 min	3-lead Holter	AF: 77.1 ± 9.7 SR: 67.3 ± 15.8	AF: 46.1% SR: 55.7%	173	76	97 (SR)	Unclear	75	79	18	1	0%
Väliaho et al., 2021 (B) [41]	Inpatients	Case-control selected cross-sectional study	Empatica E4 wrist band	MATLAB® software (version R2017b) with a novel autocorrelation (AC) feature (PPG)	1 min every 10 min, 20 min, 30 min, 60 min	3-lead Holter	AF: 77.1 ± 9.7 SR: 67.3 ± 15.8	AF: 46.1% SR: 55.7%	173	76	97 (SR)	Unclear	75	87	10	1	0%

Table 1. *Cont.*

Author, Year	Setting	Study Design	Device	Algorithm	Time Used	Gold Standard	Age (Mean ± SD)	Sex (Females %)	N	N in AF Group	N in Control Group (Type of Control Group)	Group of AFL	TP	TN	FP	FN	Unclassified/ Uninterpretable
Väliaho et al., 2021 (C) [41]	Inpatients	Case-control selected cross-sectional study	Empatica E4 wrist band	MATLAB® software (version R2017b) with a novel autocorrelation (AC) feature (PPG)	1 min every 10 min, 20 min, 30 min, 60 min	3-lead Holter	AF: 77.1 ± 9.7 SR: 67.3 ± 15.8	AF: 46.1% SR: 55.7%	173	76	97 (SR)	Unclear	72	94	3	4	0%
Väliaho et al., 2021 (D) [41]	Inpatients	Case-control selected cross-sectional study	Empatica E4 wrist band	MATLAB® software (version R2017b) with a novel autocorrelation (AC) feature (PPG)	1 min every 10 min, 20 min, 30 min, 60 min	3-lead Holter	AF: 77.1 ± 9.7 SR: 67.3 ± 15.8	AF: 46.1% SR: 55.7%	173	76	97 (SR)	Unclear	70	96	1	6	0%
Chan et al., 2016 (A) [32]	Outpatients	Cohort selected cross-sectional study	iPhone 4S	Cardio Rhythm smartphone application (Cardiio Inc.) (PPG)	51.3 s	single-lead ECG	All participants: 68.4 ± 12.2	All participants: 53.2%	1013	28	985 (non-AF)	Excluded from study	26	963	22	2	0%
Dörr et al., 2019 (A) [37]	Inpatients	Case-control selected cross-sectional study	Gear Fit 2, Samsung	Heartbeats application (Preventicus GmbH, Jena, Germany) (PPG)	1 min, 3 min and 5 min	single-lead ECG	All participants: 76.4 ± 9.5 AF: 77.4 ± 9.1 SR: 75.6 ± 9.8	All participants: 44.3% SR: 46.1% AF: 42.2%	650	237	271 (SR)	Excluded from study	222	266	5	15	21.8%
Dörr et al., 2019 (B) [37]	Inpatients	Case-control selected cross-sectional study	Gear Fit 2, Samsung	Heartbeats application (Preventicus GmbH, Jena, Germany) (PPG)	1 min, 3 min and 5 min	single-lead ECG	All participants: 76.4 ± 9.5 AF: 77.4 ± 9.1 SR: 75.6 ± 9.8	All participants: 44.3% SR: 46.1% AF: 42.2%	650	204	243 (SR)	Excluded from study	191	235	8	13	31.2%
Dörr et al., 2019 (C) [37]	Inpatients	Case-control selected cross-sectional study	Gear Fit 2, Samsung	Heartbeats application (Preventicus GmbH, Jena, Germany) (PPG)	1 min, 3 min and 5 min	single-lead ECG	All participants: 76.4 ± 9.5 AF: 77.4 ± 9.1 SR: 75.6 ± 9.8	All participants: 44.3% SR: 46.1% AF: 42.2%	650	167	202 (SR)	Excluded from study	156	198	4	11	43.2%
Lubitz et al., 2022 [31]	Outpatients	Cohort selected cross-sectional study	Fitbit device	Fitbit app (PPG)	1 week	single-lead ECG	All participants *: >75 years: 9.7% 65–74 years: 33.2% 55–64 years: 37.4% 40–54 years: 16.6% 22–39 years: 6.1%	All participants: 48.2%	1057	340	717 (non-AF)	AF group	230	706	11	110	0%
Badertscher et al., 2022 [42]	-	Cohort selected cross-sectional study	Withings Scanwatch	Withings Scanwatch detection algorithm (single-lead ECG)	30 s	12-lead ECG	All participants: 67 (54–76 years)	All participants: 48%	319	34	285 (SR)	No comment	19	247	3	6	13.8%
Bumgarner MD et al., 2018 [43]	Inpatients	Case-control selected cross-sectional study	Kardia Band	Kardia Band detection algorithm (single-lead ECG)	30 s	12-lead ECG	All participants: 68.2 ± 10.86	All participants: 17%	169	91	78 (SR)	In AF group	63	37	7	5	33.7%
Campo et al., 2022 [44]	Inpatients and outpatients	Case-control selected cross-sectional study	Withings Scanwatch	Withings Scanwatch detection algorithm (single-lead ECG)	30 s	12-lead ECG	All participants: 67.7 ± 14.8 AF: 74.3 ± 12.3 SR: 61.8 ± 14.3 Other arrhythmias: 66.5 ± 15.2 Unreadable ECGs: 78.8 ± 12.5	All participants: 61.1% AF: 42% SR: 34.5% Other arrhythmias: 40% Unreadable ECGs: 75%	258	87	155 (non-AF)	Control group	77	144	11	10	6.2%

Table 1. Cont.

Author, Year	Setting	Study Design	Device	Algorithm	Time Used	Gold Standard	Age (Mean ± SD)	Sex (Females %)	N	N in AF Group	N in Control Group (Type of Control Group)	Group of AFL	TP	TN	FP	FN	Unclassified/ Uninterpretable
Chen et al., 2020 (B) [40]	Inpatients and outpatients	Cohort selected cross-sectional study	Amazfit Health Band 1S	RealBeats Artificial Intelligence Biological Data Engine (Huami Technology) (single-lead ECG)	60 s	12-lead ECG	AF: 70.4 ± 11.5 Non-AF: 59.3 ± 14.8	AF: 43.3% Non-AF: 52.6%	401	150	25 (non-AF)	No comment	131	249	0	6	3.7%
Cunha et al., 2020 [45]	Inpatients	Cohort selected cross-sectional study	Kardia® mobile	Kardia® mobile algorithm (single-lead ECG)	30 s	12-lead ECG	-	-	129	22	78 (SR)	No comment	20	76	2	2	22.4%
Desteghe et al., 2017 (A) [46]	Inpatients	Cohort selected cross-sectional study	AliveCor	AliveCor algorithm (single-lead ECG)	30 s	12-lead ECG	All participants: 67.9 ± 14.6 AF: 73.1 ± 12.2 SR: 65.1 ± 15.0	All participants: 43.1% AF: 51.8% SR: 38.3%	265	22	243 (SR)	In AF group	12	237	6	10	0%
Desteghe et al., 2017 (B) [46]	Inpatients	Cohort selected cross-sectional study	MyDiagnostick	MyDiagnostick algorithm (single-lead ECG)	60 s	12-lead ECG	All participants: 67.9 ± 14.6 AF: 73.1 ± 12.2 SR: 65.1 ± 15.0	All participants: 43.1% AF: 51.8% SR: 38.3%	265	22	243 (SR)	In AF group	18	229	14	4	0%
Desteghe et al., 2017 (C) [46]	Inpatients	Cohort selected cross-sectional study	AliveCor	AliveCor algorithm (single-lead ECG)	30 s	6-lead ECG	-	-	113	19	94 (SR)	In AF group	15	92	2	4	0%
Desteghe et al., 2017 (D) [46]	Inpatients	Cohort selected cross-sectional study	MyDiagnostick	MyDiagnostick algorithm (single-lead ECG)	60 s	6-lead ECG	-	-	113	19	94 (SR)	In AF group	17	90	4	2	0%
Ford et al., 2022 (A) [10]	outpatients	Case-control selected cross-sectional study	Apple Watch 4	Apple Watch 4 algorithm (single-lead ECG)	30 s	12-lead ECG	All participants: 76 ± 7	All participants: 38%	125	31	94 (SR)	In AF group	6	76	0	6	29.6%
Ford et al., 2022 (B) [10]	outpatients	Case-control selected cross-sectional study	KardiaBand	KardiaBand algorithm (single-lead ECG)	30 s	12-lead ECG	All participants: 76 ± 7	All participants: 38%	125	31	94 (SR)	In AF group	26	68	5	1	20%
Fu et al., 2021 (A) [47]	-	Case-control selected cross-sectional study	Wearable Dynamic ECG Recorder	Amazfit CardiDoc application (single-lead ECG)	60 s	12-lead ECG	All participants: 59 ± 11.16 AF: 64.00 ± 9.38 SR:55.15 ± 11.01	All participants: 34% AF: 45.3% SR: 41%	114	53	61 (SR)	Excluded	47	61	0	4	1.8%
Fu et al., 2021 (B) [47]	-	Case-control selected cross-sectional study	Wearable Dynamic ECG Recorder	Amazfit CardiDoc application (single-lead ECG)	60 s	12-lead ECG	All participants: 59 ± 11.16 AF: 64.00 ± 9.38 SR:55.15 ± 11.01	All participants: 34% AF: 45.3% SR: 41%	114	53	61 (SR)	Excluded	50	61	0	2	0.9%
Fu et al., 2021 (C) [47]	-	Case-control selected cross-sectional study	Wearable Dynamic ECG Recorder	Amazfit CardiDoc application (single-lead ECG)	60 s	12-lead ECG	All participants: 59 ± 11.16 AF: 64.00 ± 9.38 SR:55.15 ± 11.01	All participants: 34% AF: 45.3% SR: 41%	114	53	61 (SR)	Excluded	50	61	0	2	0.9%
Van Haelst et al., 2018 (B) [11]	Outpatients	Cohort selected cross-sectional study	AliveCor	AliveCor algorithm (single-lead ECG)	30 s	12-lead ECG	All patients: 77.3 ± 8.0 AF: 78.8 ± 8.0 Non-AF: 75.9 ± 7.9	All participants: 57.4% AF: 51.1% No AF: 63.3%	190	75	93 (non-AF)	In AF group	73	83	10	2	19.3%
Himmelreich JCI, et al., 2019 [48]	Outpatients	Cohort selected cross-sectional study	KardiaMobile	KardiaMobile (AliveCor, Inc.) algorithm (single-lead ECG)	30 s	12-lead ECG	All participants: 64.1 ± 14.7	All participants: 46.3%	214	23	191 (SR)	In AF group	20	187	4	0	1.4%

Table 1. *Cont.*

Author, Year	Setting	Study Design	Device	Algorithm	Time Used	Gold Standard	Age (Mean ± SD)	Sex (Females %)	N	N in AF Group	N in Control Group (Type of Control Group)	Group of AFL	TP	TN	FP	FN	Unclassified/ Uninterpretable
Lown et al., 2018 (A) [49]	Outpatients	Case-control selected cross-sectional study	AliveCor	AliveCor (Kardia version 4.7.0) algorithm (single-lead ECG)	30 s	12-lead ECG	All participants: 73.9 ± 6.1	-	418	82	336 (non-AF)	In AF group	72	332	2	2	2.4%
Rajakariar et al., 2020 [50]	Inpatients	Cohort selected cross-sectional study	KardiaBand	AliveCor Kardia application V.5.0.2 (AliveCor, Mountain View, CA, USA) (single-lead ECG)	30 s	12-lead ECG	All participants: 67 ± 16 AF: 76 ± 11 SR: 64 ± 17	All participants: 43.5% AF: 48% SR: 36%	200	38	162 (SR)	No comment	36	124	13	2	12.5%
Santala et al., 2021 (1) [41]	Inpatients	Case-control selected cross-sectional study	Suunto Movesense, Suunto, Vantaa, Finland (heart belt)	Awario, Heart2Save, Kuopio, Finland (single-lead ECG)	24 h	12-lead ECG	AF: 77 ± 10 SR: 68 ± 16	AF: 48% SR: 60%	159	73	86 (SR)	No comment	73	82	4	0	0%
Santala et al., 2021 (2) (A) [51]	Inpatients	Case-control selected cross-sectional study	single-lead Necklace-embedded ECG recorder (Including Movesense ECG-sensor, Suunto, Vantaa, Finland, Necklace-ECG)	Awario, Heart2Save, Kuopio, Finland (single-lead ECG)	30 s	3-lead Holter ECG	AF (years): 72.7 ± 14.1 SR (years): 61.5 ± 18.1	AF: 56.1% SR: 53.2%	145	66	79 (SR)	No comment	54	78	0	3	6.9%
Santala et al., 2021 (2) (B) [51]	Inpatients	Case-control selected cross-sectional study	single-lead Necklace-embedded ECG recorder (Including Movesense ECG-sensor, Suunto, Vantaa, Finland, Necklace-ECG)	Awario, Heart2Save, Kuopio, Finland (single-lead ECG)	30 s	3-lead Holter ECG	AF (years): 72.7 ± 14.1 SR (years): 61.5 ± 18.1	AF: 56.1% SR: 53.2%	145	66	79 (SR)	No comment	58	75	0	1	7.6%
Santala et al., 2022 [52]	Inpatients	Case-control selected cross-sectional study	Firstbeat Bodyguard 2, Firstbeat Technologies	Awario, Heart2Save (single-lead ECG)	24 h	3-lead Holter ECG	AF: 77 ± 10 SR: 68 ± 15	AF: 47% SR: 60%	178	79	99 (SR)	No comment	79	94	5	0	0%
Abu-Alrub et al., 2022 (A) [53]	-	Case-control selected cross-sectional study	Apple Watch Series 5®	Apple Watch Series 5® (single-lead ECG)	30 s	12-lead ECG	All participants: 62 ± 7	All participants: 44%	200	100	100 (SR)	Excluded	87	86	1	7	9.5%
Abu-Alrub et al., 2022 (B) [53]	-	Case-control selected cross-sectional study	Samsung Galaxy Watch Active 3®	Samsung Galaxy Watch Active 3® (single-lead ECG)	30 s	12-lead ECG	All participants: 62 ± 7	All participants: 44%	200	100	100 (SR)	Excluded	88	81	6	5	10%
Abu-Alrub et al., 2022 (C) [53]	-	Case-control selected cross-sectional study	Withings Move ECG®	Withings Move ECG® algorithms (single-lead ECG)	30 s	12-lead ECG	All participants: 62 ± 7	All participants: 44%	200	100	100 (SR)	Excluded	78	80	3	2	18.5%

Table 1. *Cont.*

Author, Year	Setting	Study Design	Device	Algorithm	Time Used	Gold Standard	Age (Mean ± SD)	Sex (Females %)	N	N in AF Group	N in Control Group (Type of Control Group)	Group of AFL	TP	TN	FP	FN	Unclassified/ Uninterpretable
Wegner et al., 2020 (A) [54]	Inpatients	Cohort selected cross-sectional study	AliveCor Kardia ECG monitor	AliveCor Kardia ECG monitor algorithm (single-lead ECG)	30 s	12-lead ECG	All participants: 64 ± 15	All participants: 38.4%	92	27	65 (SR)	In AF group	19	45	8	0	21.7%
Wegner et al., 2020 (B) [54]	Inpatients	Cohort selected cross-sectional study	AliveCor Kardia ECG monitor	AliveCor Kardia ECG monitor algorithm (single-lead ECG)	30 s	12-lead ECG	All participants: 64 ± 15	All participants: 38.4%	92	27	65 (SR)	In AF group	15	39	3	0	38%
William et al., 2018 [55]	Inpatients	Case-control selected cross-sectional study	Kardia Mobile Cardiac Monitor	Kardia Mobile Cardiac Monitor (single-lead ECG)	30 s	12-lead ECG	All participants: 68.1 [42.6-85.6]	All participants: 32.7%	223	80	143 (SR)	In AF group	57	96	6	2	27.8%
Chan et al., 2016 (B) [32]	Outpatients	Cohort selected cross-sectional study	1st generation; AliveCor Inc.	AliveECG application (version 2.2.2) (single-lead ECG)	30 s	single-lead interpreted by cardiologists	All participants: 68.4 ± 12.2	All participants: 53.2%	1013	28 (AF)	985 (non-AF)	In control group	20	979	6	8	0%
Dörr et al., 2019 (D) [37]	Inpatients	Cohort selected cross-sectional study	AliveCor Kardia system	Heartbeats application (Preventicus GmbH, Jena, Germany) (single-lead ECG)	30 s	single-lead interpreted by cardiologists	All participants: 76.4 ± 9.5 AF: 77.4 ± 9.1 SR: 75.6 ± 9.8	All participants: 44.3% SR: 46.1% AF: 42.2%	650	319	331 (SR)	Excluded	279	262	7	1	15.5%
Orchard et al., 2016 [56]	Outpatients	Cohort selected cross-sectional study	AliveCor Heart Monitor	AliveCor Heart Monitor algorithm (single-lead ECG)	30 s	single-lead interpreted by cardiologists			972	38	934 (SR)	Excluded	36	844	8	2	8.4%
Letiska-Mieciek et al., 2022 [57]	Inpatients	Cohort selected cross-sectional study	Kardia Mobile portable device (AliveCor Inc, San Francisco, CA, USA)	AliveCor app. (single-lead ECG)	30 s	Single-lead ECG interpreted by cardiologist	All participants: 64.44 ± 10.52	All participants: 48%	50	1	49 (non-AF)	No comment	1	42	7	0	0%
Lown et al., 2018 (B) [49]	Outpatients	Case-control selected cross-sectional study	WatchBP	WatchBP algorithm (modified sphygmomanometer)		12-Lead ECG	All participants: 73.9 ± 6.1		418	82	336 (No AF)	In AF group	79	314	22	3	-
Lown et al., 2018 (C) [49]	Outpatients	Case-control selected cross-sectional study	Polar H7	PH7 (A Real-Time Atrial Fibrillation Detection Algorithm Based on the Instantaneous State of Heart Rate) (ECG data sensor)		12-Lead ECG	All participants: 73.9 ± 6.1		418	82	336 (No AF)	In AF group	79	330	6	3	-
Lown et al., 2018 (D) [49]	Outpatients	Case-control selected cross-sectional study	Bodyguard 2	BG2 (A Real-Time Atrial Fibrillation Detection Algorithm Based on the Instantaneous State of Heart Rate) (heart rate variability)		12-Lead ECG	All participants: 73.9 ± 6.1		418	82	336 (No AF)	In AF group	79	331	5	3	-

Table 1. *Cont.*

Author, Year	Setting	Study Design	Device	Algorithm	Time Used	Gold Standard	Age (Mean ± SD)	Sex (Females %)	N	N in AF Group	N in Control Group (Type of Control Group)	Group of AFL	TP	TN	FP	FN	Unclassified/ Uninterpretable
Reverberi et al., 2019 [58]	Inpatients	Case-control selected cross-sectional study	consumer-grade Bluetooth low-energy (BLE) HR monitor, of the chest-strap type	RITMIA™ (Heart Sentinel srl, Parma, Italy) (HR monitor)	-	12-lead ECG	All participants: 66.2 ± 10.7	All participants: 21.5%	182 **	99	83 (non-AF)	Excluded	96	79	4	3	-
Chen et al., 2020 (C) [40]	Inpatients and outpatients	Case-control selected cross-sectional study	Amazfit Health Band 1S (Huami Technology, Anhui, China)	RealBeats Artificial Intelligence Biological Data Engine (Huami Technology) (PPG combined with single-lead ECG)	-	12-lead ECG	AF: 70.4 ± 11.5 Non-AF: 59.3 ± 14.8	AF: 43.3% Non-AF: 52.6%	401	150	251 (non-AF)	Unclear	-	-	-	-	-

(N: number of participants; AF: Atrial Fibrillation; AFL: Atrial Flutter; SD: standard deviation; SR: Sinus Rhythm; ECG: electrocardiogram; DCNN: deep convolutional neural networks; rPPG: remote photoplethysmography; min: minutes; max: maximum; app: application; s: seconds; TP: true positive; TN: true negative; FP: false positive; FN: false negative; x (): median age (interquartile range); x []: average age [min. age–max. age]; Väliaho et al., 2019 (A): testing the AFEvidence algorithm; Chen et al., 2020 (A): testing PPG device; Chen et al., 2020 (B): testing single-lead ECG device; Chen et al. (C): testing combination of PPG and single-lead ECG; Väliaho et al., 2019 (B): testing the COSEn algorithm; Väliaho et al., 2021 (A): testing device performance when time interval between every measurement is 10 min; Väliaho et al., 2021 (B): testing device performance when time interval between every measurement is 20 min; Väliaho et al., 2021 (C): testing device performance when time interval between every measurement is 30 min; Väliaho et al., 2021 (D): testing device performance when time interval between every measurement is 60 min; Dörr et al., 2019 (A): testing performance of device when recording for 1 min; Dörr et al., 2019 (B): testing performance of device when recording for 3 min; Dörr et al., 2019 (C): testing performance of device when recording for 5 min; Dörr et al. (D): testing AliveCor; Desteghe et al., 2017 (A): testing the AliveCor in the cardiology ward population; Desteghe et al., 2017 (B): testing the MyDiagnostick in the cardiology ward population; Desteghe et al., 2017 (C): testing the AliveCor in the geriatric ward population; Desteghe et al., 2017 (D): testing the MyDiagnostick in the geriatric ward population; Ford et al., 2022 (A): testing the Apple Watch 4; Ford et al., 2022 (B): testing the KardiaBand; Fu et al., 2021 (A): testing the device in supine position; Fu et al., 2021 (B): testing the device in upright position; Fu et al., 2021 (C): testing the device after individuals climbed to the 3rd floor; Van Haelst et al., 2018 (A): testing PPG device; Van Haelst et al., 2018 (B): testing single-lead ECG device; Santala et al., 2021 (1): published in October 2021; Santala et al., 2021 (2) (A): published in May 2021 and testing the device between the palms; Santala et al., 2021 (2) (B): published in May 2021 and testing the device in the chest; Abu-Alrub et al., 2022 (A): testing the Apple Watch 5; Abu-Alrub et al., 2022 (B): testing the Samsung Galaxy Watch Active 3; Abu-Alrub et al., 2022 (C): testing the Withings Move ECG; Wegner et al., 2020 (A): testing the lead I; Wegner et al., 2020 (B): testing the novel parasternal lead; Chan et al., 2016 (A): testing the Watch BP; Lown et al., 2018 (A): testing AliveCor; Lown et al., 2018 (B): testing single-lead ECG device; Lown et al., 2018 (C): testing the Polar H7 device; Lown et al., 2018 (D): testing the Bodyguard 2 device; ** N refers to ECGs before and after cardioversion.

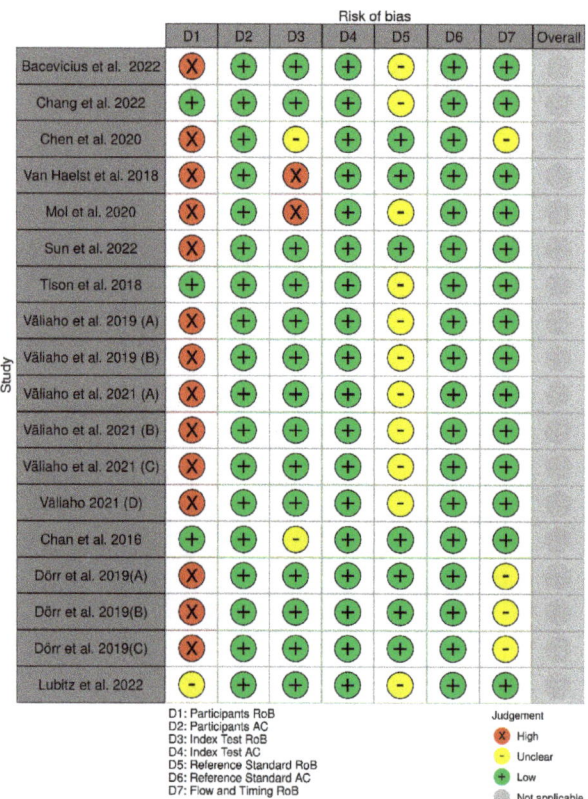

Figure 2. Assessment of risk of bias and applicability of the PPG studies. (Väliaho et al., 2019 (A): testing the AFEvidence algorithm; Väliaho et al., 2019 (B): testing the COSEn algorithm; Väliaho et al., 2021 (A): testing device performance when time interval between every measurement is 10 min; Väliaho et al., 2021 (B): testing device performance when time interval between every measurement is 20 min; Väliaho et al., 2021 (C): testing device performance when time interval between every measurement is 30 min; Väliaho et al., 2021 (D): testing device performance when time interval between every measurement is 60 min; Dörr et al., 2019 (A): testing performance of device when recording for 1 min; Dörr et al., 2019 (B): testing performance of device when recording for 3 min; Dörr et al., 2019 (C): testing performance of device when recording for 5 min).

3.3. Diagnostic Performance of Single-Lead ECG Devices
3.3.1. Study Characteristics of the Single-Lead ECG Studies

During our search, we identified 22 diagnostic accuracy studies that tested single-lead ECG devices with AI-based algorithms for the diagnosis of atrial fibrillation. Their characteristics are summarized in Table 1. Eleven studies had cohort design [11,32,40,42, 45,46,48,50,54,56,57] and the rest had case–control design [10,37,41,43,44,47,49,51–53,55]. The total number of participants was 6597. The smallest study included 50 patients [57] and the biggest study included 1013 patients [32]. Eleven studies were conducted in inpatient setting [37,41,43,45,46,50–52,54,55,57], 6 studies were conducted in outpatient setting [10,11,32,48,49,56], 2 studies were conducted in both settings [40,44] and in 3 studies the setting was not clear [42,47,53]. Eight studies tested smartwatches [10,40,42–44,47,50, 53] and the rest of studies tested other devices [11,32,37,41,45,46,48,49,51,52,54–57]. Five studies [10,46,47,51,53] tested more than one device/technology, and therefore each one included as a separate study.

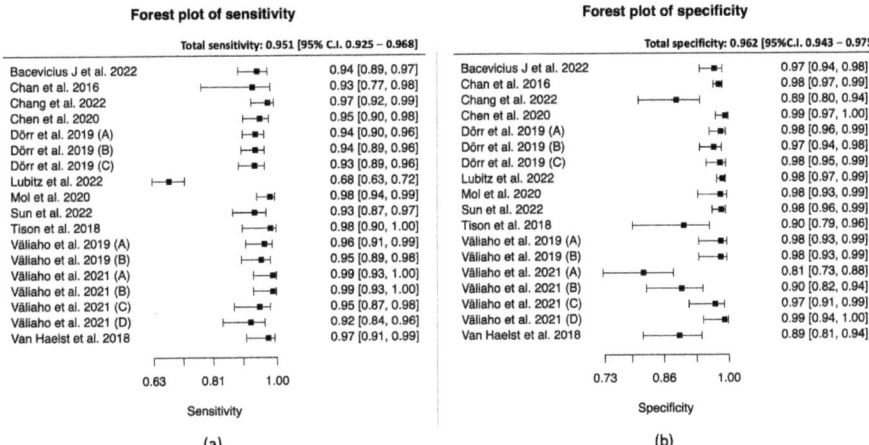

Figure 3. PPG group: (**a**) Forest plot of sensitivity; (**b**) forest plot of specificity. (Väliaho et al., 2019; (A): testing the AFEvidence algorithm, Väliaho et al., 2019; (B): testing the COSEn algorithm, Väliaho et al., 2021; (A): testing device performance when time interval between every measurement is 10 min, Väliaho et al., 2021; (B): testing device performance when time interval between every measurement is 20 min, Väliaho et al., 2021; (C): testing device performance when time interval between every measurement is 30 min, Väliaho et al., 2021; (D): testing device performance when time interval between every measurement is 60 min, Dörr et al., 2019; (A): testing performance of device when recording for 1 min, Dörr et al., 2019; (B): testing performance of device when recording for 3 min, Dörr et al., 2019; (C): testing performance of device when recording for 5 min).

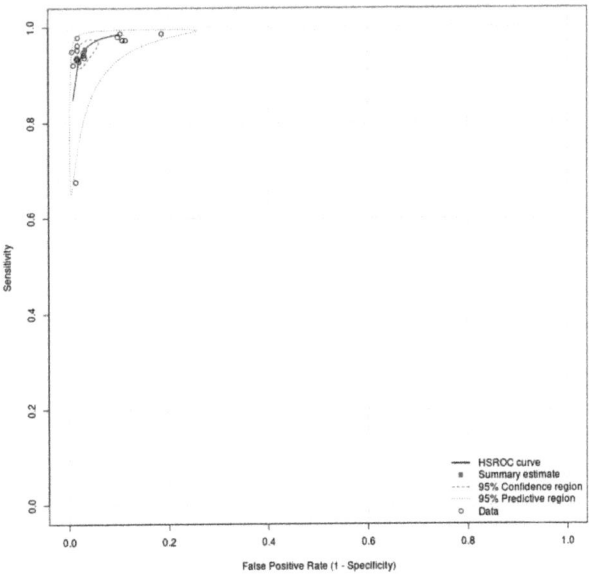

Figure 4. PPG group random effects meta-analysis.

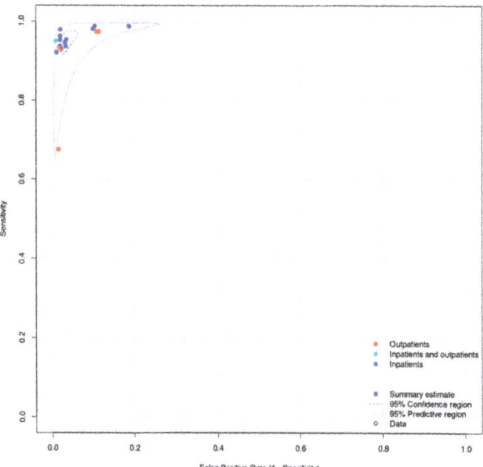

Figure 5. Subgroup analysis of the PPG studies (inpatients vs. outpatients).

3.3.2. Assessment of Risk of Bias and Applicability of the Single-Lead ECG Studies

Twelve studies [11,37,40,41,43,45,47,49,52,55] were deemed to be at high risk of bias in the participants' domain, nine studies [11,32,45,49,51,54,57] in the index test domain, four studies [45,53] in the reference standard domain, and two studies [11,45] were deemed to be at high risk of bias in the flow and timing domain (Figure 3). The studies were low in risk regarding their applicability (Figure 6).

3.3.3. Data Synthesis of the Single-Lead ECG Studies

The total sensitivity for the detection of atrial fibrillation by using single-lead ECG was 92.3% (95% C.I. 88.9–94.8%), the specificity was 96.2% (95%C.I. 94.6–97.4%), the area under the curve (AUC) for the SROC curve was 0.979, and the partial AUC was 0.939. The I^2 was 9.2% (Figures 7 and 8).

Among the studies, the AF prevalence was found to be between 2% and 61%, with median prevalence 31%. Based on these data, we used the total sensitivity and specificity to calculate the predictive false results in 1000 patients, by using different prevalence values. For a prevalence of 5%, a single-lead ECG device would have resulted in 73 (95% C.I. 49–106) false positive results and 2 (95% C.I. 1–3) false negative results in 1000 patients. For the median prevalence of our studies, 31%, a single-lead ECG device would have resulted in 53 (95% C.I. 36–77) false positive results and 12 (95% C.I. 8–17) false negative results in 1000 patients. For a high prevalence of 60%, a single-lead ECG device would have resulted in 31 (95% C.I. 21–44) false positive results and 23 (95% C.I. 16–32) false negative results in 1000 patients.

3.3.4. Subgroup Analysis (Inpatients vs. Outpatients) of the Single-Lead ECG Studies

We conducted a subgroup analysis according to the setting. In this analysis, we did not include either the studies in which the setting was not clear, or the ones that included both inpatients and outpatients.

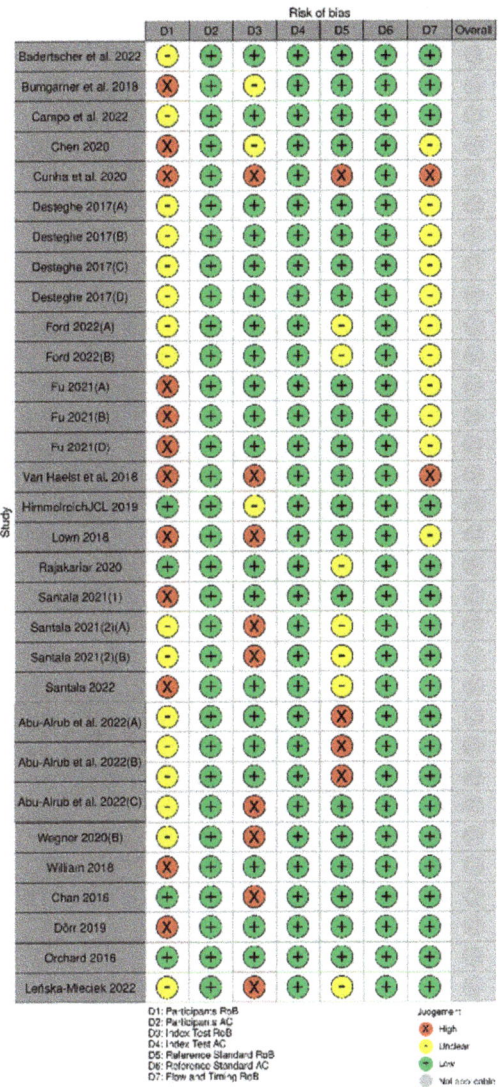

Figure 6. Assessment of risk of bias and applicability of the single-lead ECG studies. (Desteghe et al., 2017(A): testing the AliveCor in the cardiology ward population; Desteghe et al., 2017 (B): testing the MyDiagnostick in the cardiology ward population; Desteghe et al., 2017 (C): testing the AliveCor in the geriatric ward population; Desteghe et al., 2017 (D): testing the MyDiagnostick in the geriatric ward population; Ford et al., 2022 (A): testing the Apple Watch 4; Ford et al., 2022 (B): testing the KardiaBand; Fu et al., 2021 (A): testing the device in supine position, Fu et al., 2021 (B): testing the device in upright position, Fu et al., 2021 (C): testing the device after individuals climbed to the 3rd floor; Santala et al., 2021 (1): published in October 2021, Santala et al., 2021 (2) (A): published in May 2021 and testing the device between the palms, Santala et al., 2021, (2) (B): published in May 2021 and testing the device in the chest; Abu-Alrub et al., 2022(A): testing the Apple Watch 5, Abu-Alrub et al., 2022 (B): testing the Samsung Galaxy Watch Active 3, Abu-Alrub et al., 2022 (C): testing the Withings Move ECG; Wegner et al., 2020 (A): testing the lead I; Wegner et al., 2020 (B): testing the novel parasternal lead).

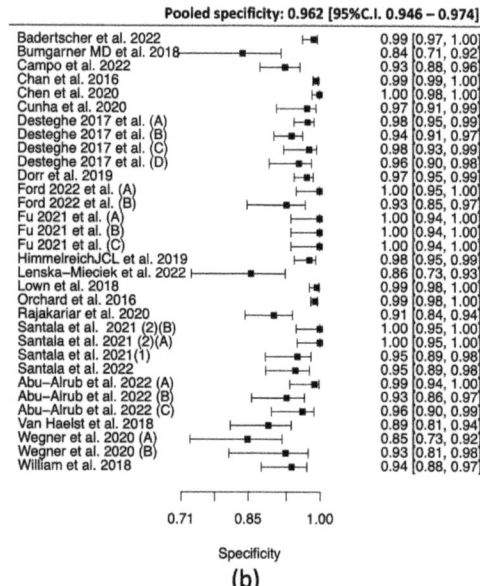

Figure 7. Single-lead ECG group: (**a**) forest plot of sensitivity, (**b**) forest plot of specificity. (Desteghe et al., 2017 (A): testing the AliveCor in the cardiology ward population; Desteghe et al., 2017 (B): testing the MyDiagnostick in the cardiology ward population; Desteghe et al., 2017 (C): testing the AliveCor in the geriatric ward population; Desteghe et al., 2017 (D): testing the MyDiagnostick in the geriatric ward population; Ford et al., 2022 (A): testing the Apple Watch 4, Ford et al., 2022 (B): testing the KardiaBand; Fu et al., 2021 (A): testing the device in supine position, Fu et al., 2021 (B): testing the device in upright position, Fu et al., 2021 (C): testing the device after individuals climbed to the 3rd floor; Santala et al., 2021 (1): published in October 2021, Santala et al., 2021 (2) (A): published in May 2021 and testing the device between the palms, Santala et al., 2021 (2) (B): published in May 2021 and testing the device in the chest; Abu-Alrub et al., 2022 (A): testing the Apple Watch 5, Abu-Alrub et al., 2022 (B): testing the Samsung Galaxy Watch Active 3, Abu-Alrub et al., 2022 (C): testing the Withings Move ECG, Wegner et al., 2020 (A): testing the lead I, Wegner et al., 2020 (B): testing the novel parasternal lead).

For the inpatients, the total sensitivity was 92.9% (95% C.I. 87.6–96) and the specificity was 94.2% (95% C.I. 91.8–95.9). The AUC was 0.974 and the partial AUC was 0.898. The I^2 was 14.4%. For the outpatients, the total sensitivity was 90.7% (95% C.I. 76.8–96.6) and the specificity was 98.1% (95% C.I. 95.1–99.3). The AUC was 0.983 and the partial AUC was 0.949. The I^2 was 26.9%. Although the sensitivity was higher in the inpatient group, the specificity was higher in the outpatients. However, the 95% confidence intervals were overlapping. In addition, there was a difference in I^2 between the subgroups. In the inpatient group, the I^2 was 14.4%, and in the outpatient group it was 26.9% (Figure 9).

3.3.5. Subgroup Analysis (Duration of Index Test) of the Single-Lead ECG Studies

We did not proceed to a formal subgroup analysis regarding the duration of the index test since most of the studies used it for 30 s (Figure 10).

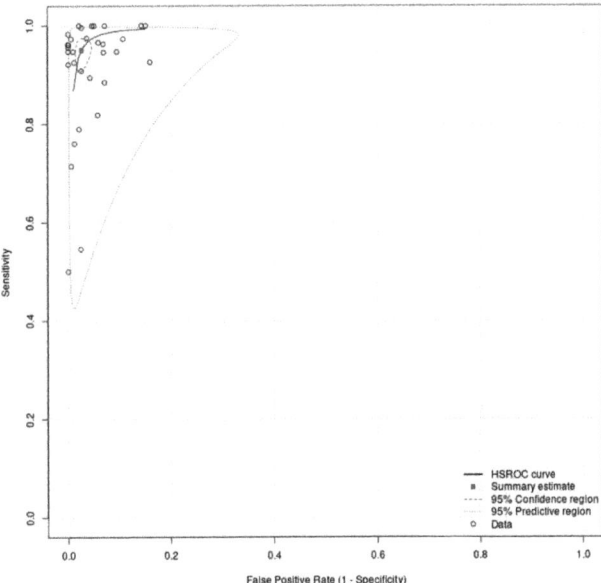

Figure 8. Single-lead ECG group: random effects meta-analysis.

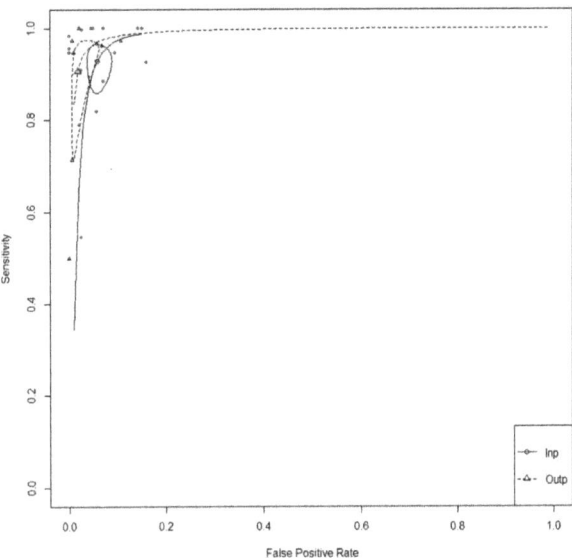

Figure 9. Single-lead ECG group: subgroup analysis (inpatients vs. outpatients).

3.3.6. Unclassified/Unreadable Results of the Single-Lead ECG Studies

Regarding the unclassified/unreadable results, we also identified significant heterogeneity in the single-lead ECG group. The reported unclassified/unreadable results ranged from 0% the minimum [32,41,46,52,57] to 38% the maximum (Table 1) [54].

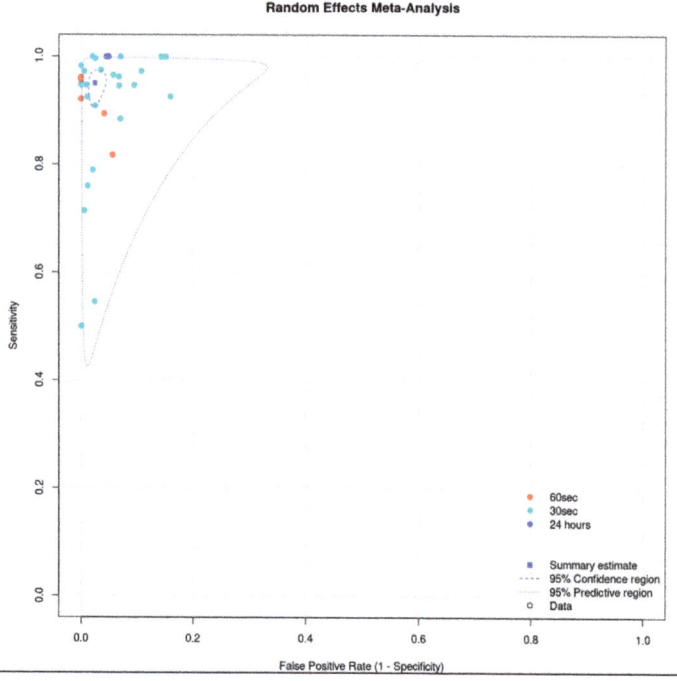

Figure 10. Single-lead ECG group: subgroup analysis (duration of index test).

3.4. Diagnostic Performance of Technologies Other Than PPG or Single-Lead ECG

As mentioned earlier, some of the studies tested technologies other than PPG and single-lead ECG. Due to there only being a few studies, we did not proceed to quantitative synthesis, but we have described them separately. Their characteristics are summarized in Table 1 and Figure 11.

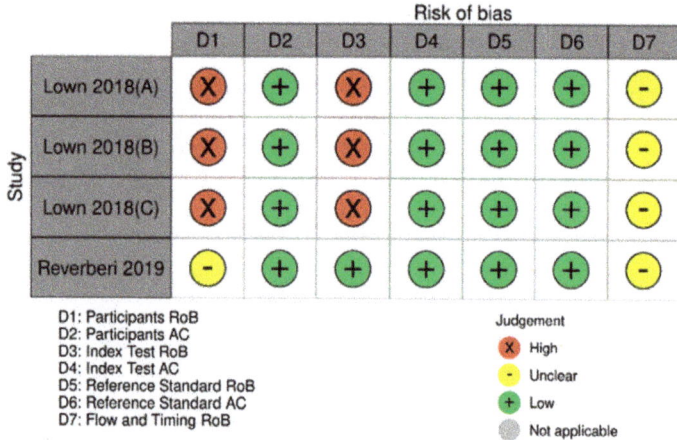

Figure 11. Miscellaneous technologies—assessment of risk of bias and applicability. (Lown et al., 2018 (A): testing the Watch BP, Lown et al., 2018 (B): testing the Polar H7 device, Lown et al., 2018 (C): testing the Bodyguard 2 device; D: domain; RoB: risk of bias; AC: applicability).

The study of Lown et al., 2018 [49], apart from single-lead ECG, tested three more devices in the same population. It tested the Watch BP device, which is a modified sphygmomanometer, and compared it with a 12-lead ECG. The resulting sensitivity was 96.34% (95% C.I. 89.68–99.24%) and the specificity was 93.45% (95% C.I. 90.25–95.85%). The same study tested two more devices that can detect AF by using heart rate variability. The Polar H7 device had a sensitivity of 96.34% (95% C.I. 89.68–99.24%) and specificity of 98.21% (95% C.I. 96.17–99.34%), and the Bodyguard 2 had a sensitivity of 96.34% (95% C.I. 89.68–99.24%) and a specificity of 98.51% (95% C.I. 96.56–99.52%).

The study of Reverberi et al., 2019 [58] is a diagnostic case–control study, which tested a chest-strap heart rate monitor in combination with the mobile application, RITMIA™, for the diagnosis of atrial fibrillation. The resulted sensitivity was 97.0% (95% C.I. 91.4–99.4%) and the specificity was 95.2% (95% C.I. 89.1–98.8%).

Finally, the study of Chen et al., 2020 [40], which was described in both the PPG and single-lead ECG groups, also tested the combination of both technologies. Specifically, during this test, the PPG mode was on, and if AF was detected, then participants were notified to perform a single-lead ECG. If the single-lead ECG was also positive for AF, then the result was considered positive. Otherwise, the final result was considered negative. The sensitivity for this mode was 80% (95% C.I. 72.52–85.90) and the specificity was 96.81% (95% C.I. 93.58–98.51).

4. Discussion

In this metanalysis, the two main technologies used to automatically detect AF (PPG and single-lead ECG) demonstrated very high diagnostic accuracy. Although the PPG technology proved to be more sensitive than the single-lead ECG, their 95% confidence intervals were overlapping. On the other hand, the two technologies had equal specificity.

In the PPG group, we noticed that four studies [31,33,36,42] showed significantly lower specificity compared to the rest (Figure 3). A further review of the studies demonstrated that, in most cases, the duration of the index test was prolonged, which may increase the false positive results. On contrary, the prolonged period of the index test can decrease the unclassified/unreadable results, since most of the studies with 0% unclassified/unreadable results used the devices for a longer period of time, and specifically from 10 min [35] to 1 week [41]. In the subgroup analysis between inpatients and outpatients in the PPG group, we did not observe any differences in the SROC curve; however, the small number of studies did not allow us to proceed to a quantitative synthesis.

In the single-lead ECG group, the lower pooled sensitivity could be partially explained by the lower duration of the index test. In most of the studies, it was applied for 30 to 60 s, compared to the PPG which was applied for at least 1 min. In addition, operation of a single-lead ECG requires action by the individual, and therefore unsupervised recordings could result in more poor-quality tracings. In this group, we performed two subgroup analyses. In the inpatients versus outpatients subgroup, the 95% confidence intervals were overlapping, and in the duration of the index test analysis (30 s vs. 60 s), we did not observe any clusters in the SROC curve. In relation to the unclassified/unreadable results, we observed significant heterogeneity in this group as well. Similarly with the PPG group, we noticed that most of the single-lead ECG studies with 0% unclassified/unreadable results used the index test for a prolonged period of time and/or allowed multiple measurements.

In both of the above groups, risk of bias was high or unknown in the participants selection domain, mainly due to case–control design in combination with ambiguity of the selection process. The rest of the domains were deemed mostly low risk of bias, and the applicability of the diagnostic test was satisfactory.

Other technologies, such as the modified sphygmomanometer and the heart rate variability, demonstrated very high sensitivity and specificity in their respective studies; however, the data were not enough to conduct a metanalysis. The study of Chen et al., 2020 [40] is especially interesting, because it tested the combination of PPG and single-lead ECG. During this study, individuals were being tested by continuous PPG, and they were asked to perform a single-lead ECG only when the PPG outcome was "possible AF". Only if the single-lead ECG confirmed the diagnosis, then the individual was notified that they may suffer from AF. This study showed very high specificity but not as high sensitivity (~80%). Since more and more devices offer the possibility of both PPG and single-lead ECG, its combination can be proved valuable. All the technologies resulted in unclassified/unreadable results, which demonstrated significant heterogeneity among the studies.

Our findings are comparable with previous similar metanalyses [5–7,59] and suggest that widely available AI-based devices can accurately detect AF and can be used as a screening tool. So far, screening for AF is a controversial area. ESC guidelines support screening in targeted populations [3]; however, the American guidelines advise that the evidence is limited [60]. Long-term continuous screening in high-risk populations proved effective in detection of AF in a randomized study [61]. Another randomized trial showed that screening for AF led to fewer events for the combined primary outcome which included stroke, systemic embolism, bleeding leading to hospitalization and all-cause death [62]. Simulation studies using contemporary screening methods in elderly populations showed that screening is cost-effective, reduces stroke episodes, but increases bleeding risk and events [63,64].

In this context, our findings suggest that easily accessible AI-based devices can be convenient and non-invasive tools for AF screening. Compared to the traditional methods, these devices allow long-term passive monitoring, which is a paramount advantage given the paroxysmal and often asymptomatic nature of AF. Also, it provides individuals with the opportunity to record a trace at any time which can be useful when, for example, they develop symptoms. Most importantly, the AI-based devices do not require a health care professional at the stage of rhythm diagnosis; therefore, the devices allow more time for physicians to focus on the rest of the management.

5. Strengths and Limitations

Our study was designed and conducted according to the PRISMA guidelines. The review was very extended, since it identified almost 15,000 studies, and more than 1000 studies were reviewed based on their full text. The screening was conducted by two blinded and independent investigators, and the statistical analysis was performed for the two main technologies separately. Furthermore, we proceeded to subgroup analysis and described technologies other than the main two. We also calculated the false results for different prevalence values, which eventually is directly applicable to daily clinical practice.

On the other hand, our study demonstrates certain weaknesses. First of all, part of our study's drawbacks arises from the limitations of the included studies. To start with the unclassified/unreadable results, there was significant heterogeneity among the studies. Many authors excluded them completely, some included them as false, and others included them as true or false depending on the reference standard. In our study, these results were excluded from the calculation of sensitivity and specificity and were described separately. Also, in many studies, atrial flutter and fibrillation were considered as the same disease, with the argument that their complications and treatment are very similar. However, others either excluded patients with atrial flutter completely or included them in the control group. Lastly, there was heterogeneity in the control groups, since some studies used only patients in sinus rhythm as control, and others used patients with any rhythm other than AF. Another issue was the use of multiple different devices and AI algorithms. On several occasions, the name or the version of the device and/or the AI algorithm were not even reported. Many authors tested the same devices with different algorithms, or they tested an amended version of the commercial algorithm. This heterogeneity constitutes a burden in the validation of devices and algorithms since it is difficult to appreciate the impact of their variability.

In addition, the executive part of our study appears to have certain limitations. First of all, the data extraction was performed mainly by one researcher, due to limited time and resources. Also, we had to amend our protocol, especially regarding the choice of reference standard test. Apart from the 12-lead ECG, we included other reference standard tests, since more tests are now accepted as gold standards for the diagnosis of atrial fibrillation. Furthermore, due to the complexity of diagnostic metanalysis, we could not proceed to more advanced statistical analyses, such as further subgroup and network metanalysis. Similarly, we did not calculate the reporting bias due to the complexity of metanalysis of diagnostic accuracy studies.

6. Conclusions

In summary, our findings support that both PPG and single-lead ECG devices have excellent sensitivity and specificity for the automated diagnosis of atrial fibrillation and can be used as screening tools. A prolonged period of monitoring may result in more false positive results, but less unclassified/unreadable outcomes. Further validation studies need to be conducted for alternative technologies, such as modified sphygmomanometry and combination of PPG and single-lead ECG. Further clinical trials are necessary to evaluate the cost-effectiveness, and risks and benefits, especially in younger populations where AI-based devices are widely available.

Funding: This research received no external funding.

Data Availability Statement: Data are contained within the article.

Conflicts of Interest: The authors declare no conflict of interest.

References

1. Freedman, B.; Potpara, T.S.; Lip, G.Y.H. Stroke prevention in atrial fibrillation. *Lancet* **2016**, *388*, 806–817. [CrossRef] [PubMed]
2. Mairesse, G.H.; Moran, P.; Van Gelder, I.C.; Elsner, C.; Rosenqvist, M.; Mant, J.; Banerjee, A.; Gorenek, B.; Brachmann, J.; Varma, N.; et al. Screening for atrial fibrillation: A European Heart Rhythm Association (EHRA) consensus document endorsed by the Heart Rhythm Society (HRS), Asia Pacific Heart Rhythm Society (APHRS), and Sociedad Latinoamericana de Estimulación Cardíaca y Electrofisiología (SOLAECE). *EP Eur.* **2017**, *19*, 1589–1623. [CrossRef]
3. Hindricks, G.; Potpara, T.; Dagres, N.; Arbelo, E.; Bax, J.J.; Blomström-Lundqvist, C.; Boriani, G.; Castella, M.; Dan, G.-A.; Dilaveris, P.E.; et al. 2020 ESC Guidelines for the diagnosis and management of atrial fibrillation developed in collaboration with the European Association for Cardio-Thoracic Surgery (EACTS): The Task Force for the diagnosis and management of atrial fibrillation of the European Society of Cardiology (ESC) Developed with the special contribution of the European Heart Rhythm Association (EHRA) of the ESC. *Eur. Heart J.* **2021**, *42*, 373–498. [CrossRef]
4. Li, K.H.C.; White, F.A.; Tipoe, T.; Liu, T.; Wong, M.C.; Jesuthasan, A.; Baranchuk, A.; Tse, G.; Yan, B.P. The Current State of Mobile Phone Apps for Monitoring Heart Rate, Heart Rate Variability, and Atrial Fibrillation: Narrative Review. *JMIR Mhealth Uhealth* **2019**, *7*, e11606. [CrossRef] [PubMed]
5. Taggar, J.S.; Coleman, T.; Lewis, S.; Heneghan, C.; Jones, M. Accuracy of methods for detecting an irregular pulse and suspected atrial fibrillation: A systematic review and meta-analysis. *Eur. J. Prev. Cardiol.* **2015**, *23*, 1330–1338. [CrossRef]
6. Yang, T.Y.; Huang, L.; Malwade, S.; Hsu, C.-Y.; Chen, Y.C. Diagnostic Accuracy of Ambulatory Devices in Detecting Atrial Fibrillation: Systematic Review and Meta-analysis. *JMIR Mhealth Uhealth* **2021**, *9*, e26167. [CrossRef]
7. Nazarian, S.; Lam, K.; Darzi, A.; Ashrafian, H. Diagnostic Accuracy of Smartwatches for the Detection of Cardiac Arrhythmia: Systematic Review and Meta-analysis. *J. Med. Internet Res.* **2021**, *23*, e28974. [CrossRef]
8. Kavsaoğlu, A.R.; Polat, K.; Hariharan, M. Non-invasive prediction of hemoglobin level using machine learning techniques with the PPG signal's characteristics features. *Appl. Soft Comput.* **2015**, *37*, 983–991. [CrossRef]
9. Pereira, T.; Tran, N.; Gadhoumi, K.; Pelter, M.M.; Do, D.H.; Lee, R.J.; Colorado, R.; Meisel, K.; Hu, X. Photoplethysmography based atrial fibrillation detection: A review. *NPJ Digit. Med.* **2020**, *3*, 3. [CrossRef]
10. Ford, C.; Xie, C.X.; Low, A.; Rajakariar, K.; Koshy, A.N.; Sajeev, J.K.; Roberts, L.; Pathik, B.; Teh, A.W. Comparison of 2 Smart Watch Algorithms for Detection of Atrial Fibrillation and the Benefit of Clinician Interpretation. *JACC Clin. Electrophysiol.* **2022**, *8*, 782–791. [CrossRef]
11. Van Haelst, R. The diagnostic accuracy of smartphone applications to detect atrial fibrillation: A head-to-head comparison between Fibricheck and AliveCor. Master Thesis, KU Leuven University, Leuven, Belgium, 2016. Available online: https://www.icho-info.be/application/content/downloadthesis/id/1320 (accessed on 10 July 2023).
12. Benezet-Mazuecos, J.; García-Talavera, C.S.; Rubio, J.M. Smart devices for a smart detection of atrial fibrillation. *J. Thorac. Dis.* **2018**, *10* (Suppl. S33), S3824–S3827. [CrossRef] [PubMed]
13. Welcome to the Preferred Reporting Items for Systematic Reviews and Meta-Analyses (PRISMA) Website! Available online: http://www.prisma-statement.org/ (accessed on 28 September 2023).

14. Available online: https://www.crd.york.ac.uk/prospero/display_record.php?RecordID=357232 (accessed on 28 September 2023).
15. Available online: https://www.cochrane.org/news/cochrane-recommends-covidence-new-reviews (accessed on 28 September 2023).
16. PWhiting, P.F.; Rutjes, A.W.S.; Westwood, M.E.; Mallett, S.; Deeks, J.J.; Reitsma, J.B.; Leeflang, M.M.G.; Sterne, J.A.C.; Bossuyt, P.M.M. QUADAS-2: A Revised Tool for the Quality Assessment of Diagnostic Accuracy Studies. *Ann. Intern. Med.* **2011**, *155*, 529–536. [CrossRef] [PubMed]
17. Available online: https://onlinelibrary.wiley.com/doi/full/10.1002/jrsm.1439 (accessed on 28 September 2023).
18. Zhou, Y.; Dendukuri, N. Statistics for quantifying heterogeneity in univariate and bivariate meta-analyses of binary data: The case of meta-analyses of diagnostic accuracy. *Stat. Med.* **2014**, *33*, 2701–2717. [CrossRef]
19. Shen, Q.; Li, J.; Cui, C.; Wang, X.; Gao, H.; Liu, C.; Chen, M. A wearable real-time telemonitoring electrocardiogram device compared with traditional Holter monitoring. *J. Biomed. Res.* **2021**, *35*, 238–246. [CrossRef]
20. Selder, J.L.; Breukel, L.; Blok, S.; van Rossum, A.C.; Tulevski, I.I.; Allaart, C.P. A mobile one-lead ECG device incorporated in a symptom-driven remote arrhythmia monitoring program. The first 5982 Hartwacht ECGs. *Neth. Heart J.* **2019**, *27*, 38–45. [CrossRef]
21. Koh, K.T.; Law, W.C.; Zaw, W.M.; Foo, D.H.P.; Tan, C.T.; Steven, A.; Samuel, D.; Fam, T.L.; Chai, C.H.; Wong, Z.S.; et al. Smartphone electrocardiogram for detecting atrial fibrillation after a cerebral ischaemic event: A multicentre randomized controlled trial. *EP Eur.* **2021**, *23*, 1016–1023. [CrossRef] [PubMed]
22. Hiraoka, D.; Inui, T.; Kawakami, E.; Oya, M.; Tsuji, A.; Honma, K.; Kawasaki, Y.; Ozawa, Y.; Shiko, Y.; Ueda, H.; et al. Diagnosis of Atrial Fibrillation Using Machine Learning with Wearable Devices after Cardiac Surgery: Algorithm Development Study. *JMIR Form. Res.* **2022**, *6*, e35396. [CrossRef] [PubMed]
23. Avram, R.; Ramsis, M.; Cristal, A.D.; Nathan, V.; Zhu, L.; Kim, J.; Kuang, J.; Gao, A.; Vittinghoff, E.; Rohdin-Bibby, L.; et al. Validation of an algorithm for continuous monitoring of atrial fibrillation using a consumer smartwatch. *Heart Rhythm.* **2021**, *18*, 1482–1490. [CrossRef]
24. Scholten, J.; Jansen, W.P.; Horsthuis, T.; Mahes, A.D.; Winter, M.M.; Zwinderman, A.H.; Keijer, J.T.; Minneboo, M.; de Groot, J.R.; Bokma, J.P. Six-lead device superior to single-lead smartwatch ECG in atrial fibrillation detection. *Am. Heart J.* **2022**, *253*, 53–58. [CrossRef]
25. Brasier, N.; Raichle, C.J.; Dörr, M.; Becke, A.; Nohturfft, V.; Weber, S.; Bulacher, F.; Salomon, L.; Noah, T.; Birkemeyer, R.; et al. Detection of atrial fibrillation with a smartphone camera: First prospective, international, two-centre, clinical validation study (DETECT AF PRO). *EP Eur.* **2019**, *21*, 41–47. [CrossRef]
26. Palà, E.; Bustamante, A.; Clúa-Espuny, J.L.; Acosta, J.; González-Loyola, F.; Dos Santos, S.; Ribas-Segui, D.; Ballesta-Ors, J.; Penalba, A.; Giralt, M.; et al. Blood-biomarkers and devices for atrial fibrillation screening: Lessons learned from the AFRICAT (Atrial Fibrillation Research In CATalonia) study. *PLoS ONE* **2022**, *17*, e0273571. [CrossRef] [PubMed]
27. Rischard, J.; Waldmann, V.; Moulin, T.; Sharifzadehgan, A.; Lee, R.; Narayanan, K.; Garcia, R.; Marijon, E. Assessment of Heart Rhythm Disorders Using the AliveCor Heart Monitor: Beyond the Detection of Atrial Fibrillation. *JACC Clin. Electrophysiol.* **2020**, *6*, 1313–1315. [CrossRef] [PubMed]
28. Mannhart, D.; Lischer, M.; Knecht, S.; Lavallaz, J.d.F.d.; Strebel, I.; Serban, T.; Vögeli, D.; Schaer, B.; Osswald, S.; Mueller, C.; et al. Clinical Validation of 5 Direct-to-Consumer Wearable Smart Devices to Detect Atrial Fibrillation: BASEL Wearable Study. *JACC Clin. Electrophysiol.* **2023**, *9*, 232–242. [CrossRef] [PubMed]
29. Lau, J.K.; Lowres, N.; Neubeck, L.; Brieger, D.B.; Sy, R.W.; Galloway, C.D.; Albert, D.E.; Freedman, S.B. iPhone ECG application for community screening to detect silent atrial fibrillation: A novel technology to prevent stroke. *Int. J. Cardiol.* **2013**, *165*, 193–194. [CrossRef] [PubMed]
30. Tison, G.H.; Sanchez, J.M.; Ballinger, B.; Singh, A.; Olgin, J.E.; Pletcher, M.J.; Vittinghoff, E.; Lee, E.S.; Fan, S.M.; Gladstone, R.A.; et al. Passive Detection of Atrial Fibrillation Using a Commercially Available Smartwatch. *JAMA Cardiol.* **2018**, *3*, 409–416. [CrossRef]
31. Lubitz, S.A.; Faranesh, A.Z.; Selvaggi, C.; Atlas, S.J.; McManus, D.D.; Singer, D.E.; Pagoto, S.; McConnell, M.V.; Pantelopoulos, A.; Foulkes, A.S. Detection of Atrial Fibrillation in a Large Population Using Wearable Devices: The Fitbit Heart Study. *Circulation* **2022**, *146*, 1415–1424. [CrossRef]
32. Chan, P.; Wong, C.; Poh, Y.C.; Pun, L.; Leung, W.W.; Wong, Y.; Wong, M.M.; Poh, M.; Chu, D.W.; Siu, C.; et al. Diagnostic Performance of a Smartphone-Based Photoplethysmographic Application for Atrial Fibrillation Screening in a Primary Care Setting. *J. Am. Heart Assoc.* **2016**, *5*, e003428. [CrossRef]
33. Chang, P.-C.; Wen, M.-S.; Chou, C.-C.; Wang, C.-C.; Hung, K.-C. Atrial fibrillation detection using ambulatory smartwatch photoplethysmography and validation with simultaneous holter recording. *Am. Heart J.* **2022**, *247*, 55–62. [CrossRef]
34. Sun, Y.; Yang, Y.-Y.; Wu, B.-J.; Huang, P.-W.; Cheng, S.-E.; Chen, C.-C. Contactless facial video recording with deep learning models for the detection of atrial fibrillation. *Sci. Rep.* **2022**, *12*, 281. [CrossRef]
35. Mol, D.; Riezebos, R.K.; Marquering, H.A.; Werner, M.E.; Lobban, T.C.; de Jong, J.S.; de Groot, J.R. Performance of an automated photoplethysmography-based artificial intelligence algorithm to detect atrial fibrillation. *Cardiovasc. Digit. Health J.* **2020**, *1*, 107–110. [CrossRef]
36. Väliaho, E.-S.; Kuoppa, P.; A Lipponen, J.; Martikainen, T.J.; Jäntti, H.; Rissanen, T.T.; Kolk, I.; Castrén, M.; Halonen, J.; Tarvainen, M.P.; et al. Wrist band photoplethysmography in detection of individual pulses in atrial fibrillation and algorithm-based detection of atrial fibrillation. *EP Eur.* **2019**, *21*, 1031–1038. [CrossRef] [PubMed]

37. Dörr, M.; Nohturfft, V.; Brasier, N.; Bosshard, E.; Djurdjevic, A.; Gross, S.; Raichle, C.J.; Rhinisperger, M.; Stöckli, R.; Eckstein, J. The WATCH AF Trial: SmartWATCHes for Detection of Atrial Fibrillation. *JACC Clin. Electrophysiol.* **2019**, *5*, 199–208. [CrossRef] [PubMed]
38. Väliaho, E.-S.; Lipponen, J.A.; Kuoppa, P.; Martikainen, T.J.; Jäntti, H.; Rissanen, T.T.; Castrén, M.; Halonen, J.; Tarvainen, M.P.; Laitinen, T.M.; et al. Continuous 24-h Photoplethysmogram Monitoring Enables Detection of Atrial Fibrillation. *Front. Physiol.* **2022**, *12*, 778775. [CrossRef] [PubMed]
39. Bacevicius, J.; Abramikas, Z.; Dvinelis, E.; Audzijoniene, D.; Petrylaite, M.; Marinskiene, J.; Staigyte, J.; Karuzas, A.; Juknevicius, V.; Jakaite, R.; et al. High Specificity Wearable Device with Photoplethysmography and Six-Lead Electrocardiography for Atrial Fibrillation Detection Challenged by Frequent Premature Contractions: DoubleCheck-AF. *Front. Cardiovasc. Med.* **2022**, *9*, 869730. [CrossRef] [PubMed]
40. Chen, E.; Jiang, J.; Su, R.; Gao, M.; Zhu, S.; Zhou, J.; Huo, Y. A new smart wristband equipped with an artificial intelligence algorithm to detect atrial fibrillation. *Heart Rhythm.* **2020**, *17*, 847–853. [CrossRef]
41. Santala, E.O.; Halonen, J.; Martikainen, S.; Jäntti, H.; Rissanen, T.T.; Tarvainen, M.P.; Laitinen, T.P.; Laitinen, T.M.; Väliaho, E.-S.; Hartikainen, J.E.K.; et al. Automatic Mobile Health Arrhythmia Monitoring for the Detection of Atrial Fibrillation: Prospective Feasibility, Accuracy, and User Experience Study. *JMIR Mhealth Uhealth* **2021**, *9*, e29933. [CrossRef]
42. Badertscher, P.; Lischer, M.; Mannhart, D.; Knecht, S.; Isenegger, C.; Lavallaz, J.D.F.d.; Schaer, B.; Osswald, S.; Kühne, M.; Sticherling, C. Clinical validation of a novel smartwatch for automated detection of atrial fibrillation. *Heart Rhythm. O2* **2022**, *3*, 208–210. [CrossRef]
43. Bumgarner, J.M.; Lambert, C.T.; Hussein, A.A.; Cantillon, D.J.; Baranowski, B.; Wolski, K.; Lindsay, B.D.; Wazni, O.M.; Tarakji, K.G. Smartwatch Algorithm for Automated Detection of Atrial Fibrillation. *J. Am. Coll. Cardiol.* **2018**, *71*, 2381–2388. [CrossRef]
44. Campo, D.; Elie, V.; de Gallard, T.; Bartet, P.; Morichau-Beauchant, T.; Genain, N.; Fayol, A.; Fouassier, D.; Pasteur-Rousseau, A.; Puymirat, E.; et al. Atrial Fibrillation Detection With an Analog Smartwatch: Prospective Clinical Study and Algorithm Validation. *JMIR Form. Res.* **2022**, *6*, e37280. [CrossRef]
45. Cunha, S.; Antunes, E.; Antoniou, S.; Tiago, S.; Relvas, R.; Fernandez-Llimós, F.; da Costa, F.A. Raising awareness and early detection of atrial fibrillation, an experience resorting to mobile technology centred on informed individuals. *Res. Soc. Adm. Pharm.* **2020**, *16*, 787–792. [CrossRef]
46. Desteghe, L.; Raymaekers, Z.; Lutin, M.; Vijgen, J.; Dilling-Boer, D.; Koopman, P.; Schurmans, J.; Vanduynhoven, P.; Dendale, P.; Heidbuchel, H. Performance of handheld electrocardiogram devices to detect atrial fibrillation in a cardiology and geriatric ward setting. *EP Eur.* **2017**, *19*, 29–39. [CrossRef]
47. Fu, W.; Li, R. Diagnostic performance of a wearing dynamic ECG recorder for atrial fibrillation screening: The HUAMI heart study. *BMC Cardiovasc. Disord.* **2021**, *21*, 558. [CrossRef] [PubMed]
48. Himmelreich, J.C.; Karregat, E.P.; Lucassen, W.A.; van Weert, H.C.; de Groot, J.R.; Handoko, M.L.; Nijveldt, R.; Harskamp, R. Diagnostic Accuracy of a Smartphone-Operated, Single-Lead Electrocardiography Device for Detection of Rhythm and Conduction Abnormalities in Primary Care. *Ann. Fam. Med.* **2019**, *17*, 403. [CrossRef] [PubMed]
49. Lown, M.; Yue, A.M.; Shah, B.N.; Corbett, S.J.; Lewith, G.; Stuart, B.; Garrard, J.; Brown, M.; Little, P.; Moore, M. Screening for Atrial Fibrillation Using Economical and Accurate Technology (From the SAFETY Study). *Am. J. Cardiol.* **2018**, *122*, 1339–1344. [CrossRef] [PubMed]
50. Rajakariar, K.; Koshy, A.N.; Sajeev, J.K.; Nair, S.; Roberts, L.; Teh, A.W. Accuracy of a smartwatch based single-lead electrocardiogram device in detection of atrial fibrillation. *Heart* **2020**, *106*, 665. [CrossRef]
51. Santala, O.E.; Lipponen, J.A.; Jäntti, H.; Rissanen, T.T.; Halonen, J.; Kolk, I.; Pohjantähti-Maaroos, H.; Tarvainen, M.P.; Väliaho, E.; Hartikainen, J.; et al. Necklace-embedded electrocardiogram for the detection and diagnosis of atrial fibrillation. *Clin. Cardiol.* **2021**, *44*, 620–626. [CrossRef]
52. Santala, O.E.; A Lipponen, J.; Jäntti, H.; Rissanen, T.T.; Tarvainen, M.P.; Laitinen, T.P.; Laitinen, T.M.; Castrén, M.; Väliaho, E.-S.; A Rantula, O.; et al. Continuous mHealth Patch Monitoring for the Algorithm-Based Detection of Atrial Fibrillation: Feasibility and Diagnostic Accuracy Study. *JMIR Cardio.* **2022**, *6*, e31230. [CrossRef]
53. Abu-Alrub, S.; Strik, M.; Ramirez, F.D.; Moussaoui, N.; Racine, H.P.; Marchand, H.; Buliard, S.; Haïssaguerre, M.; Ploux, S.; Bordachar, P. Smartwatch Electrocardiograms for Automated and Manual Diagnosis of Atrial Fibrillation: A Comparative Analysis of Three Models. *Front. Cardiovasc. Med.* **2022**, *9*, 836375. [CrossRef]
54. Wegner, F.K.; Kochhäuser, S.; Ellermann, C.; Lange, P.S.; Frommeyer, G.; Leitz, P.; Eckardt, L.; Dechering, D.G. Prospective blinded Evaluation of the smartphone-based AliveCor Kardia ECG monitor for Atrial Fibrillation detection: The PEAK-AF study. *Eur. J. Intern. Med.* **2020**, *73*, 72–75. [CrossRef]
55. William, A.D.; Kanbour, M.; Callahan, T.; Bhargava, M.; Varma, N.; Rickard, J.; Saliba, W.; Wolski, K.; Hussein, A.; Lindsay, B.D.; et al. Assessing the accuracy of an automated atrial fibrillation detection algorithm using smartphone technology: The iREAD Study. *Heart Rhythm.* **2018**, *15*, 1561–1565. [CrossRef]
56. Orchard, J.; Lowres, N.; Ben Freedman, S.; Ladak, L.; Lee, W.; Zwar, N.; Peiris, D.; Kamaladasa, Y.; Li, J.; Neubeck, L. Screening for atrial fibrillation during influenza vaccinations by primary care nurses using a smartphone electrocardiograph (iECG): A feasibility study. *Eur. J. Prev. Cardiol.* **2016**, *23* (Suppl. S2), 13–20. [CrossRef] [PubMed]

57. Leńska-Mieciek, M.; Kuls-Oszmaniec, A.; Dociak, N.; Kowalewski, M.; Sarwiński, K.; Osiecki, A.; Fiszer, U. Mobile Single-Lead Electrocardiogram Technology for Atrial Fibrillation Detection in Acute Ischemic Stroke Patients. *J. Clin. Med.* **2022**, *11*, 665. [CrossRef] [PubMed]
58. Reverberi, C.; Rabia, G.; De Rosa, F.; Bosi, D.; Botti, A.; Benatti, G. The RITMIA^{TM} Smartphone App for Automated Detection of Atrial Fibrillation: Accuracy in Consecutive Patients Undergoing Elective Electrical Cardioversion. *Biomed. Res. Int.* **2019**, *2019*, 4861951. [CrossRef] [PubMed]
59. Lead-I ECG Devices for Detecting Symptomatic Atrial Fibrillation Using Single Time Point Testing in Primary Care. 2019. Available online: www.nice.org.uk/guidance/dg35 (accessed on 28 September 2023).
60. Us Preventive Services Task Force; Davidson, K.W.; Barry, M.J.; Mangione, C.M.; Cabana, M.; Caughey, A.B.; Davis, E.M.; Donahue, K.E.; Doubeni, C.A.; Epling, J.W.; et al. Screening for Atrial Fibrillation: US Preventive Services Task Force Recommendation Statement. *JAMA* **2022**, *327*, 360–367. [CrossRef]
61. Sanna, T.; Diener, H.-C.; Passman, R.S.; Di Lazzaro, V.; Bernstein, R.A.; Morillo, C.A.; Rymer, M.M.; Thijs, V.; Rogers, T.; Beckers, F.; et al. Cryptogenic Stroke and Underlying Atrial Fibrillation. *N. Engl. J. Med.* **2014**, *370*, 2478–2486. [CrossRef]
62. Svennberg, E.; Friberg, L.; Frykman, V.; Al-Khalili, F.; Engdahl, J.; Rosenqvist, M. Clinical outcomes in systematic screening for atrial fibrillation (STROKESTOP): A multicentre, parallel group, unmasked, randomised controlled trial. *Lancet* **2021**, *398*, 1498–1506. [CrossRef]
63. Chen, W.; Khurshid, S.; Singer, D.E.; Atlas, S.J.; Ashburner, J.M.; Ellinor, P.T.; McManus, D.D.; Lubitz, S.A.; Chhatwal, J. Cost-effectiveness of Screening for Atrial Fibrillation Using Wearable Devices. *JAMA Health Forum* **2022**, *3*, e222419. [CrossRef]
64. Khurshid, S.; Chen, W.; Singer, D.E.; Atlas, S.J.; Ashburner, J.M.; Choi, J.G.; Hur, C.; Ellinor, P.T.; McManus, D.D.; Chhatwal, J.; et al. Comparative clinical effectiveness of population-based atrial fibrillation screening using contemporary modalities: A decision-analytic model. *J. Am. Heart Assoc.* **2021**, *10*, e020330. [CrossRef]

Disclaimer/Publisher's Note: The statements, opinions and data contained in all publications are solely those of the individual author(s) and contributor(s) and not of MDPI and/or the editor(s). MDPI and/or the editor(s) disclaim responsibility for any injury to people or property resulting from any ideas, methods, instructions or products referred to in the content.

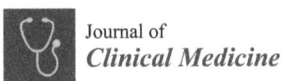

Systematic Review

Comparative Analysis of Morbidity and Mortality Outcomes in Elderly and Nonelderly Patients Undergoing Elective TEVAR: A Systematic Review and Meta-Analysis

Angelos Frisiras [1,†], Emmanuel Giannas [1,†], Stergios Bobotis [1], Ilektra Kanella [1], Arian Arjomandi Rad [2], Alessandro Viviano [3], Kyriakos Spiliopoulos [4], Dimitrios E. Magouliotis [5] and Thanos Athanasiou [6,*]

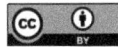

Citation: Frisiras, A.; Giannas, E.; Bobotis, S.; Kanella, I.; Arjomandi Rad, A.; Viviano, A.; Spiliopoulos, K.; Magouliotis, D.E.; Athanasiou, T. Comparative Analysis of Morbidity and Mortality Outcomes in Elderly and Nonelderly Patients Undergoing Elective TEVAR: A Systematic Review and Meta-Analysis. *J. Clin. Med.* **2023**, *12*, 5001. https://doi.org/10.3390/jcm12155001

Academic Editor: Teruhiko Imamura

Received: 11 June 2023
Revised: 14 July 2023
Accepted: 27 July 2023
Published: 29 July 2023

Copyright: © 2023 by the authors. Licensee MDPI, Basel, Switzerland. This article is an open access article distributed under the terms and conditions of the Creative Commons Attribution (CC BY) license (https:// creativecommons.org/licenses/by/ 4.0/).

[1] Faculty of Medicine, Imperial College London, Charing Cross Hospital, London W6 8RF, UK; angelos.frisiras18@imperial.ac.uk (A.F.); emmanouil.giannas18@imperial.ac.uk (E.G.); stergios.bobotis18@imperial.ac.uk (S.B.); ilektra.kanella18@imperial.ac.uk (I.K.)
[2] Medical Sciences Division, University of Oxford, Oxford OX1 3AZ, UK; arian.arjomandirad@gmail.com
[3] Department of Cardiothoracic Surgery, Imperial College NHS Trust, Hammersmith Hospital, London W12 0HS, UK; alessandro.viviano@nhs.net
[4] Department of Cardiothoracic Surgery, University of Thessaly, Biopolis, 41 110 Larissa, Greece; spiliopoulos@uth.gr
[5] Unit of Quality Improvement, Department of Cardiothoracic Surgery, University of Thessaly, Biopolis, 41 110 Larissa, Greece; dimitrios.magouliotis.18@alumni.ucl.ac.uk
[6] Department of Surgery and Cancer, Imperial College London, St Mary's Hospital, London W2 1NY, UK
* Correspondence: t.athanasiou@imperial.ac.uk
† These authors contributed equally to this work.

Abstract: Objective: Due to an ever-increasing ageing population and limited available data around the use of thoracic endovascular aortic repair (TEVAR) in elderly patients, investigating its efficacy and safety in this age cohort is of vital importance. We thus reviewed the existing literature on this topic to assess the feasibility of TEVAR in elderly patients with severe thoracic aortic pathologies. Methods: We identified all original research studies that assessed TEVAR in elderly patients published up to 2023. Morbidity, as assessed by neurological and respiratory complications, endoleaks, and length of stay, was the primary endpoint. Short-term mortality and long-term survival were the secondary endpoints. The Mantel–Haenszel random and fixed effects methods were used to calculate the odds ratios for each outcome. Further sensitivity and subgroup analyses were performed to validate the outcomes. Results: Twelve original studies that evaluated elective TEVAR outcomes in elderly patients were identified. Seven studies directly compared the use of TEVAR between an older and a younger patient group. Apart from a shorter hospital stay in older patients, no statistically significant difference between the morbidity outcomes of the two different cohorts was found. Short-term mortality and long-term survival results favoured the younger population. Conclusions: The present meta-analysis indicates that, due to a safe perioperative morbidity profile, TEVAR should not be contraindicated in patients based purely on old age. Further research using large patient registries to validate our findings in elderly patients with specific aortic pathologies and both elective and emergency procedures is necessary.

Keywords: TEVAR; thoracic aorta; endovascular repair; elderly; age; morbidity; mortality

1. Introduction

Thoracic endovascular aortic repair (TEVAR) has achieved rapid adoption as a treatment modality for thoracic aortic disease since its introduction in 1992. The minimally invasive nature of TEVAR and its short-term safety and efficacy have led to its expanding utilization as the primary treatment approach for various aortic pathologies, including penetrating atherosclerotic ulcers and aortic transections [1]. TEVAR has been associated with decreased in-hospital mortality rates, reduced intraoperative blood loss, and perioperative morbidity compared to open surgical repair [2]. The minimally invasive nature of TEVAR and its short-term safety and efficacy have led to its increasing implementation as the mainstay of treatment for thoracic aortic aneurysms (TAAs) and thoracic aortic dissections (TADs) [3].

While there is substantial evidence supporting the use of TEVAR in nonelderly patients with a low-risk factor profile, concerns have been raised about its suboptimal outcomes in certain populations, particularly the elderly. Multiple studies have shown increased postoperative morbidity, such as stroke and pulmonary complications [4–6], and poor mortality outcomes [5,7] in the elderly population when compared to younger counterparts. Furthermore, increasing age has been described as an independent risk factor for higher mortality among patients undergoing TEVAR [3]. This could be attributed to the increased comorbidities, frailty, and age-related physiological changes observed in the elderly population, posing unique challenges in the management of thoracic aortic disease. Consequently, the available data on the morbidity and mortality outcomes of TEVAR in the elderly are limited due to the small number of such patients who have undergone the procedure and received a systematic follow-up.

Thus, the question of whether TEVAR should be offered to this age group remains unanswered. This is particularly important as, due to an ever-increasing ageing population, it is projected that by 2050 more than 50% of aortic dissections will occur in patients over 75 years old [8,9]. In light of the changing demographic landscape, there is an increasing need for compelling evidence to determine the efficacy of TEVAR across different age groups and whether it should be offered to the elderly population.

In this context, we designed a systematic review and meta-analysis aiming to evaluate TEVAR morbidity and mortality outcomes in elderly patients. This was achieved by comparing the morbidity and mortality outcomes of TEVAR between elderly and nonelderly patients. The primary endpoint was perioperative morbidity defined as (1) endoleaks, (2) neurological complications, (3) respiratory complications, and (4) length of hospital stay (LoS), and secondary outcomes included in-hospital mortality and long-term survival following TEVAR.

2. Materials and Methods

2.1. Literature Search

This study was conducted in accordance with a protocol agreed upon by all authors and the Preferred Reporting Items for Systematic Reviews and Meta-Analysis (PRISMA) guidelines [8]. The Medline (PubMed) literature was systematically searched for studies reporting on outcomes in elderly patients undergoing TEVAR. The last day of the search was the 4 February 2023. The following MeSH terms were used in our search: "TEVAR", "octogenarians", "elderly", "age", "nonagenarians", "outcomes", "complications", and "mortality". Articles were also identified using the function "related studies" on the PubMed platform. Duplicate articles were removed. Included studies were (1) original reports with ≥ 10 patients, (2) written in the English language, (3) performed on human subjects, and (4) reported on elderly patients undergoing TEVAR. Abstracts, letters to the editor, and case reports were excluded. A kappa-coefficient analysis regarding the level of agreement for the inclusion of the selected studies was performed.

2.2. Data Extraction

Data extraction was performed independently by two reviewers (AF and SB) into a comprehensive Excel spreadsheet. In cases of discrepancy, studies were discussed in group meetings with the senior authors (DEM and TA) until a consensus was reached. The following information was extracted from each study: first author, year of publication, study-population characteristics, study design, baseline patient characteristics, number of patients operated using TEVAR, the age limit for defining the elderly population, and postoperative outcomes.

2.3. Patient Characteristics

This study attempted to compare the outcomes of elective TEVAR in elderly and nonelderly patients. Studies which reported on outcomes of urgent TEVAR only and on debranching TEVAR were excluded. The majority of the studies included, however, did not distinguish or conduct subgroup analysis between elective and emergency TEVAR. The elderly patients were defined as the experimental group and nonelderly patients as the control group. From the included studies, eight studies used 80 years of age for defining elderly [4,9–15], three studies used 75 years of age [1,16,17], and one subgrouped patients in >75 and >80 age groups [5]. Studies that used cutoff points below the age of 75 were excluded from the analysis.

The baseline preoperative patient characteristics of the included studies are presented in Table 1. All patients included in this study suffered from a thoracic aortic pathology which was treated using the TEVAR procedure. More specifically, these included thoracic aortic aneurysms (TAA), aortic dissections, other [penetrating aortic ulcer (PAU), traumatic aortic injury (TAI), or intramural haematoma (IMH)]. The detailed aortic pathology of patients in each study is presented in Table 2.

Seven studies directly compared TEVAR outcomes between elderly and nonelderly patients [1,4,5,10,12,14,17], with three studies comparing emergency and elective TEVAR procedures [5,9,11]. In addition, six studies conducted KM analysis investigating the overall survival (OS) in elderly patients undergoing TEVAR [1,4,5,13,15,16]. A minimum of three studies per outcome were needed for data synthesis and analysis. In cases where less than three studies reported on a complication, such as renal complications, a comparison was not possible.

2.4. Endpoints of Interest

2.4.1. Primary Endpoint

The primary endpoint of this study was to assess and compare the perioperative morbidity of TEVAR between elderly and nonelderly patients. As mortality trends often favour younger populations, the decision to select morbidity outcomes as the primary endpoint was made. Morbidity was defined based on the following outcomes: (1) neurological complications (2), endoleaks, (3) respiratory complications, and (4) length of hospital stay. Due to the heterogeneity of definitions of neurological complications provided by the papers examined, the umbrella term 'neurological complications' was tilized, which involved cerebrovascular accidents (CVAs) and paralysis/paraplegia. Studies that reported separately on the aforementioned outcomes were combined and reported under 'neurological complications'.

2.4.2. Secondary Endpoint

The secondary endpoint of this study was mortality, defined as a (1) short-term mortality, specifically either 30-day or in-hospital mortality, and (2) overall survival following TEVAR procedures. Both 30-day mortality/in-hospital mortality and overall survival were compared in elderly and nonelderly patients.

Table 1. Baseline preoperative patient characteristics. Age presented as mean (±SD) or median (IQR). E: elderly, NE: nonelderly, HTN: hypertension, CVD: cerebrovascular disease, DM: diabetes mellitus, CKD: chronic kidney disease, COPD: chronic obstructive pulmonary disease, CAD: coronary artery disease, ND: nondocumented. References: [3,6,7,9–17].

	n		Age, yrs		Preoperative Baseline Patient Characteristics													
					Male (%)		HTN (%)		CVD (%)		DM (%)		CKD (%)		Smoking (%)		COPD (%)		CAD (%)	
	E	NE	E	NE	E	NE	E	NE	E	NE	E	NE	E	NE	E	NE	E	NE	E	NE
Alnahhal 2022 [16]	676	3432	83 (80–86)	64 (54–72)	333 (49)	2132 (62)	597 (88)	2707 (79)	77 (11)	315 (9)	109 (16)	531 (15)	137 (20)	600 (17)	292 (43)	137 (20)	163 (24)	708 (21)	300 (44)	901 (26)
Dakour-Aridi 2021 [6]	390	1652	83 (81–86)	68 (60–74)	251 (51)	984 (60)	360 (92)	1,475 (89)	42 (11)	204 (12)	63 (16)	262 (16)	186 (49)	549 (35)	231 (59)	720 (44)	123 (32)	500 (30)	74 (19)	312 (19)
Akhmerov 2021 [17]	25	ND	84.8 ± 3.7	ND	16 (64)	ND	24 (96)	ND	ND	ND	4 (16)	ND	ND	ND	18 (72)	ND	2 (8)	ND	ND	ND
Yamauchi 2019 [15]	57	ND	84.1 ± 3.4	ND	29 (51)	ND	46 (81)	ND	3 (5)	ND	8 (14)	ND	3 (5)	ND	ND	ND	8 (14)	ND	12 (21)	ND
Buckenham 2015 [14]	19	245	84.0 ± 3.1	59 ± 17.2	11 (58)	164 (67)	13 (68)	151 (62)	3 (16)	17 (7)	1 (5)	20 (8)	0 (0)	24 (10)	7 (37)	140 (57)	ND	ND	ND	ND
Preventza 2010 [13]	101	ND	83.6 ± 3.1	ND	61 (60)	ND	85 (84)	ND	2 (2)	ND	23 (23)	ND	24 (24)	ND	76 (75)	ND	33 (33)	ND	12 (12)	ND
Kpodonou 2008 [12]	44	205	84.0 ± 2.7	66.0 ± 11.0	27 (61)	120 (59)	34 (77)	155 (76)	1 (2)	12 (6)	ND	ND	15 (34)	45 (21)	38 (86)	150 (73)	4 (9)	40 (20)	4 (9)	17 (8)
De Rango 2016 [7]	57	84	67.3 ± 16.7		30 (53)	71 (85)	43 (75)	52 (62)	1 (2)	6 (7)	4 (7)	7 (8)	10 (18)	10 (12)	ND	ND	21 (37)	28 (33)	ND	ND
Kern 2006 [18]	18	24	78.6	62 ± 2.8	67	21	15 (83)	14 (58)	5 (28)	3 (13)	ND	ND	2 (11)	3 (13)	ND	ND	6 (33)	8 (33)	6 (33)	8 (33)
Czerny 2010 [3]	56	170	67	ND	39 (70)	53 (72)	ND	ND	ND	ND	3 (5)	13 (8)	ND	ND	ND	ND	26 (46)	51 (30)	15 (27)	39 (23)
Patel 2008 [19]	52	ND	80.6 ± 4.0	ND	26 (50)	ND	41 (79)	ND	6 (15)	ND	7 (14)	ND	ND	ND	33 (64)	ND	21 (40)	ND	29 (56)	ND
Karimi 2016 [11]	41	ND	83.0 ± 3.0	ND	24 (59)	ND	39 (95)	ND	6 (15)	ND	7 (18)	ND	11 (27)	ND	31 (76)	ND	13 (32)	ND	8 (20)	ND

Table 2. Baseline preoperative aortic pathology. E: elderly, NE: nonelderly, TAA: thoracic aortic aneurysm, AD: aortic dissection, Other: penetrating aortic ulcer (PAU), traumatic aortic injury (TAI), intramural haematoma (IMH). References: [1,4,5,9–17].

	E			NE			Total		
Study	TAA	AD	Other	TAA	AD	Other	TAA	AD	Other
Alnahhal 2022 [16]	415	169	92	1328	1244	860	1743	1413	952
Dakour-Aridi 2021 [6]	336	54	0	1063	589	0	1399	643	0
Akhmerov 2021 [17]	15	7	3	N/A	N/A	N/A	15	7	3
Yamauchi 2019 [15]	50	6	1	N/A	N/A	N/A	50	6	1
Buckenham 2015 [14]	N/A	N/A	N/A	N/A	N/A	N/A	132	77	55
Preventza 2010 [13]	75	11	15	N/A	N/A	N/A	75	11	15
Kpodonou 2008 [12]	26	9	9	84	58	34	110	67	43
De Rango 2016 [7]	38	5	13	35	23	26	73	28	38
Kern 2006 [18]	N/A	N/A	N/A	N/A	N/A	N/A	N/A	N/A	N/A
Czerny 2010 [3]	N/A	N/A	N/A	N/A	N/A	N/A	100	57	69
Patel 2008 [19]	24	7	19	N/A	N/A	N/A	24	7	19
Karimi 2016 [11]	24	0	17	N/A	N/A	N/A	24	0	17

Study quality and risk of bias assessment were performed using the Risk of Bias in Non-Randomized Studies of Interventions tool (ROBINS-I) to evaluate non-RCTs [19]. No RCTs reporting on outcomes in the elderly following TEVAR were identified in the literature. Two reviewers (EG and AF) rated the studies independently, and the final decisions were achieved by consensus in cases of any disagreement.

2.5. Subgroup Analysis: Elective vs. Emergency

Where available, data on the outcomes of emergency and elective TEVAR were used for a sensitivity analysis to explore how the outcomes in the elderly population were affected by the nature of the operation. The only outcome in which there was sufficient data to enable such a subgroup analysis regarding emergency and elective operations was short-term mortality.

2.6. Statistical and Sensitivity Analysis

The Mantel–Haenszel random and fixed effects methods were used to combine the odds ratio (OR) for outcomes of interest allowing for comparison between elderly and nonelderly populations. Due to the heterogeneity of the studies' populations and surgical techniques, a random effect analysis was necessary to account for the variance within each study and between them. For funnel plots, the fixed-effect method was chosen because their purpose is not to estimate an overall effect size but rather to visually inspect the distribution of study results and identify potential bias [20]. Two strategies were used to assess the heterogeneity of the data. Firstly, publication bias was explored graphically using funnel plots. Secondly, sensitivity analysis was performed using the leave-one-out method. This involves conducting a meta-analysis on each subgroup of studies per outcome by excluding exactly one study.

Pooled overall survival analysis was performed using the published Kaplan–Meier graphs from the included studies using a two-stage approach [18]. In stage one, raw data coordinates, time, and survival probability were extracted for elderly patients from the Kaplan–Meier curves of 9 studies. Kpodonou et al. were excluded from OS analysis as the number of patients at risk at specific time points was not available and individual patient data could not be extracted. During stage two, individual patient data were reconstructed using data coordinates based on the raw data coordinates from the first stage and the numbers at risk at certain time points. The reconstructed individual patient data from all the included studies were then pooled and a Kaplan–Meier graph was produced. The threshold for statistical significance was set as a p-value of less than 0.05. Data and statistical analysis were performed using RevMan V5.4 (The Cochrane Collaboration) and IBM SPSS Statistics (Armonk, New York, United States).

3. Results

The total number of studies included in this analysis was 12 (Figure 1). All the included studies were retrospective cohort studies, published between 2006 and 2022. The quality assessment for the included studies is demonstrated in Figure 2. The baseline preoperative patient characteristics of the included studies are presented in Table 1. The level of agreement between the two reviewers was "almost perfect" (kappa = 0.946, 95% CI:0.934, 0.958).

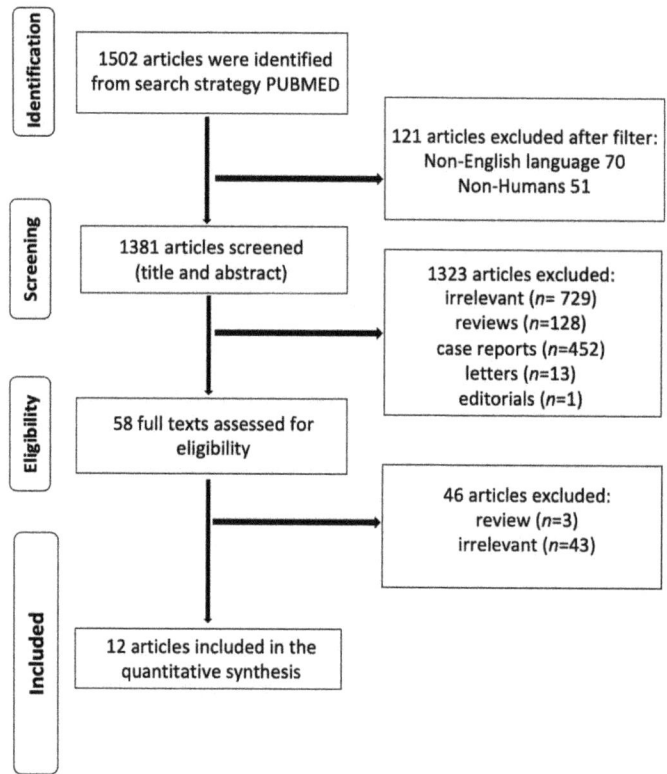

Figure 1. Flow Chart of the current systematic review and meta-analysis.

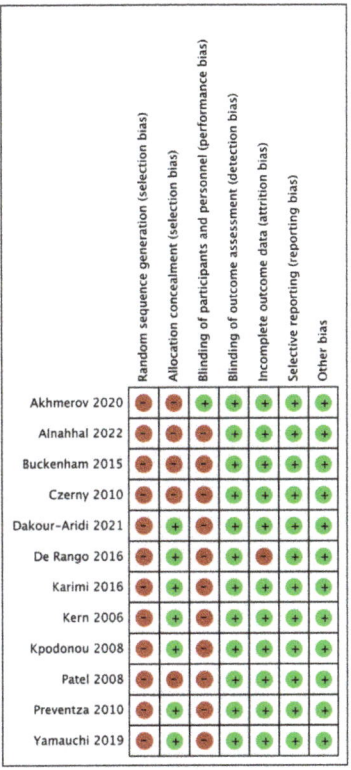

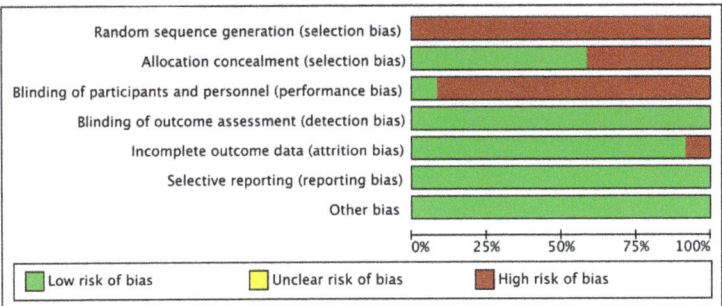

Figure 2. (a) Risk of Bias in Non-Randomized Studies of Interventions. (b) Risk of Bias in Non-Randomized Studies of Interventions tool with summary plot. References: [3,6,7,11–19].

3.1. Primary Endpoint—Morbidity

3.1.1. Neurological Complications

Five included studies investigated the number of neurological complications between the elderly and nonelderly populations. Thus, a total of 1186 elderly and 5618 nonelderly patients were compared for this outcome. Figure 3a demonstrates that the incidence of neurological complications was not significantly different between the two cohorts (OR = 0.91 [95% CI 0.63–1.31]).

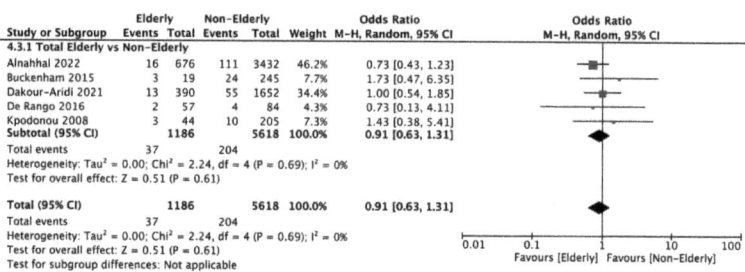

(a)

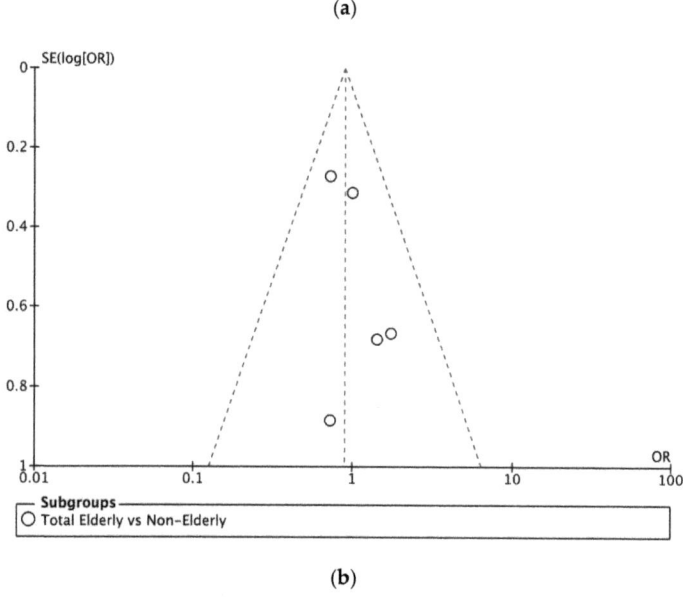

(b)

Figure 3. (a) Comparison of neurological complications between elderly and nonelderly patients undergoing TEVAR. (b) Funnel plot assessing the publication bias for neurological complications in elderly patients. References: [6,7,12,14,16].

3.1.2. Endoleaks

Endoleaks in both populations were reported in three of the included studies, amounting to a total number of 118 elderly and 399 younger patients. As shown in Figure 4a, no significant difference in the incidence of endoleaks between elderly and nonelderly populations was observed (OR = 1.53, [95% CI = 0.52–4.55]).

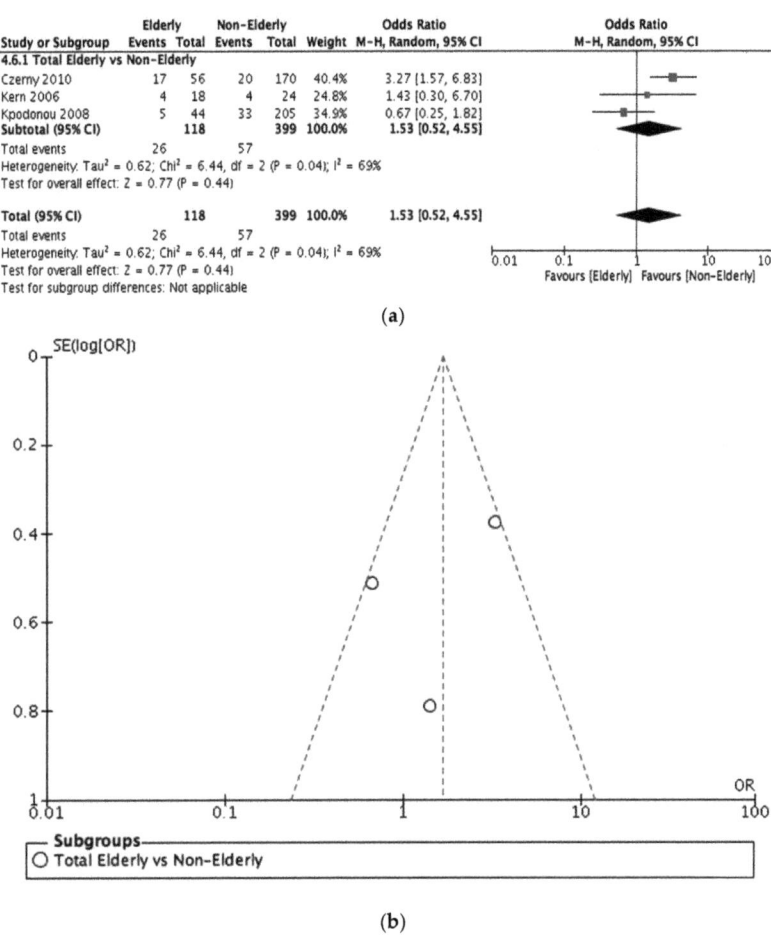

Figure 4. (a) Comparison of rate of endoleaks between elderly vs. nonelderly patients undergoing TEVAR. (b) Funnel plot assessing the publication bias for the rate of endoleaks. References: [3,12,18].

3.1.3. Respiratory Complications

Data on respiratory complications among both age cohorts were documented in four studies. This led to a comparison of 1128 elderly and 5313 nonelderly patients. There was no significant difference in the incidence of respiratory complications (OR = 1.18, 95% CI = 0.59–2.35) (Figure 5a).

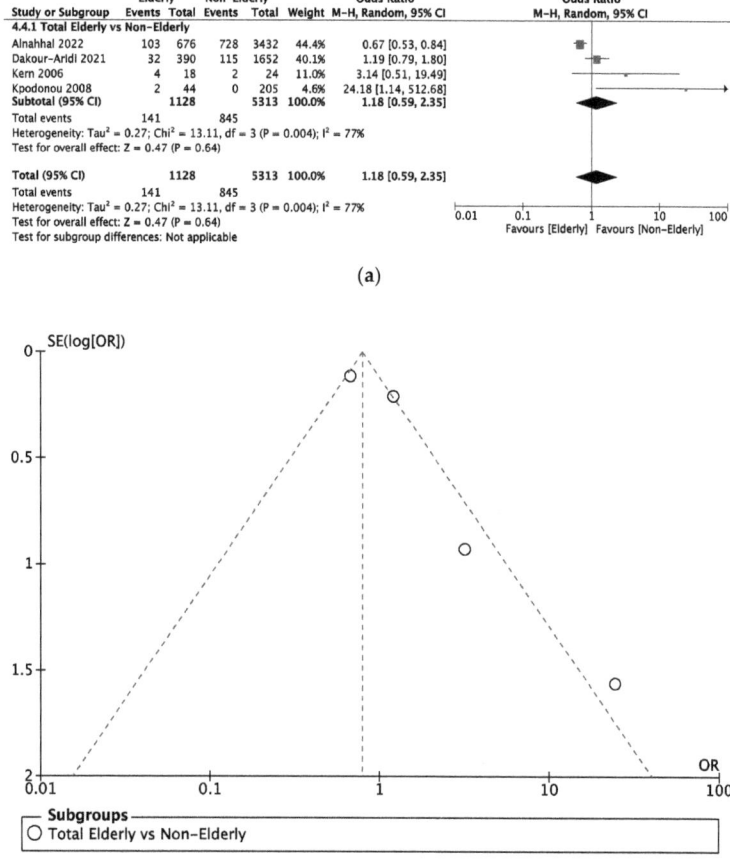

Figure 5. (a) Comparison of respiratory complications between elderly vs. nonelderly patients undergoing TEVAR. (b) Funnel plot assessing the publication bias for respiratory complications. References: [6,12,16,18].

3.2. Length of Hospital Stay

The duration of hospital stay in both age groups was reported in four studies. Hence, 757 elderly patients and 3906 nonelderly were pooled for this outcome. Figure 6a depicts that there was a tendency towards a shorter length of hospital stay in the elderly cohort (OR = −1.26, [95% −2.34 −0.17]).

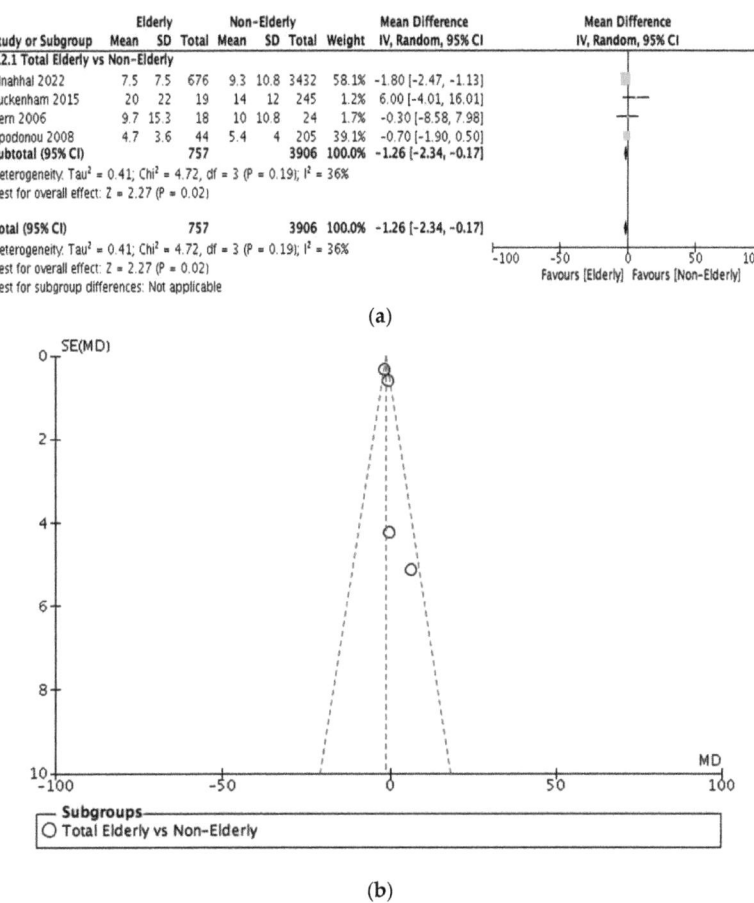

Figure 6. (a) Comparison of length of hospital stay between elderly vs. nonelderly patients undergoing TEVAR. (b) Funnel plot assessing the publication bias for length of hospital stay. References: [12,14,16,18].

3.3. Secondary Endpoint
Short-Term Mortality

As this endpoint was documented in seven studies for both cohorts, a comparison of short-term mortality was carried out between 1288 elderly patients and 5925 younger patients. Figure 7a shows that short-term mortality favoured the nonelderly population compared to elderly patients (OR = 1.81, [95% CI 1.18–2.76]).

The number of studies reporting on elective versus emergency TEVAR procedures in the elderly was three. This translated to a total of 152 patients undergoing elective operations and 47 patients undergoing emergency TEVAR. A comparison regarding short-term mortality between elective and emergency TEVAR procedures in elderly patients revealed a significantly higher mortality in emergency repairs (OR = 0.09, [95% CI 0.02–0.35]) (Figure 8a).

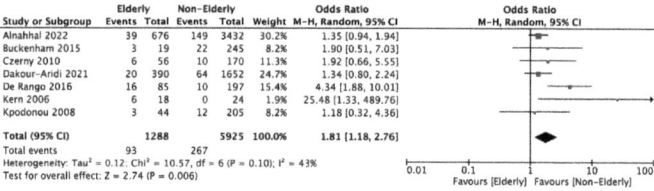

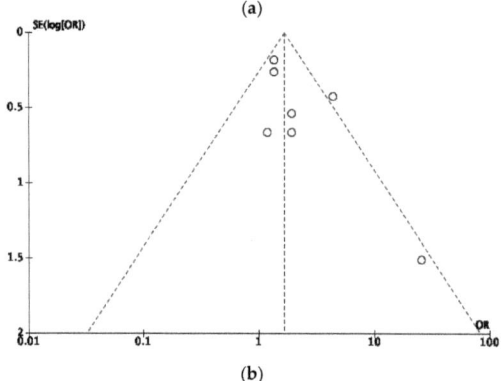

Figure 7. (a) Comparison of short-term mortality between elderly vs. nonelderly patients. (b) Funnel plot assessing the publication bias for short-term mortality in elderly patients. References: [3,6,7,12,14,16,18].

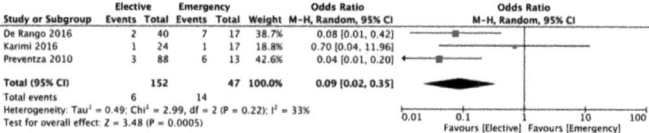

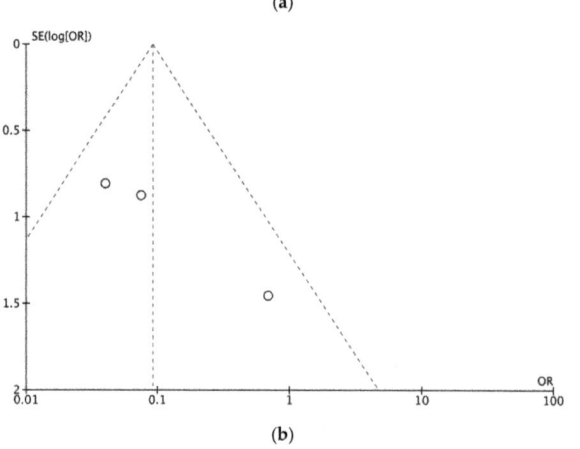

Figure 8. (a) Comparison of short-term mortality between elderly patients undergoing elective vs. emergency TEVAR procedures. (b) Funnel plot assessing the publication bias for short-term mortality in elective vs. emergency TEVAR procedures. References: [7,11,13].

3.4. Secondary Endpoint

Overall Survival

Figure 9 demonstrates the pooled Kaplan–Meier curves for overall survival in a cohort of 2823 patients from six studies, with median follow-up ranging from 12 to 25 months. The cohort was stratified into elderly (n = 633) and nonelderly (n = 1897) and Kaplan–Meier curves were constructed to analyse overall survival. Patients in the elderly group had a mean OS of 42.9 months compared to 50.6 months for nonelderly patients (42.9; CI 39.7–46.2 vs. 50.6; CI 48.9–52.3, $p < 0.001$).

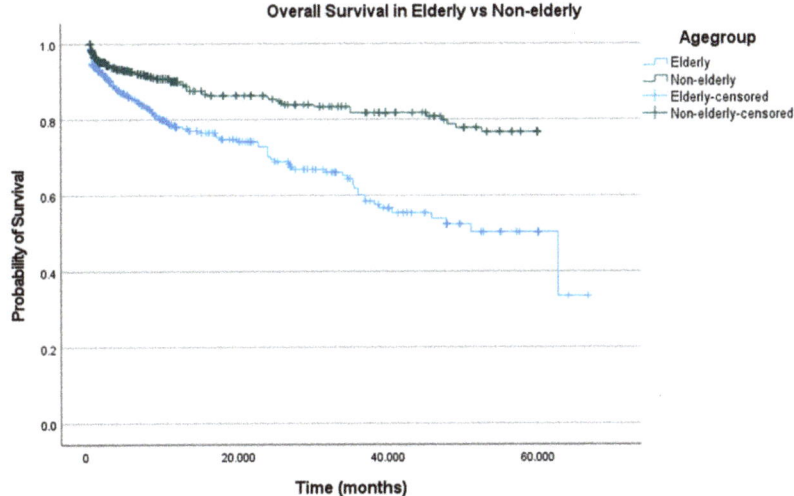

Figure 9. Cumulative Kaplan–Meier curve for overall survival (OS) of elderly vs. nonelderly patients undergoing TEVAR.

3.5. Sensitivity Analysis

Funnel plots investigating publication bias for each outcome are presented in Figures 3–8. The funnel plots for the incidence of neurological complications, endoleaks, and hospital stay in elderly vs. nonelderly patients (Figures 3b, 4b and 6b) show homogenous groups of studies. Figure 5b exhibits heterogeneity between the three studies investigating respiratory complications. Figures 7b and 8b for short-term mortality resemble symmetrical inverted funnels (95% CI) with only one study being outside in the first case.

No significant difference was found in the leave-one-out method when comparing elderly vs. nonelderly patients in the following primary endpoints: 30-day mortality, neurological complications, and respiratory complications. A significant difference was observed when excluding the studies by Kpodonou, Alnahhal, and Kern et al. [10,14,17] regarding mean hospital stay, and when excluding the study by Kpodonou et al. [10] regarding endoleaks. In the comparison of 30-day mortality between elective and urgent TEVAR, leaving out the study by Dakour-Aridi [4] also led to a statistically significant difference in the sensitivity analysis.

4. Discussion

This systematic review and meta-analysis demonstrated that the morbidity associated with TEVAR did not differ significantly between elderly and nonelderly patients. A shorter length of hospital stay was also identified in the older age group. Regarding our secondary endpoints, short-term mortality was found to be lower in the nonelderly population. In addition, younger patients also exhibited higher long-term overall survival rates with lower long-term mortality rates.

Neurological complications often have significant long-term health implications for patients, especially for elderly ones, and are commonly reported by studies [21,22]. Our findings did not show any statistically significant difference in post-TEVAR neurological complications between the two cohorts. Older age was also not found to be a significant predictor for stroke in a multivariable regression model of a prospective observational study [21]. Similar findings were reported by a large retrospective study investigating patients with type B dissections. The researchers' risk analysis concluded that increasing age was not independently associated with a higher incidence of neurological complications [20]. Examples of risk factors which have been linked to higher rates of strokes and other neurological events in the existing literature include LSA coverage, prior stroke, and coronary artery disease, long duration of the procedure, aortic rupture, and female gender [20–22].

Endoleaks represent a common reason for reintervention following endovascular aortic repair, contributing to significant postoperative morbidity [23,24]. No significant difference in the rates of post-TEVAR endoleaks was found between the two age groups in this review. The lack of sufficient data distinguishing between the different types of endoleaks (I, II, or III) and documenting how long after TEVAR they were detected prevented us from carrying out further subgroup analyses. All three different types and both early and late endoleaks have been reported post-TEVAR in the literature [25,26]. Varying rates of reinterventions have been found following each endoleak type, with type II requiring the least secondary procedures [23]. A more detailed documentation of this important post-TEVAR outcome in the elderly population is, hence, needed in research studies. Nevertheless, evaluation of our results suggests no significant added risk for elderly patients undergoing TEVAR regarding the development of endoleaks.

Respiratory complications and postoperative length of hospital stay in the elderly after TEVAR are less reported in the literature. In a large US nationwide study, TEVAR was associated with decreased respiratory complications and LoS compared to open aortic repair, even though the TEVAR population was significantly older [27]. Hence, TEVAR appears to be an attractive alternative treatment option to open surgery for elderly patients, due to a lower respiratory morbidity risk. Potential reasons for the favourable LoS in the older age group after TEVAR need to be explored. Data from the endovascular repair of abdominal aortic aneurysms have shown that older age was associated with higher rates of nonhome discharge [28]. Thus, older patients who are going to be transferred to other facilities due to known comorbidities or frailty might potentially get discharged earlier than younger patients. Dissections, emergency procedures and previous cardiac history have been identified as significant predictors of prolonged hospital stay after TEVAR [29]. Considering the limited available studies for these outcomes, it is evident that more research is necessary.

Short-term mortality, either reported as 30-day or in-hospital mortality, was the endpoint most commonly documented by studies comparing post-TEVAR outcomes between elderly and younger patients ($n = 7$). Previous studies have also demonstrated that the short-term mortality of elderly patients post-TEVAR is higher compared to the nonelderly. Using data from large multinational registries, Hellgren et al. identified a higher short-term death rate in patients over 80 years old undertaking TEVAR for a variety of aortic pathologies [30]. In addition, Naazie et al. conducted a risk analysis on patients undergoing TEVAR for descending aortic aneurysms and reported that age over 75 years old is associated with higher mortality [31]. Apart from increasing age, other factors, such as female sex, coronary artery disease, ASA class, and urgency of the procedure, have also been found to be predictors of a higher early death rate [31]. Elderly patients also had lower overall survival compared to their nonelderly counterparts. Our findings regarding both short- and long-term mortality could be attributed to the generally higher prevalence of comorbidities, frailty, and cardiovascular disease risk factors among the older population [32]. However, it is important to consider the methodological limitations of the included studies, such as the absence of random treatment allocation and potential selection bias favouring elderly patients with lower comorbidities. Consequently, there is a possibility that long-term mortality rates in the elderly have been underestimated due to these limitations.

As the incidence of aortic pathologies in elderly patients continues to rise [6,7] and the applications of TEVAR for various aortic pathologies constantly expand, the evaluation of TEVAR use in older patients is becoming even more important for clinical practice. Due to its minimally invasive nature, an increasing number of patients are becoming eligible for procedural repair. Evidently, from 2003–2004 to 2011–2012, the proportion of procedural management of ruptured TAAs in patients over 80 years old performed with TEVAR increased from 18% to 86% [33]. Our analysis showed that, while increasing age is associated with higher mortality rates post-TEVAR, this trend was not observed in morbidity outcomes. With no added risk for adverse perioperative morbidity outcomes, we demonstrate that increasing age should not be a contraindication for TEVAR on its own. Quality-of-life investigations, which depict the impact of the aforementioned physical complications on patients' overall health, are also gaining steady ground in the assessment of elderly patients. As identified by a systematic review examining thoracic aorta interventions, the postaortic surgery health-related quality of life of elderly cohorts was similar to a matched population [34]. This finding indicates a satisfactory return to the preinterventional baseline for most patients, an important consideration after every operation in older patients. Elderly patients should, hence, be considered for endovascular repair for aortic pathologies, predominantly in elective cases, unless other risk factors associated with worse TEVAR morbidity outcomes are identified.

The population included in this review consisted of patients undergoing TEVAR for a variety of aortic pathologies. As most studies did not report separate outcome results for each diagnosis; a comprehensive analysis of how post-TEVAR morbidity and mortality varied with different aortic presentations could not be conducted. Comparisons of patient outcomes undergoing TEVAR for aortic aneurysms and dissections have yielded variable results. Although some studies report similar postoperative morbidity and mortality [35,36], inferior outcomes in patients suffering from aneurysms have also been found [37,38]. Another important consideration when assessing TEVAR use is whether the endovascular repair was carried out electively or as an emergency procedure. The lack of subgroup analyses on urgent vs. elective TEVAR in the studies included in this review meant that postoperative complications after acute and nonacute presentations could not be compared. Even for short-term mortality, the outcome most commonly reported, only three studies provided separate data for both elective and urgent aortic pathologies [5,9,11]. Death rates were lower after elective procedures, an observation generally supported by the existing literature [39–43]. Thus, in studies consisting of elderly populations, more detailed reporting of distinct post-TEVAR outcomes for the most common aortic presentations and for elective and emergency procedures is recommended.

The limitations of this meta-analysis greatly depend on the individual studies used, which were retrospective cohort studies, as no relevant RCTs were identified during the literature search. Due to the nature of the comparison, an RCT between the two age groups might not be feasible. Hence, future research using large TEVAR registries should be prioritised. Until then, this systematic review and meta-analysis remains the best level of evidence around TEVAR use in the elderly. In addition, as mentioned, renal complications and the effect of different aortic conditions, and the urgency of the procedure on outcomes after TEVAR, were not explored. There was also a lack of available information about other important procedural details, such as renal complications, type of anaesthesia, and duration of the TEVAR procedure. We strongly recommend that future studies report on these variables, as they can influence surgical outcomes. Patient data were derived from Kaplan–Meier curves, and not individual patient information, thus further limiting us from conducting even more subgroup analyses based on various patient characteristics. Different selection criteria between studies and confounding variables are also significant factors that could not be controlled.

5. Conclusions

The overall findings of this systematic review and meta-analysis suggested that morbidity following TEVAR, assessed by the incidence of neurological complications, respiratory complications, and endoleaks, was similar in elderly and nonelderly patients. Short-term mortality and long-term overall survival post-TEVAR favoured, as expected, the younger population. Due to its safe perioperative morbidity profile, it can be concluded that patients should not be excluded from elective TEVAR interventions purely based on age criteria.

Author Contributions: Conceptualization, A.F., E.G., S.B., I.K., D.E.M. and T.A.; methodology, A.F., E.G., S.B., I.K., D.E.M. and T.A.; software, A.F., E.G., S.B., I.K., A.A.R. and A.V.; validation, A.V., K.S., D.E.M. and T.A.; formal analysis, A.F., E.G., S.B. and I.K.; investigation, A.F., E.G., S.B. and I.K.; resources, A.F., E.G., S.B., I.K. and A.A.R.; data curation, A.A.R. and D.E.M.; writing—original draft preparation, A.F., E.G., S.B., I.K., A.A.R., D.E.M. and T.A.; writing—review and editing, A.F., E.G., S.B., I.K., A.A.R., D.E.M., A.V., K.S. and T.A.; visualization, D.E.M. and A.A.R.; supervision, D.E.M. and T.A.; project administration, D.E.M., A.V. and T.A.; funding acquisition, T.A. All authors have read and agreed to the published version of the manuscript.

Funding: This research received no external funding.

Institutional Review Board Statement: Not applicable.

Informed Consent Statement: Not applicable.

Data Availability Statement: The data that support the findings of this study are available from the corresponding author, upon reasonable request.

Conflicts of Interest: The authors declare no conflict of interest.

References

1. Nation, D.; Wang, G. TEVAR: Endovascular Repair of the Thoracic Aorta. *Semin. Interv. Radiol.* **2015**, *32*, 265–271. [CrossRef] [PubMed]
2. Liu, J.; Xia, J.; Yan, G.; Zhang, Y.; Ge, J.; Cao, L. Thoracic endovascular aortic repair versus open chest surgical repair for patients with type B aortic dissection: A systematic review and meta-analysis. *Ann. Med.* **2019**, *51*, 360–370. [CrossRef] [PubMed]
3. Czerny, M.; Funovics, M.; Ehrlich, M.; Hoebartner, M.; Sodeck, G.; Dumfarth, J.; Schoder, M.; Juraszek, A.; Dziodzio, T.; Loewe, C.; et al. Risk Factors of Mortality in Different Age Groups After Thoracic Endovascular Aortic Repair. *Ann. Thorac. Surg.* **2010**, *90*, 534–538. [CrossRef]
4. Jonker, F.; Verhagen, H.; Heijmen, R.; Lin, P.; Trimarchi, S.; Lee, W.; Moll, F.; Athamneh, H.; Muhs, B. Endovascular Treatment of Ruptured Thoracic Aortic Aneurysm in Patients Older than 75 Years. *Eur. J. Vasc. Endovasc. Surg.* **2011**, *41*, 48–53. [CrossRef] [PubMed]
5. Jonker, F.H.; Verhagen, H.J.; Heijmen, R.H.; Lin, P.H.; Trimarchi, S.; Lee, W.A.; Moll, F.L.; Athamneh, H.; Muhs, B.E. Endovascular Repair of Ruptured Thoracic Aortic Aneurysms: Predictors of Procedure-Related Stroke. *Ann. Vasc. Surg.* **2011**, *25*, 3–8. [CrossRef]
6. Dakour-Aridi, H.; Yin, K.; Hussain, F.; Locham, S.; Azizzadeh, A.; Malas, M.B. Outcomes of intact thoracic endovascular aortic repair in octogenarians. *J. Vasc. Surg.* **2021**, *74*, 882–892.e1. [CrossRef]
7. De Rango, P.; Isernia, G.; Simonte, G.; Cieri, E.; Marucchini, A.; Farchioni, L.; Verzini, F.; Lenti, M. Impact of age and urgency on survival after thoracic endovascular aortic repair. *J. Vasc. Surg.* **2016**, *64*, 25–32. [CrossRef]
8. LeMaire, S.A.; Russell, L. Epidemiology of thoracic aortic dissection. *Nat. Rev. Cardiol.* **2011**, *8*, 103–113. [CrossRef]
9. Howard, D.P.J.; Sideso, E.; Handa, A.; Rothwell, P.M. Incidence, risk factors, outcome and projected future burden of acute aortic dissection. *Ann. Cardiothorac. Surg.* **2014**, *3*, 278–284. [CrossRef]
10. Page, M.J.; McKenzie, J.E.; Bossuyt, P.M.; Boutron, I.; Hoffmann, T.C.; Mulrow, C.D.; Moher, D. The PRISMA 2020 statement: An updated guideline for reporting systematic reviews. *Int. J. Surg.* **2021**, *88*, 105906. [CrossRef]
11. Karimi, A.; McCord, M.R.; Beaver, T.M.; Martin, T.D.; Hess, P.J.; Beck, A.W.; Feezor, R.J.; Klodell, C.T. Operative and Mid-Term Outcomes of Thoracic Aortic Operation in Octogenarians and Beyond. *J. Card. Surg.* **2016**, *31*, 334–340. [CrossRef]
12. Kpodonu, J.; Preventza, O.; Ramaiah, V.G.; Shennib, H.; Wheatley, G.H., III; Rodriguez-Lopez, J.A.; Williams, J.; Diethrich, E.B. Endovascular repair of the thoracic aorta in octogenarians. *Eur. J. Cardiothorac Surg.* **2008**, *34*, 630–634. [CrossRef]
13. Preventza, O.; Bavaria, J.; Ramaiah, V.; Moser, G.W.; Szeto, W.; Wheatley, G.; Moeller, P.; Rodriquez-Lopez, J.; Diethrich, E. Thoracic Endo-grafting is a Viable Option for the Octogenarian. *Ann. Thorac. Surg.* **2010**, *90*, 78–82. [CrossRef] [PubMed]
14. Buckenham, T.; Pearch, B.; Wright, I. Endoluminal thoracic aortic repair in the octogenarian and nonagenarian: The New Zealand experience. *J. Med. Imaging Radiat. Oncol.* **2015**, *59*, 39–46. [CrossRef]

15. Yamauchi, T.; Kubota, S.; Hasegawa, K.; Ueda, H. Clinical results and medical costs of thoracic endovascular aortic repair in pa-tients over 80 years of age. *J. Artif. Organs* **2019**, *22*, 61–67. [CrossRef]
16. Alnahhal, K.I.; Narayanan, M.K.; Lingutla, R.; Parikh, S.; Iafrati, M.; Kumar, S.; Salehi, P. Outcomes of Thoracic Endovascular Aortic Repair in Octogenarians. *Vasc. Endovasc. Surg.* **2022**, *56*, 158–165. [CrossRef]
17. Akhmerov, A.; Shah, A.S.; Gupta, N.; Tulloch, A.W.; Gewertz, B.; Azizzadeh, A. Thoracic Endovascular Aortic Repair in Octogenarians and Nonagenarians. *Ann. Vasc. Surg.* **2020**, *68*, 299–304. [CrossRef]
18. Kern, J.A.; Matsumoto, A.H.; Tribble, C.G.; Gazoni, L.M.; Peeler, B.B.; Harthun, N.L.; Chong, T.; Cherry, K.J.; Dake, M.D.; Angle, J.S.; et al. Thoracic Aortic Endografting Is the Treatment of Choice for Elderly Patients with Thoracic Aortic Disease. *Ann. Surg.* **2006**, *243*, 815–823. [CrossRef] [PubMed]
19. Patel, H.J.; Williams, D.M.; Upchurch, G.R.; Dasika, N.L.; Passow, M.C.; Prager, R.L.; Deeb, G.M. A Comparison of Open and Endovascular Descending Thoracic Aortic Repair in Patients Older Than 75 Years of Age. *Ann. Thorac. Surg.* **2008**, *85*, 1597–1604. [CrossRef] [PubMed]
20. Dettori, J.R.; Norvell, D.C.; Chapman, J.R. Fixed-Effect vs Random-Effects Models for Meta-Analysis: 3 Points to Consider. *Glob. Spine J.* **2022**, *12*, 1624–1626. [CrossRef]
21. Sterne, J.A.; Hernán, M.A.; Reeves, B.C.; Savović, J.; Berkman, N.D.; Viswanathan, M.; Higgins, J.P. ROBINS-I: A tool for assessing risk of bias in non-randomized studies of interven-tions. *BMJ* **2016**, *355*, i4919. [CrossRef]
22. Liu, N.; Zhou, Y.; Lee, J.J. IPDfromKM: Reconstruct individual patient data from published Kaplan-Meier survival curves. *BMC Med. Res. Methodol.* **2021**, *21*, 111. [CrossRef] [PubMed]
23. Buth, J.; Harris, P.L.; Hobo, R.; van Eps, R.; Cuypers, P.; Duijm, L.; Tielbeek, X. Neurologic complications associated with endovascular repair of thoracic aortic pathology: Incidence and risk factors. A study from the European Collaborators on Stent/Graft Techniques for Aortic Aneurysm Repair (EUROSTAR) Registry. *J. Vasc. Surg.* **2007**, *46*, 1103–1111. [CrossRef] [PubMed]
24. Reutersberg, B.; Gleason, T.; Desai, N.; Ehrlich, M.; Evangelista, A.; Braverman, A.; Myrmel, T.; Chen, E.P.; Estrera, A.; Schermerhorn, M.; et al. Neurological event rates and associated risk factors in acute type B aortic dissections treated by thoracic aortic endovascular repair. *J. Thorac. Cardiovasc. Surg.* **2022**. online ahead of print. [CrossRef]
25. Piazza, M.; Squizzato, F.; Milan, L.; Miccoli, T.; Grego, F.; Antonello, M. Incidence and predictors of neurological complications following thoracic endovascular aneurysm repair in the global registry for endovascular aortic treatment. *Eur. J. Vasc. Endovasc. Surg.* **2019**, *58*, 512–519. [CrossRef] [PubMed]
26. Morales, J.P.; Greenberg, R.K.; Lu, Q.; Cury, M.; Hernandez, A.V.; Mohabbat, W.; Moon, M.C.; Morales, C.A.; Bathurst, S.; Schoenhagen, P. Endoleaks Following Endovascular Repair of Thoracic Aortic Aneurysm: Etiology and Outcomes. *J. Endovasc. Ther.* **2008**, *15*, 631–638. [CrossRef]
27. Bischoff, M.S.; Geisbüsch, P.; Kotelis, D.; Müller-Eschner, M.; Hyhlik-Dürr, A.; Böckler, D. Clinical significance of type II endoleaks after thoracic endovascular aortic repair. *J. Vasc. Surg.* **2013**, *58*, 643–650. [CrossRef]
28. Biancari, F.; Mariscalco, G.; Mariani, S.; Saari, P.; Satta, J.; Juvonen, T. Endovascular Treatment of Degenerative Aneurysms Involving Only the Descending Thoracic Aorta. *J. Endovasc. Ther.* **2016**, *23*, 387–392. [CrossRef]
29. Mustafa, S.T.; Sadat, U.; Majeed, M.U.; Wong, C.M.; Michaels, J.; Thomas, S.M. Endovascular Repair of Nonruptured Thoracic Aortic Aneurysms: Systematic Review. *Vascular* **2010**, *18*, 28–33. [CrossRef]
30. Hughes, K.; Guerrier, J.; Obirieze, A.; Ngwang, D.; Rose, D.; Tran, D.; Cornwell, E.; Obisesan, T.; Preventza, O. Open versus endovascular repair of thoracic aortic an-eurysms. *Vasc. Endovasc. Surg.* **2014**, *48*, 383–387. [CrossRef]
31. Boitano, L.T.; Iannuzzi, J.C.; Tanious, A.; Mohebali, J.; Schwartz, S.I.; Chang, D.C.; Clouse, W.D.; Conrad, M.F. Preoperative Predictors of Discharge Destination after Endovascular Repair of Abdominal Aortic Aneurysms. *Ann. Vasc. Surg.* **2019**, *57*, 109–117. [CrossRef]
32. Belkin, N.; Jackson, B.M.; Foley, P.J.; Damrauer, S.M.; Kalapatapu, V.; Golden, M.A.; Fairman, R.M.; Kelz, R.R.; Wang, G.J. Length of Stay after Thoracic Endovascular Aortic Repair Depends on Indication and Acuity. *Ann. Vasc. Surg.* **2019**, *55*, 157–165. [CrossRef]
33. Hellgren, T.; Beck, A.W.; Behrendt, C.-A.; Becker, D.; Beiles, B.; Boyle, J.R.; Jormalainen, M.; Koncar, I.; Espada, C.L.; Setacci, C.; et al. Thoracic Endovascular Aortic Repair Practice in 13 Countries. *Ann. Surg.* **2020**, *276*, e598–e604. [CrossRef]
34. Naazie, I.N.; Das Gupta, J.; Azizzadeh, A.; Arbabi, C.; Zarkowsky, D.; Malas, M.B. Risk calculator predicts 30-day mortality after thoracic endovascular aortic repair for intact descending thoracic aortic aneurysms in the Vascular Quality Initiative. *J. Vasc. Surg.* **2022**, *75*, 833–841. [CrossRef] [PubMed]
35. Costantino, S.; Paneni, F.; Cosentino, F. Ageing, metabolism and cardiovascular disease. *J. Physiol.* **2016**, *594*, 2061–2073. [CrossRef]
36. Ultee, K.H.; Zettervall, S.L.; Soden, P.A.; Buck, D.B.; Deery, S.E.; Shean, K.E.; Verhagen, H.J.; Schermerhorn, M.L. The impact of endovascular repair on management and outcome of ruptured thoracic aortic aneurysms. *J. Vasc. Surg.* **2017**, *66*, 343–352. [CrossRef] [PubMed]
37. Jarral, O.A.; Kidher, E.; Patel, V.M.; Nguyen, B.; Pepper, J.; Athanasiou, T. Quality of life after intervention on the thoracic aorta. *Eur. J. Cardio-Thorac. Surg.* **2015**, *49*, 369–389. [CrossRef]
38. Clough, R.E.; Patel, A.S.; Lyons, O.T.; Bell, R.E.; Zayed, H.A.; Carrell, T.W.; Taylor, P.R. Pathology specific early outcome after thoracic endo-vascular aortic repair. *Eur. J. Vasc. Endovasc. Surg.* **2014**, *48*, 268–275. [CrossRef] [PubMed]

39. Gallo, M.; Berg, J.C.v.D.; Torre, T.; Riggi, M.; Demertzis, S.; Ferrari, E. Long-Term Outcomes and Risk Factors Analysis for Patients Undergoing Thoracic Endovascular Aorta Repair (TEVAR), According to the Aortic Pathologies. *Ann. Vasc. Surg.* 2023. *online ahead of print*. [CrossRef]
40. Haji-Zeinali, A.M.; Mansouri, P.; Hosseini, N.R.; Abbasi, K.; Shirzad, M.; Jameie, M.; Haji-Zeinali, M.M. Five-Year Survival and Complications of Thoracic Endovascular Aortic Repair (TEVAR): A Single Tertiary Center Registry for All-Comers Patients. *Cardiovasc. Revascularization Med.* **2023**, *51*, 23–30. [CrossRef]
41. Patterson, B.; Holt, P.; Nienaber, C.; Cambria, R.; Fairman, R.; Thompson, M. Aortic pathology determines midterm outcome after endovascular repair of the thoracic aorta: Report from the Medtronic thoracic endovascular registry (MOTHER) database. *Circulation* **2013**, *127*, 24–32. [CrossRef] [PubMed]
42. Schaffer, J.M.; Lingala, B.; Miller, D.C.; Woo, Y.J.; Mitchell, R.S.; Dake, M.D. Midterm survival after thoracic endovascular aortic repair in more than 10,000 Medicare patients. *J. Thorac. Cardiovasc. Surg.* **2015**, *149*, 808–823. [CrossRef] [PubMed]
43. Fiorucci, B.; Kölbel, T.; Rohlffs, F.; Heidemann, F.; Carpenter, S.W.; Debus, E.S.; Tsilimparis, N. The role of thoracic endovascular repair in elective, symptomatic and ruptured thoracic aortic diseases. *Eur. J. Cardio-Thorac. Surg.* **2019**, *56*, 197–203. [CrossRef] [PubMed]

Disclaimer/Publisher's Note: The statements, opinions and data contained in all publications are solely those of the individual author(s) and contributor(s) and not of MDPI and/or the editor(s). MDPI and/or the editor(s) disclaim responsibility for any injury to people or property resulting from any ideas, methods, instructions or products referred to in the content.

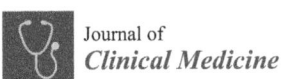

Systematic Review

The Postoperative Effect of Sugammadex versus Acetylcholinesterase Inhibitors in Colorectal Surgery: An Updated Meta-Analysis

Sascha Vaghiri [1,†], Dimitrios Prassas [1,†], Sarah Krieg [2], Wolfram Trudo Knoefel [1] and Andreas Krieg [1,*]

[1] Department of Surgery (A), Heinrich-Heine-University and University Hospital Duesseldorf, Moorenstr. 5, Bldg. 12.46, 40225 Duesseldorf, Germany; sascha.vaghiri@med.uni-duesseldorf.de (S.V.); dimitrios.prassas@med.uni-duesseldorf.de (D.P.)

[2] Clinic for Gastroenterology, Hepatology and Infectious Diseases, Heinrich-Heine-University and University Hospital Duesseldorf, 40225 Duesseldorf, Germany; sarah.krieg@med.uni-duesseldorf.de

* Correspondence: andreas.krieg@med.uni-duesseldorf.de

† These authors contributed equally to this work.

Abstract: Background: the aim of this meta-analysis was to evaluate the postoperative effects of neuromuscular blockade reversal with sugammadex compared with acetylcholinesterase inhibitors in colorectal surgery. Methods: A systematic literature search was performed for studies comparing the postoperative course of patients receiving neuromuscular blockade reversal with either sugammadex or acetylcholinesterase inhibitors (control) after colorectal surgery. Data from eligible studies were extracted, qualitatively assessed, and included in a meta-analysis. Odds ratios and standardized mean differences with 95% confidence intervals (CIs) were calculated. Results: Five studies with a total of 1969 patients were included (sugammadex n = 1137, control n = 832). Sugammadex reversal resulted in a significantly faster return of defecation or flatus after surgery compared to acetylcholinesterase inhibitors (SMD 13.01, 95% CI 6.55–19.46, p = < 0.0001). There were no significant differences between the two groups in other clinical outcomes such as surgical morbidity and length of hospital stay. Conclusion: The present data support the beneficial impact of sugammadex on gastrointestinal motility after colorectal surgery. However, the effect of sugammadex on the prevention of surgical complications and a prolonged hospital stay is diminishing. Larger randomized controlled trials with standardized study protocols are needed to validate the results presented here.

Keywords: sugammadex; acetylcholinesterase inhibitors; colorectal surgery; operative outcome; gastrointestinal motility

1. Introduction

Postoperative ileus (POI) is unfortunately a common phenomenon after gastrointestinal surgery and contributes to high morbidity, prolonged hospital stay, increased readmission rates, and thus high hospital costs [1,2]. Even in the era of improved recovery programs, POI rates between 15% and 30% are reported after colorectal surgery [3,4]. Nowadays, muscle relaxation with neuromuscular blocking agents (NMBAs) is widely used to improve surgical conditions and reduce the rate of postoperative adverse events [5,6]. Residual effects of neuromuscular blockade and muscle weakness are associated with postoperative pulmonary complications (POPCs) and impaired clinical recovery in the postanesthesia care unit (PACU) [7,8]. Acetylcholinesterase inhibitors such as neostigmine or pyridostigmine have traditionally been used to reverse the effects of NMBAs [9]. Potential cholinergic side effects of acetylcholinesterase inhibitors due to peripheral muscarinic activation are treated via the concomitant administration of anticholinergics (e.g., atropine or glycopyrrolate) [10]. Sugammadex is a modified γ-cyclodextrin that forms a stable 1:1 complex with aminosteroidal neuromuscular blockers such as rocuronium or vecuronium, reducing their availability to nicotinic receptors [11]. In a Cochrane-based meta-analysis of 41 included studies, sugammadex was found to have a faster potential to antagonize the rocuronium-induced neuromuscular blockade (regardless of the depth of blockade) and 40% fewer adverse events compared with neostigmine [12]. However, there are conflicting results in the literature regarding postoperative defecation when sugammadex or neostigmine is administered as their effect on bowel motility and recovery has still not been fully elaborated upon [13,14]. This could be partly related to the fact that no unified and reproducible outcome measures of gastrointestinal motility function throughout the literature exists [15]. Therefore, our primary objective was to critically evaluate the role of sugammadex compared to "classical" acetylcholinesterase inhibitors in the postoperative course of patients undergoing colorectal surgery by means of a systematic review and meta-analysis. Special attention will be paid to all reported parameters of postoperative gastrointestinal motility.

2. Material and Methods

Prior to the study initiation, the study protocol was registered in the International Prospective Register of Systematic Reviews (PROSPERO CRD 42022383245). This meta-analysis was conducted in accordance with the current PRISMA statement (Preferred Reporting Items for Systematic Reviews and Meta-Analyses) [16] and the latest version of the Cochrane Handbook for Systematic Reviews of Interventions [17].

2.1. Eligibility Criteria and Group Definition

All studies comparing postoperative clinical outcomes after the reversal of neuromuscular blockade with sugammadex or an acetylcholinesterase inhibitor (defined as the comparator) in patients undergoing colorectal surgery were included. To avoid heterogeneity, only studies in which 100% of patients underwent colorectal surgery for any reason were included. Particular attention was paid to postoperative gastrointestinal motility parameters such as ileus, time to first bowel movement or flatus, and time to first solid food intake. Other outcomes of interest included postoperative morbidity and mortality, number of pulmonary events, length of postoperative hospital stay, and rate of readmission to the hospital or intensive care unit. To be included in the analysis, studies had to report at least one of the outcomes listed above. Publications that were randomized controlled trials (RCTs) or prospective or retrospective comparative cohort studies were included in the analysis. Disagreements or differing conclusions in the selection of studies were resolved either via consensus or consultation with an independent third author (S.K.).

2.2. Literature Search

A systematic electronic search of the Pubmed (Medline) and Scopus databases without time or language restrictions was performed to identify articles comparing outcomes in patients with colorectal surgery after the reversal of neuromuscular blockade with sugammadex or an acetylcholinesterase inhibitor. The following search terms were used in combination with the Boolean operators AND or OR: "sugammadex", "Bridion®", "neuromuscular reversal", "neostigmine", "acetylcholine", "pyridostigmine", and "colorectal". In addition, the reference list of retrieved articles (including systematic reviews, case reports, editorials, or experimental studies) was reviewed to identify potentially relevant citations for analysis. Two reviewers (S.V. and D.P.) performed the primary search and independently assessed each abstract and eligible study for relevance for inclusion in the meta-analysis. A third reviewer (S.K.) was consulted as needed. The final literature search was performed on 20 January 2023.

2.3. Data Extraction and Outcome Measures

Two authors (S.V. and D.P.) independently recorded all available and relevant data from studies meeting the inclusion criteria on a self-generated electronic data extraction sheet. Study- and patient-specific information included country of origin, year of publication, study design, exclusion criteria, enrollment period, type and composition of neuromuscular reversal drug, number of patients enrolled per group and their demographics (age, sex, body mass index (BMI), ASA class, and comorbidities), surgical indication, proportion of laparoscopic and open surgery procedures, duration of anesthesia (min), and follow-up period. The primary endpoint was time (hours) to first documented postoperative bowel movement or flatus. The secondary postoperative endpoints analyzed were ileus (as individually defined by the authors), time to first solid oral intake (hours), postoperative nausea and vomiting (PONV), reported adverse pulmonary events (pooled composite of pneumonia, hypoxemia, postoperative supplemental oxygen, acute respiratory distress syndrome, pulmonary embolism, and emergency sugammadex use), urinary tract infection, anastomotic leak, bleeding, postoperative wound infection, length of postoperative hospital stay (days), PACU stay (minutes), reoperation rate (within 30 days), hospital and ICU readmission rate, and mortality. Again, discrepancies in data extraction were resolved via consensus or reassessment by an independent third author (S.K.).

2.4. Quality Assessment

The quality of the included non-randomized trials was independently assessed by the authors using the ROBINS-I tool [18], which covers seven different domains of bias at three time points in each trial: before intervention (confounding and selection of participants), during intervention (classification of interventions), and after intervention (bias due to deviations from planned interventions, missing data, measurement of outcomes, and selection of reported outcomes). Based on these domains, a final assessment of the overall risk of bias for each included study was possible in the categories "low risk", "moderate risk", "high risk", and "critical risk". The Grading of Recommendations, Assessment, Development, and Evaluation (GRADE) method [19] with four assigned levels of evidence (high, moderate, low, and very low) was used to adequately document the strength of evidence for the significant outcomes [19,20].

2.5. Statistical Analyses

Statistical analysis was performed using RevMan software (version 5.3; Copenhagen: The Nordic Cochrane Centre, The Cochrane Collaboration, 2014). Pairwise meta-analyses were performed. For each endpoint of interest, summary treatment effect estimates with 95% confidence intervals (CIs) were calculated. For dichotomous endpoints, the odds ratio (OR) was chosen as the effect measure. For continuous outcomes, standardized mean differences (SMDs) were calculated. The methods proposed by Luo et al. [21] and Wan et al. [22] were used to calculate the mean and standard deviation (SD) from the available median and interquartile range data. The degree of heterogeneity among the included studies was interpreted as follows after applying the Cochrane Q test (chi-square test; Chi^2) and measuring inconsistency (I^2): 0–30% low heterogeneity, 30–50% moderate heterogeneity, and 50–90% substantial heterogeneity [17,23]. If heterogeneity was low or moderate ($I^2 < 50\%$), summary estimates were calculated using a fixed-effects method. Where appropriate, subgroup analyses were performed to examine heterogeneity in the results. Publication bias tests and funnel plots were not performed due to the small number of studies included in the meta-analysis, as recommended [17].

3. Results

3.1. Study and Patient Characteristics

The initial database search using the predefined keywords yielded 365 potentially relevant abstracts. Of these, 14 full-text articles were screened for eligibility and finally 5 non-randomized observational studies (1 multi-center prospective and 4 single-center retrospective) comparing the outcome of neuromuscular blockade reversal with sugammadex and acetylcholinesterase inhibitors were included in the qualitative and quantitative data analysis [24–28]. The PRISMA flowchart for the literature search is shown in Figure 1. Of the total 1969 patients included (1114 men/855 women), 1137 were assigned to the sugammadex group and 832 were assigned to the acetylcholinesterase inhibitor group (control). Two studies used pyridostigmine as the acetylcholinesterase inhibitor [24,26], and three studies used neostigmine [25,27,28]. Three studies included both malignant and non-malignant cases [25,27,28], while two studies included only patients with colorectal cancer [24,26]. The rate of laparoscopic surgery ranged from 20–100% in the sugammadex group to 22–100% in the control group. Inpatient [25,26] and up to 30 days [24,27,28] follow-up data were presented. The study by Serrano et al. [27] was a prespecified substudy of the POWER trial [29]. Tables 1–3 provide a detailed summary of the study and clinical characteristics.

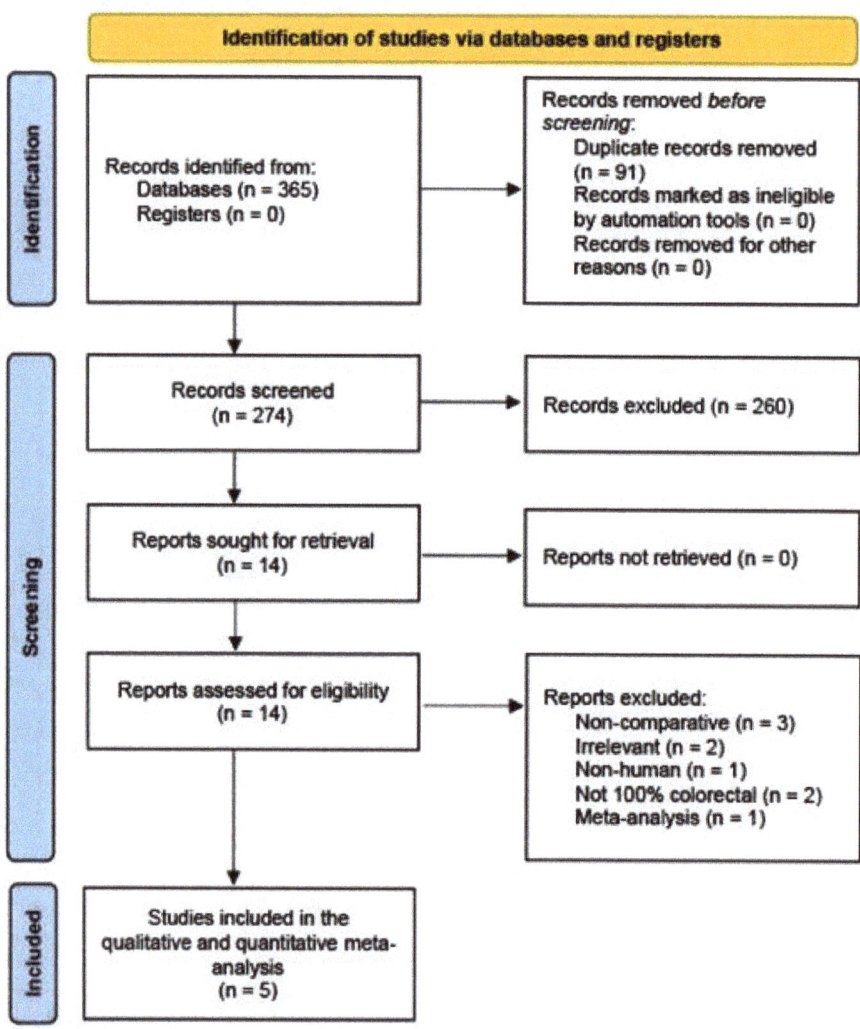

Figure 1. Flowchart for identifying and selecting studies for review analysis.

Table 1. Study characteristics.

Author	Year	Origin	Study Design	Recruitment Period	Sample Size	Exclusion Criteria	Colorectal Cases (%)	Reversal agents	Follow-Up Period	Primary Outcome
Chae et al. [24]	2019	Republic of Korea	Single-center, retrospective	2012–2017	314	Age < 21 years, neuromuscular disease, impaired hepatic and renal function, combined or emergency procedures, non-malignant disease	314 (100)	Sugammadex vs. Pyridostigmine	30 days	Total and postoperative length of hospital stay; delayed discharge rate and readmission rate
Hunt et al. [25]	2020	USA	Single-center, retrospective	2014–2017	224	Age < 18 years, preoperative renal or hepatic failure, bowel obstruction, conversion laparotomy, postoperative mechanical ventilation, emergency surgery, ASA class > III, combination of sugammadex and neostigmine, glycopyrrolate use with sugammadex but without neostigmine, epidural anesthesia, bowel obstruction, open surgery, no documented postoperative bowel movement	224 (100)	Sugammadex vs. Neostigmine/ Glycopyrrolate	In hospital	Time to first bowel movement (in hours) after reversal
Oh et al. [26]	2021	Republic of Korea	Single-center, retrospective	2014–2018	420	Robotic surgery, combined surgeries, non-malignant disease, direct postoperative ICU transfer, incomplete medical records, neuromuscular blockade other than rocuronium, deep neuromuscular blockade	420 (100)	Sugammadex vs. Pyridostigmine	In hospital	Postoperative respiratory adverse events
Serrano et al. [27]	2021	Spain	Multi-center, prospective (sub-study of POWER trial)	2017	676	Age < 18 years, emergency surgery, non-ERAS adherence	676 (100)	Sugammadex vs. Neostigmine	30 days	Moderate-severe postoperative complications, length of hospital stay
Traeger et al. [28]	2022	Australia	Single-center, retrospective	2019–2021	335	Age < 18 years, pelvic exenteration, robotic surgery, no reversal agent, combination of sugammadex and neostigmine, pyridostigmine prescription	335 (100)	Sugammadex vs. Neostigmine/ Glycopyrrolate	30 days	Gastrointestinal recovery (GI-2): time of first bowel movement and tolerance of solid diet

Table 2. Patient characteristics.

Author	Reversal Agent	No. of Patients	Age (Years)	Sex (Male/Female)	BMI (kg/m^2)	ASA Class (%)	Diabetes Mellitus (%)	Smoking History (%)	Cardiac Disease (%)	Pulmonary Disease (%)	Arterial Hypertension (%)
Chae et al. [24]	Sugammadex	157	62.5 ± 11.5 *	86/71	23.8 ± 3.3 *	ASA I 67 (43) ASA II 90 (57)	30 (19)	NS	76 (48)	6 (4)	NS
	Pyridostigmine	157	63.1 ± 11.8	83/74	23.4 ± 3.4	ASA I 77 (49) ASA II 80 (51)	26 (17)	NS	70 (45)	2 (1)	NS
Hunt et al. [25]	Sugammadex	96	60.68 (14.64) *	36/60	29.3 (6.09) *	ASA I–III 96 (100)	NS	16 (16.7)	NS	NS	NS
	Neostigmine/ Glycopyrrolate	128	60.34 (14.08)	58/70	29.6 (6.19)	ASA I–III 128 (100)	NS	36 (28.1)	NS	NS	NS
Oh et al. [26]	Sugammadex	210	68.0 [61.0;75.0] #	129/81	24.0 ± 3.3 *	ASA III–IV 32 (15.2)	NS	49 (23.3)	NS	27 (12.9)	NS
	Pyridostigmine	210	68.0 [60.0;74.0]	133/77	24.2 ± 3.4	ASA III–IV 28 (13.3)	NS	45 (21.4)	NS	21 (10.0)	NS
Serrano et al. [27]			All patients	All patients	All patients	All patients	All patients	All patients	All patients	All patients	All patients
	Sugammadex	563	67.9 (12.8) *	398/278	27.0 (4.7) *	ASA I 54 (8.0) ASA II 360 (53.3) ASA III 245 (36.2) ASA IV 17 (2.5)	141 (20.9)	126 (18.6)	108 (15.9)	104 (15.4)	348 (51.5)
	Neostigmine	113									
Traeger et al. [28]	Sugammadex	111	67 (57–76 [18–94]) †	62/49	28.7 (24.7–32.9 [18.2–73.0]) †	ASA I 3 (2.7) ASA II 41 (36.9) ASA III 62 (55.9) ASA IV 5 (4.5)	26 (23.4)	57 (51.4)	4 (3.6)	17 (15.3)	63 (56.8)
	Neostigmine/ Glycopyrrolate	224	64 (53–72 [19–90])	129/95	26.8 (23.4–30.4 [15.9–58.8])	ASA I 5 (2.2) ASA II 118 (52.7) ASA III 101 (45.1) ASA IV 0 (0)	39 (17.4)	112 (50)	7 (3.1)	15 (6.7)	93 (41.5)

BMI: body mass index, ASA: American Society of Anesthesiology. NS: not stated, * mean ± standard deviation, # median [IQR], † median (IQR [range]).

Table 3. Surgical and anesthesiologic features.

Author	Reversal Agent	NMBA	Anesthesia Time (min)	Laparoscopic Approach (%)	Cancer Surgery (%)
Chae et al. [24]	Sugammadex	Rocuronium	176.0 ± 46.7 *	32 (20)	157 (100)
	Pyridostigmine	Rocuronium	175.1 ± 41.0	34 (22)	157 (100)
Hunt et al. [25]	Sugammadex	Rocuronium or Vercuronium	229.8 (166.2) #	96 (100)	52 (54.2)
	Neostigmine/ Glycopyrrolate	Rocuronium or Vercuronium	214.2 (127.8)	128 (100)	67 (52.3)
Oh et al. [26]	Sugammadex	Rocuronium	202.5 [177.0; 240.0] #	210 (100)	210 (100)
	Pyridostigmine	Rocuronium	201.5 [170.0; 238.0]	210 (100)	210 (100)
Serrano et al. [27]	Sugammadex Neostigmine	All patients NS	All patients NS	All patients 471 (69.7)	All patients NS
Traeger et al. [28]	Sugammadex	NS	170 (120–215 [29–443]) †	74 (66.7)	73 (65.8)
	Neostigmine/ Glycopyrrolate	NS	157 (110–194 [42–378])	111 (50.9)	123 (54.9)

NMBA: neuromuscular blocking agent, NS: not stated, * mean ± standard deviation, # median (IQR), † median (IQR [range]).

3.2. Study Quality and Risk of Bias

The risk of bias (Figure 2) was moderate in all included studies according to the Robins I tool [18]. However, the most important limiting factor in terms of bias was the non-randomized and observational study design of all of the studies. In addition, the definition of gastrointestinal motility outcomes varied widely among the included studies, and not all outcomes of interest were available in each study. Based on the GRADE method [19], the level of evidence for the primary endpoint was rated as being very low (Table 4).

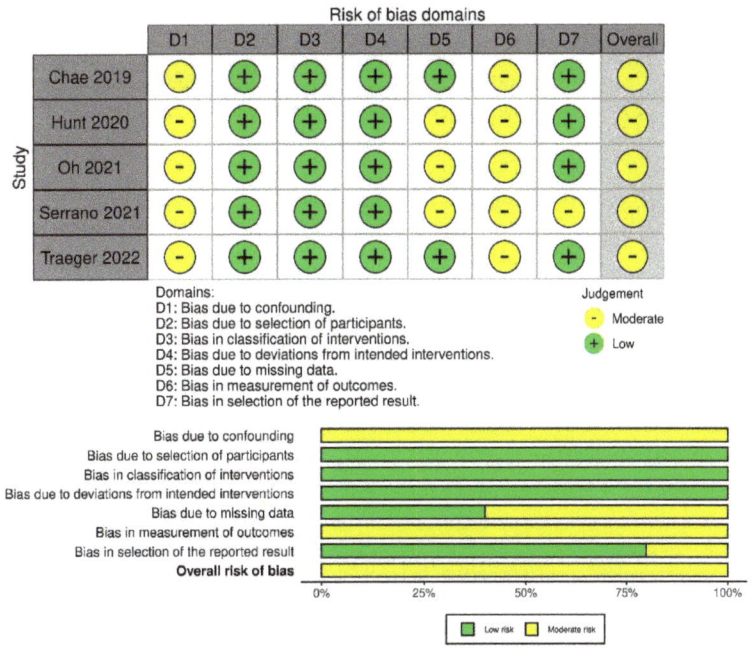

Figure 2. Summary of risk of bias and graphical representation of included studies [24–28] based on the ROBINS-I tool.

Table 4. Level of certainty of the evidence as assessed by the GRADE approach for the primary endpoint.

Outcomes	No. of Studies	No. of Included Patients		SMD/OR [95% CI]	Quality Assessment					Quality
		Sugammadex	Control		Risk of Bias [a]	Inconsistency	Indirectness	Imprecision	Publication Bias	
Time to first postoperative bowel movement or flatus	2 [25,28]	207	352	SMD 13.01 [6.55–19.46]	Serious (−1)	Serious (−1)	No indirectness	No imprecision	NA	Very low

OR: odds ratio, SMD: standardized mean difference, NA: not available. [a] Risk of bias assessed using the ROBINS-I tool.

3.3. Gastrointestinal Motility Outcomes

3.3.1. Time to First Bowel Movement or Flatus

Time to first bowel movement or flatus as the primary endpoint was reported in two studies with 559 patients [25,28]. In the sugammadex group, the time to first postoperative bowel movement or flatus was significantly shorter than in the control group (SMD 13.01, 95% CI 6.55–19.46, $p < 0.0001$). Importantly, heterogeneity was low ($I^2 = 0\%$, Chi2 test: $p = 0.58$) (Figure 3).

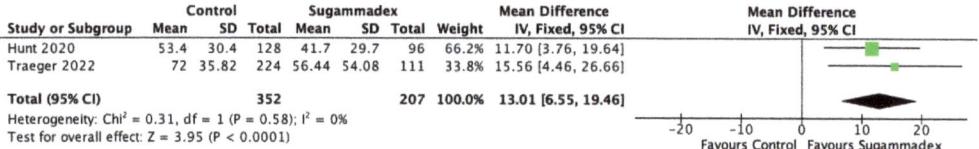

Figure 3. Forest plot comparing time to first bowel movement or flatus between sugammadex-reversed cases and controls from the studies published by Hunt et al. [25] and Traeger et al. [28].

3.3.2. Time to First Oral Diet Intake

Two studies reported on the time to first oral food intake [24,28]. Meta-analysis revealed no statistically significant difference between the two groups regarding the time to first postoperative oral food intake (SMD 4.27, 95% CI −5.29–13.84, $p = 0.38$). The degree of heterogeneity was low ($I^2 = 16\%$, Chi2 test: $p = 0.27$) (Figure 4).

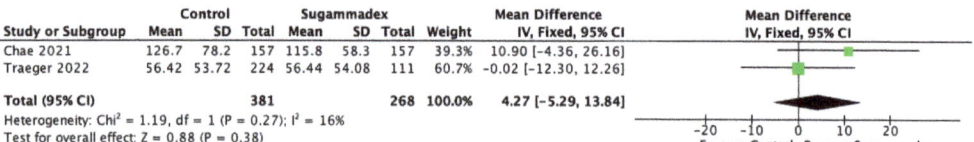

Figure 4. Forest plot comparing time to first oral food intake between sugammadex and control from the studies published by Chae et al. [24] and Traeger et al. [28].

3.3.3. Ileus

Postoperative ileus was reported in four studies [24,25,27,28]. A meta-analysis of the pooled data showed no significant difference between the sugammadex and acetylcholinesterase inhibitor groups in terms of postoperative ileus rate (OR 1.44, 95% CI 0.66–3.11, $p = 0.36$). The data for this outcome were highly heterogeneous ($I^2 = 81\%$, Chi2-test: $p = 0.001$). The source of heterogeneity was identified in the study by Chae et al. [24]. However, the subsequent subgroup with low heterogeneity ($I^2 = 2\%$, Chi2 test: $p = 0.36$) still demonstrated no difference in the reported ileus rates between both groups (OR 0.99, 95% CI 0.69–1.44, $p = 0.97$) (Figure 5).

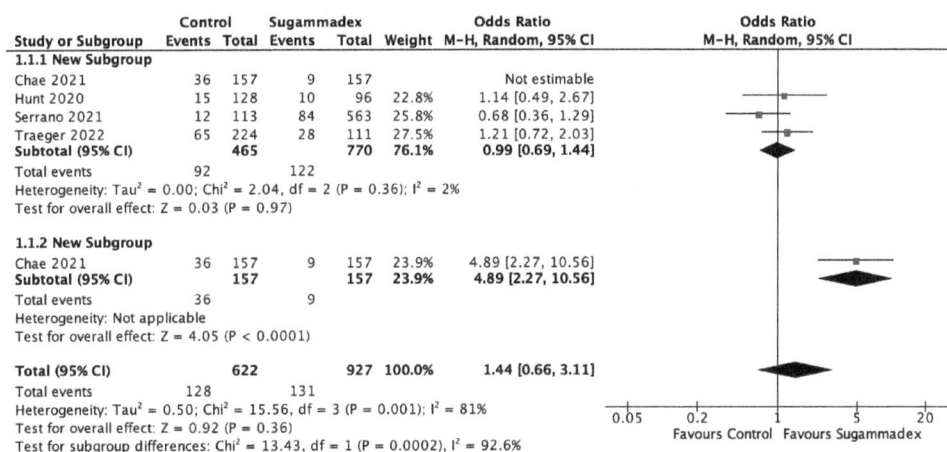

Figure 5. Forest plot comparing ileus rates in sugammadex-antagonized cases and controls from the studies published by Chae et al. [24], Hunt et al. [25], Serrano et al. [27] and Traeger et al. [28].

3.4. Non-Gastrointestinal Motility Outcomes

Analysis of secondary endpoints other than gastrointestinal motility (urinary tract infection, pulmonary morbidity, PONV, postoperative hospitalization, anastomotic leak, bleeding, wound infection, ICU stay, repeat surgery, repeat hospitalization, repeat ICU stay, and mortality) showed no statistically significant difference between the sugammadex and control groups. A detailed summary is shown in Table 5.

Table 5. Non-gastrointestinal motility outcomes.

Outcomes	No. of Included Studies	No. of Included Patients	SMD/OR [95% CI]	p-Value	Heterogeneity Level	
					I^2 (%)	p-Value
Urinary tract infection	2 [24,27]	990	0.37 [0.07–2.04]	0.25	0	0.63
Pulmonary morbidity	3 [24,26,27]	1410	0.77 [0.46–1.29]	0.32	0	0.41
PONV	2 [25,26]	644	0.91 [0.59–1.41]	0.67	0	0.59
Length of postoperative hospital stay	4 [24–26,28]	1293	−0.03 [−0.27–0.21]	0.80	0	0.87
Anastomotic leak	2 [27,28]	970	1.11 [0.31–3.94]	0.87	61	0.11
Bleeding	2 [24,27]	990	0.76 [0.24–2.43]	0.64	3	0.31
Surgical site infection	2 [24,27]	990	0.65 [0.40–1.07]	0.09	0	0.74
PACU stay	2 [24,26]	734	−0.95 [−3.04–1.14]	0.37	0	0.91
Reoperation	3 [26–28]	1431	0.89 [0.54–1.48]	0.66	0	0.73
ICU readmission	2 [24,28]	649	1.16 [0.44–3.06]	0.76	32	0.23
Hospital readmission	3 [24,27,28]	1325	1.07 [0.68–1.67]	0.78	0	0.80
Mortality	2 [24,27]	990	1.89 [0.19–18.81]	0.59	61	0.11

ICU: intensive care unit, OR: odds ratio, PACU: postanesthesia care unit, PONV: postoperative nausea and vomiting, SMD: standardized mean difference.

4. Discussion

Although the level of evidence seems to be very low, the results of our meta-analysis suggest that the reversal of the neuromuscular blockade with sugammadex compared with acetylcholinesterase inhibitors accelerates postoperative bowel motility in colorectal surgery. However, other surrogate markers of gastrointestinal motility such as ileus or time to first solid food intake were not affected by the type of reversal agent. In addition, no significant effect on clinical outcomes, including pulmonary events, postoperative complications and mortality, or length of hospital stay was observed in patients receiving sugammadex.

To our knowledge, this is the first meta-analysis comparing sugammadex and classic acetylcholinesterase inhibitors exclusively in colorectal surgery, with a special focus on gastrointestinal motility parameters. With the increasing number of colorectal procedures, enhanced recovery after surgery (ERAS) pathways with a multimodality approach toward minimizing postoperative ileus [30] are becoming increasingly important as they have been shown to reduce postoperative complications and length of hospital stay [31].

The pharmacological effect of sugammadex lies in its ability to create a tight 1:1 complex with aminosteroid neuromuscular blocking agents. This complex results in a decrease in free NMBA plasma concentration, promoting a gradient shift from the peripheral compartment (including neuromuscular junction) into plasma [11,32]. Furthermore, the potential impact of sugammadex on gastrointestinal motility is linked to the affinity to bind with steroid hormones [28,33]. In contrast, the administration of anticholinergics to prevent the cholinergic side effects of acetylcholinesterase inhibitors may unintentionally cause adverse gastrointestinal effects such as constipation or ileus [11].

Deljou et al. [34] also demonstrated in a large cohort of transabdominal surgery patients that reversal with sugammadex was associated with a faster occurrence of the first postoperative bowel movement compared to neostigmine/glycopyrrolate, whereas the length of hospital stay showed no statistical difference between the two reversal groups. However, this retrospective study did not report the overall rate of colorectal surgery, limiting the power in this subgroup. The same results were observed in another study by Cho et al. [35], who analyzed the recovery time of gastrointestinal motility in 736 patients after open pancreaticoduodenectomy. Sugammadex administration resulted in a lower incidence of delayed flatus passage and delayed tolerance to oral food intake compared to neostigmine administration.

Time to first bowel movement was also studied in three randomized trials with conflicting results. While An et al. [36] showed that the use of sugammadex in laparoscopic cholecystectomy was associated with earlier first postoperative flatus, the studies by Claroni et al. [37] and Sen at al. [33] failed to demonstrate a significant effect of sugammadex on gastrointestinal motility in robotic cystectomy and thyroid surgery, respectively. One explanation for the incongruent and heterogeneous results regarding intestinal motility in our meta-analysis and in the literature may be the different definition of ileus. In contrast to Chae et al. [24] and Serrano et al. [27] who did not specify the definition of ileus, Hunt and co-workers [25] reported ileus rates based on clinical records and documentation, and Traeger et al. [28] defined ileus as the failure to reach GI-2 (consisting of time to defecate and oral solid food intake without nausea) after four postoperative days. Furthermore, the development of postoperative ileus is triggered by a complex neuro-immuno-inflammatory response and the μ-opioid receptor activation pathway [13,38]. Therefore, reduced surgical trauma and opioid-sparing postoperative analgesia may be more effective in ileus prophylaxis than the reversal of the neuromuscular blockade with sugammadex or acetylcholinesterase inhibitors [13]. Interestingly, it has been demonstrated that patients undergoing right-sided colectomy have a higher incidence of postoperative ileus compared to patients with left hemicolectomy [39]. The type and side of resection were reported in four included studies [25–28], but based on the provided data, a subgroup analysis was not possible for determining the reversal effect after right- and left-sided colectomy. Another important flaw is the lack of complementary information regarding time point and duration of sugammadex or acetylcholinesterase inhibitor administration, and not all studies mentioned the exact dosage of the applied reversal agents in their protocols [26–28], thus restricting definite conclusions and recommendations. Sugammadex was associated with a significant lower incidence of pulmonary reverse events, as demonstrated in a large multicenter cohort study [40]. However, in a recently published study by Alday et al. [7] with 126 patients undergoing major abdominal surgery including 80 colorectal cases, no difference was found in terms of pulmonary function in the sugammadex and neostigmine groups. In line with this observation, we also could not find a significant advantage of sugmmadex in preventing pulmonary morbidity in colorectal surgery with 1410 included patients.

In a recently published meta-analysis, Chen et al. [41] for the first time compared the postoperative outcomes of sugammadex with a control drug for neuromuscular reversal after colorectal surgery. The authors showed that there was no statistically significant difference between the two groups in total hospital length of stay and rates of adverse respiratory events. However, despite its novelty, this study has some major weaknesses in terms of study selection and results: (1) The authors included studies with varying proportions of colorectal procedures (63.3–100%). Although the majority of patients underwent colorectal surgery, the results were from a heterogeneous study population. (2) The included study by Piccioni et al. [42] investigated the outcome of patients treated with sugammadex versus a placebo, whereas all of the other analyzed studies compared the effect of sugammadex with classical non-selective cholinesterase inhibitors such as pyridostigmine or neostigmine. (3) The authors focused mainly on postoperative respiratory events and length of hospital stay, whereas other important pillars of the ERAS concept such as postoperative nutrition and ileus were not considered in the meta-analysis.

Based on the results presented, the validity of the recommendation for clinical practice is clearly limited, especially considering the retrospective design of four of the included studies, which may be subject to bias and misinterpretation. The quality of the data may vary within these retrospective studies, and thus unwanted variables may influence the result. Even though the studies included 100% colorectal surgical procedures, they show a noteworthy heterogeneity of study protocols and gastrointestinal motility outcome definitions. In order to address this important issue and with respect to the variable definitions, all provided bowel function outcome measures were included in the meta-analysis. Of note, the proposed composite GI-2 outcome as a validated and evidence-based measure [15] was only mentioned in one study [28].

Furthermore, the exclusion criteria of the individual studies vary considerably, not only with regard to the neuromuscular blocking agent and its combination preparation, but also with regard to the surgical indication. The proportion of open versus laparoscopic procedures and the extent of surgical resection as an important factor in the development of ileus are not evenly distributed.

In addition, the economic benefit of sugammadex remains controversial [43–45]. In a recent study from Taiwan, for example, despite better postoperative recovery, the benefits of sugammadex did not outweigh the higher costs compared with neostigmine [46]. Moreover, different healthcare systems and costs must be taken into account when considering the use of sugammadex. Although a newly approved drug is initially protected by a patent, once the patent expires, other companies can manufacture and sell the drug as a generic under a different name. The price will then be determined by competition and will usually fall. This scenario can of course be applied to sugammadex; so, it is likely that the introduction of generics will make sugammadex cheaper and more widely available in the future.

5. Conclusions

The use of sugammadex to reverse neuromuscular blockade during colorectal surgery was associated with faster postoperative defecation or flatus compared with acetylcholinesterase inhibitors. However, sugammadex did not show significant superiority in other gastrointestinal motility parameters and clinical endpoints such as length of postoperative hospital stay and complications. Due to the lack of high-quality randomized trials and varying definitions of outcome measures for the postoperative return of bowel movement, the results must be interpreted with caution and the value of sugammadex in colorectal surgery requires further investigation.

Author Contributions: Conceptualization, S.V., D.P. and A.K.; methodology, S.V. and D.P.; software, D.P.; validation, S.V., D.P. and S.K.; formal analysis, S.V., D.P. and A.K.; investigation, S.V., D.P. and S.K.; resources, S.V. and D.P.; data curation, S.V., D.P. and S.K.; writing–original draft preparation, S.V., D.P. and A.K.; writing–review and editing, A.K. and W.T.K.; visualization, D.P.; supervision,

A.K.; project administration, A.K. All authors have read and agreed to the published version of the manuscript.

Funding: The article processing charge was funded by the Open Access fond of the Heinrich-Heine-University Duesseldorf.

Institutional Review Board Statement: This article does not contain any studies with human participants or animals. For this type of study, no ethical approval was required or obtained.

Informed Consent Statement: For this type of study, informed consent was not required.

Data Availability Statement: Not applicable.

Conflicts of Interest: The authors declare that they have no conflict of interest.

References

1. Senagore, A.J. Pathogenesis and Clinical and Economic Consequences of Postoperative Ileus. *Am. J. Health Syst. Pharm.* **2007**, *64*, S3–S7. [CrossRef] [PubMed]
2. Tevis, S.E.; Carchman, E.H.; Foley, E.F.; Harms, B.A.; Heise, C.P.; Kennedy, G.D. Postoperative Ileus–More than Just Prolonged Length of Stay? *J. Gastrointest. Surg.* **2015**, *19*, 1684–1690. [CrossRef] [PubMed]
3. Venara, A.; Meillat, H.; Cotte, E.; Ouaissi, M.; Duchalais, E.; Mor-Martinez, C.; Wolthuis, A.; Regimbeau, J.M.; Ostermann, S.; Hamel, J.F.; et al. Incidence and Risk Factors for Severity of Postoperative Ileus After Colorectal Surgery: A Prospective Registry Data Analysis. *World J. Surg.* **2020**, *44*, 957–966. [CrossRef] [PubMed]
4. Dai, X.; Ge, X.; Yang, J.; Zhang, T.; Xie, T.; Gao, W.; Gong, J.; Zhu, W. Increased Incidence of Prolonged Ileus after Colectomy for Inflammatory Bowel Diseases under ERAS Protocol: A Cohort Analysis. *J. Surg. Res.* **2017**, *212*, 86–93. [CrossRef]
5. Brusasco, C.; Germinale, F.; Dotta, F.; Benelli, A.; Guano, G.; Campodonico, F.; Ennas, M.; Di Domenico, A.; Santori, G.; Introini, C.; et al. Low Intra-Abdominal Pressure with Complete Neuromuscular Blockage Reduces Post-Operative Complications in Major Laparoscopic Urologic Surgery: A before-after Study. *J. Clin. Med.* **2022**, *11*, 7201. [CrossRef]
6. Lowen, D.J.; Hodgson, R.; Tacey, M.; Barclay, K.L. Does Deep Neuromuscular Blockade Provide Improved Outcomes in Low Pressure Laparoscopic Colorectal Surgery? A Single Blinded Randomized Pilot Study. *ANZ J. Surg.* **2022**, *92*, 1447–1453. [CrossRef]
7. Alday, E.; Muñoz, M.; Planas, A.; Mata, E.; Alvarez, C. Effects of Neuromuscular Block Reversal with Sugammadex versus Neostigmine on Postoperative Respiratory Outcomes after Major Abdominal Surgery: A Randomized-Controlled Trial. *Can. J. Anaesth.* **2019**, *66*, 1328–1337. [CrossRef]
8. Murphy, G.S.; Szokol, J.W.; Avram, M.J.; Greenberg, S.B.; Shear, T.; Vender, J.S.; Gray, J.; Landry, E. Postoperative Residual Neuromuscular Blockade Is Associated with Impaired Clinical Recovery. *Anesth. Analg.* **2013**, *117*, 133–141. [CrossRef]
9. Colović, M.B.; Krstić, D.Z.; Lazarević-Pašti, T.D.; Bondžić, A.M.; Vasić, V.M. Acetylcholinesterase Inhibitors: Pharmacology and Toxicology. *Curr. Neuropharmacol.* **2013**, *11*, 315–335. [CrossRef]
10. Mirakhur, R.K.; Briggs, L.P.; Clarke, R.S.; Dundee, J.W.; Johnston, H.M. Comparison of Atropine and Glycopyrrolate in a Mixture with Pyridostigmine for the Antagonism of Neuromuscular Block. *Br. J. Anaesth.* **1981**, *53*, 1315–1320. [CrossRef]
11. Keating, G.M. Sugammadex: A Review of Neuromuscular Blockade Reversal. *Drugs* **2016**, *76*, 1041–1052. [CrossRef] [PubMed]
12. Hristovska, A.-M.; Duch, P.; Allingstrup, M.; Afshari, A. Efficacy and Safety of Sugammadex versus Neostigmine in Reversing Neuromuscular Blockade in Adults. *Cochrane Database Syst. Rev.* **2017**, *8*, CD012763. [CrossRef] [PubMed]
13. Kim, D.K. Limited Advantage of Sugammadex Reversal over the Traditional Neuromuscular Reversal Technique in Terms of Postoperative Recovery of Bowel Function. *Korean J. Anesthesiol.* **2020**, *73*, 87–88. [CrossRef] [PubMed]
14. Traeger, L.; Kroon, H.M.; Bedrikovetski, S.; Moore, J.W.; Sammour, T. The Impact of Acetylcholinesterase Inhibitors on Ileus and Gut Motility Following Abdominal Surgery: A Clinical Review. *ANZ J. Surg.* **2022**, *92*, 69–76. [CrossRef]
15. Chapman, S.J.; Thorpe, G.; Vallance, A.E.; Harji, D.P.; Lee, M.J.; Fearnhead, N.S. Association of Coloproctology of Great Britain and Ireland Gastrointestinal Recovery Group Systematic Review of Definitions and Outcome Measures for Return of Bowel Function after Gastrointestinal Surgery. *BJS Open* **2019**, *3*, 1–10. [CrossRef] [PubMed]
16. Moher, D.; Liberati, A.; Tetzlaff, J.; Altman, D.G. PRISMA Group Preferred Reporting Items for Systematic Reviews and Meta-Analyses: The PRISMA Statement. *PLoS Med.* **2009**, *6*, e1000097. [CrossRef] [PubMed]
17. Cochrane Handbook for Systematic Reviews of Interventions. Available online: https://training.cochrane.org/handbook (accessed on 2 February 2023).
18. Sterne, J.A.; Hernán, M.A.; Reeves, B.C.; Savović, J.; Berkman, N.D.; Viswanathan, M.; Henry, D.; Altman, D.G.; Ansari, M.T.; Boutron, I.; et al. ROBINS-I: A Tool for Assessing Risk of Bias in Non-Randomised Studies of Interventions. *BMJ* **2016**, *355*, i4919. [CrossRef]
19. Guyatt, G.H.; Oxman, A.D.; Kunz, R.; Woodcock, J.; Brozek, J.; Helfand, M.; Alonso-Coello, P.; Glasziou, P.; Jaeschke, R.; Akl, E.A.; et al. GRADE Guidelines: 7. Rating the Quality of Evidence–Inconsistency. *J. Clin. Epidemiol.* **2011**, *64*, 1294–1302. [CrossRef]
20. Malmivaara, A. Methodological Considerations of the GRADE Method. *Ann. Med.* **2015**, *47*, 1–5. [CrossRef]

21. Luo, D.; Wan, X.; Liu, J.; Tong, T. Optimally Estimating the Sample Mean from the Sample Size, Median, Mid-Range, and/or Mid-Quartile Range. *Stat. Methods Med. Res.* **2018**, *27*, 1785–1805. [CrossRef]
22. Wan, X.; Wang, W.; Liu, J.; Tong, T. Estimating the Sample Mean and Standard Deviation from the Sample Size, Median, Range and/or Interquartile Range. *BMC Med. Res. Methodol.* **2014**, *14*, 135. [CrossRef] [PubMed]
23. Higgins, J.P.T.; Thompson, S.G.; Deeks, J.J.; Altman, D.G. Measuring Inconsistency in Meta-Analyses. *BMJ* **2003**, *327*, 557–560. [CrossRef] [PubMed]
24. Chae, Y.J.; Joe, H.B.; Oh, J.; Lee, E.; Yi, I.K. Thirty-Day Postoperative Outcomes Following Sugammadex Use in Colorectal Surgery Patients; Retrospective Study. *J. Clin. Med.* **2019**, *8*, 97. [CrossRef] [PubMed]
25. Hunt, M.E.; Yates, J.R.; Vega, H.; Heidel, R.E.; Buehler, J.M. Effects on Postoperative Gastrointestinal Motility After Neuromuscular Blockade Reversal With Sugammadex Versus Neostigmine/Glycopyrrolate in Colorectal Surgery Patients. *Ann. Pharmacother.* **2020**, *54*, 1165–1174. [CrossRef] [PubMed]
26. Oh, C.; Jo, Y.; Sim, S.; Yun, S.; Jeon, S.; Chung, W.; Yoon, S.-H.; Lim, C.; Hong, B. Post-Operative Respiratory Outcomes Associated with the Use of Sugammadex in Laparoscopic Colorectal Cancer Surgery: A Retrospective, Propensity Score Matched Cohort Study. Available online: https://www.signavitae.com/articles/10.22514/sv.2020.16.0116#CiteAndShare (accessed on 2 February 2023).
27. Serrano, A.B.; DÍaz-Cambronero, Ó.; Melchor-RipollÉs, J.; Abad-Gurumeta, A.; Ramirez-Rodriguez, J.M.; MartÍnez-Ubieto, J.; SÁnchez-Merchante, M.; Rodriguez, R.; JordÁ, L.; Gil-Trujillo, S.; et al. Neuromuscular Blockade Management and Postoperative Outcomes in Enhanced Recovery Colorectal Surgery: Secondary Analysis of POWER Trial. *Minerva Anestesiol.* **2021**, *87*, 13–25. [CrossRef] [PubMed]
28. Traeger, L.; Hall, T.D.; Bedrikovetski, S.; Kroon, H.M.; Dudi-Venkata, N.N.; Moore, J.W.; Sammour, T. Effect of Neuromuscular Reversal with Neostigmine/Glycopyrrolate versus Sugammadex on Postoperative Ileus Following Colorectal Surgery. *Tech. Coloproctol.* **2022**, *27*, 217–226. [CrossRef]
29. Ripollés-Melchor, J.; Ramírez-Rodríguez, J.M.; Casans-Francés, R.; Aldecoa, C.; Abad-Motos, A.; Logroño-Egea, M.; García-Erce, J.A.; Camps-Cervantes, Á.; Ferrando-Ortolá, C.; Suarez de la Rica, A.; et al. Association between Use of Enhanced Recovery After Surgery Protocol and Postoperative Complications in Colorectal Surgery: The Postoperative Outcomes Within Enhanced Recovery After Surgery Protocol (POWER) Study. *JAMA Surg.* **2019**, *154*, 725–736. [CrossRef]
30. Gustafsson, U.O.; Scott, M.J.; Hubner, M.; Nygren, J.; Demartines, N.; Francis, N.; Rockall, T.A.; Young-Fadok, T.M.; Hill, A.G.; Soop, M.; et al. Guidelines for Perioperative Care in Elective Colorectal Surgery: Enhanced Recovery After Surgery (ERAS®) Society Recommendations: 2018. *World J. Surg.* **2019**, *43*, 659–695. [CrossRef]
31. Greco, M.; Capretti, G.; Beretta, L.; Gemma, M.; Pecorelli, N.; Braga, M. Enhanced Recovery Program in Colorectal Surgery: A Meta-Analysis of Randomized Controlled Trials. *World J. Surg.* **2014**, *38*, 1531–1541. [CrossRef]
32. Nag, K.; Singh, D.R.; Shetti, A.N.; Kumar, H.; Sivashanmugam, T.; Parthasarathy, S. Sugammadex: A Revolutionary Drug in Neuromuscular Pharmacology. *Anesth. Essays Res.* **2013**, *7*, 302–306. [CrossRef]
33. Sen, A.; Erdivanli, B.; Tomak, Y.; Pergel, A. Reversal of Neuromuscular Blockade with Sugammadex or Neostigmine/Atropine: Effect on Postoperative Gastrointestinal Motility. *J. Clin. Anesth.* **2016**, *32*, 208–213. [CrossRef] [PubMed]
34. Deljou, A.; Schroeder, D.R.; Ballinger, B.A.; Sprung, J.; Weingarten, T.N. Effects of Sugammadex on Time of First Postoperative Bowel Movement: A Retrospective Analysis. *Mayo Clin. Proc. Innov. Qual. Outcomes* **2019**, *3*, 294–301. [CrossRef] [PubMed]
35. Cho, H.-Y.; Kim, H.; Yoon, S.; Lee, H.-J.; Kim, H.; Lee, H.-C.; Kim, W.-H.; Jang, J.-Y. Effect of Sugammadex on the Recovery of Gastrointestinal Motility after Open Pancreaticoduodenectomy: A Single-Center Retrospective Study. *Minerva Anestesiol.* **2021**, *87*, 1100–1108. [CrossRef] [PubMed]
36. An, J.; Noh, H.; Kim, E.; Lee, J.; Woo, K.; Kim, H. Neuromuscular Blockade Reversal with Sugammadex versus Pyridostigmine/Glycopyrrolate in Laparoscopic Cholecystectomy: A Randomized Trial of Effects on Postoperative Gastrointestinal Motility. *Korean J. Anesthesiol.* **2020**, *73*, 137–144. [CrossRef] [PubMed]
37. Claroni, C.; Covotta, M.; Torregiani, G.; Marcelli, M.E.; Tuderti, G.; Simone, G.; Scotto di Uccio, A.; Zinilli, A.; Forastiere, E. Recovery from Anesthesia after Robotic-Assisted Radical Cystectomy: Two Different Reversals of Neuromuscular Blockade. *J. Clin. Med.* **2019**, *8*, 1774. [CrossRef]
38. Bragg, D.; El-Sharkawy, A.M.; Psaltis, E.; Maxwell-Armstrong, C.A.; Lobo, D.N. Postoperative Ileus: Recent Developments in Pathophysiology and Management. *Clin. Nutr.* **2015**, *34*, 367–376. [CrossRef]
39. Seo, S.H.B.; Carson, D.A.; Bhat, S.; Varghese, C.; Wells, C.I.; Bissett, I.P.; O'Grady, G. Prolonged Postoperative Ileus Following Right- versus Left-Sided Colectomy: A Systematic Review and Meta-Analysis. *Color. Dis.* **2021**, *23*, 3113–3122. [CrossRef]
40. Kheterpal, S.; Vaughn, M.T.; Dubovoy, T.Z.; Shah, N.J.; Bash, L.D.; Colquhoun, D.A.; Shanks, A.M.; Mathis, M.R.; Soto, R.G.; Bardia, A.; et al. Sugammadex versus Neostigmine for Reversal of Neuromuscular Blockade and Postoperative Pulmonary Complications (STRONGER): A Multicenter Matched Cohort Analysis. *Anesthesiology* **2020**, *132*, 1371–1381. [CrossRef]
41. Chen, A.T.; Patel, A.; McKechnie, T.; Lee, Y.; Doumouras, A.G.; Hong, D.; Eskicioglu, C. Sugammadex in Colorectal Surgery: A Systematic Review and Meta-Analysis. *J. Surg. Res.* **2022**, *270*, 221–229. [CrossRef]
42. Piccioni, F.; Mariani, L.; Bogno, L.; Rivetti, I.; Tramontano, G.T.A.; Carbonara, M.; Ammatuna, M.; Langer, M. An Acceleromyographic Train-of-Four Ratio of 1.0 Reliably Excludes Respiratory Muscle Weakness after Major Abdominal Surgery: A Randomized Double-Blind Study. *Can. J. Anaesth.* **2014**, *61*, 641–649. [CrossRef]

43. Wachtendorf, L.J.; Tartler, T.M.; Ahrens, E.; Witt, A.S.; Azimaraghi, O.; Fassbender, P.; Suleiman, A.; Linhardt, F.C.; Blank, M.; Nabel, S.Y.; et al. Comparison of the Effects of Sugammadex versus Neostigmine for Reversal of Neuromuscular Block on Hospital Costs of Care. *Br. J. Anaesth.* **2023**, *130*, 133–141. [CrossRef] [PubMed]
44. Ren, M.; Wang, Y.; Luo, Y.; Fang, J.; Lu, Y.; Xuan, J. Economic Analysis of Sugammadex versus Neostigmine for Reversal of Neuromuscular Blockade for Laparoscopic Surgery in China. *Health Econ. Rev.* **2020**, *10*, 35. [CrossRef] [PubMed]
45. Carron, M.; Baratto, F.; Zarantonello, F.; Ori, C. Sugammadex for Reversal of Neuromuscular Blockade: A Retrospective Analysis of Clinical Outcomes and Cost-Effectiveness in a Single Center. *Clinicoecon. Outcomes Res.* **2016**, *8*, 43–52. [CrossRef] [PubMed]
46. Lan, W.; Tam, K.-W.; Chen, J.-T.; Cata, J.P.; Cherng, Y.-G.; Chou, Y.-Y.; Chien, L.-N.; Chang, C.-L.; Tai, Y.-H.; Chu, L.-M. Cost-Effectiveness of Sugammadex Versus Neostigmine to Reverse Neuromuscular Blockade in a University Hospital in Taiwan: A Propensity Score-Matched Analysis. *Healthcare* **2023**, *11*, 240. [CrossRef] [PubMed]

Disclaimer/Publisher's Note: The statements, opinions and data contained in all publications are solely those of the individual author(s) and contributor(s) and not of MDPI and/or the editor(s). MDPI and/or the editor(s) disclaim responsibility for any injury to people or property resulting from any ideas, methods, instructions or products referred to in the content.

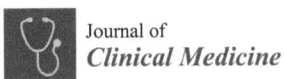

Brief Report

Is There a High Risk for GI Bleeding Complications in Patients Undergoing Abdominal Surgery?

Dörte Wichmann [1,*,†], Olena Orlova [2,†], Alfred Königsrainer [1] and Markus Quante [1]

[1] Department of General, Visceral and Transplant Surgery, University Hospital Tübingen, Hoppe-Seyler-Str. 3, 72076 Tübingen, Germany
[2] Medical Clinic, Mühlacker Hospital, Hermann-Hesse-Strasse 34, 75417 Mühlacker, Germany
* Correspondence: doerte.wichmann@med.uni-tuebingen.de; Tel.: +49-7071-2968143
† These authors contributed equally to this work.

Abstract: Introduction: Gastrointestinal bleeding (GIB) can cause life-threatening situations. Here, endoscopy is the first-line diagnostic and therapeutic mode in patients with GIB among further therapeutic approaches such as embolization or medical treatment. Although GIB is considered the most common indication for emergency endoscopy in clinical practice, data on GIB in abdominal surgical patients are still scarce. Patients and methods: For the present study, all emergency endoscopies performed on hospitalized abdominal surgical patients over a 2-year period (1 July 2017–30 June2019) were retrospectively analyzed. Primary endpoint was 30-day mortality. Secondary endpoints were length of hospital stay, cause of bleeding, and therapeutic success of endoscopic intervention. Results: During the study period, bleeding events with an indication for emergency endoscopy occurred in 2.0% (129/6455) of all surgical inhouse patients, of whom 83.7% (n = 108) underwent a surgical procedure. In relation to the total number of respective surgical procedures during the study period, the bleeding incidence was 8.9% after hepatobiliary surgery, 7.7% after resections in the upper gastrointestinal tract, and 1.1% after colonic resections. Signs of active or past bleeding in the anastomosis area were detected in ten patients (6.9%). The overall 30-day mortality was 7.75%. Conclusions: The incidence of relevant gastrointestinal bleeding events in visceral surgical inpatients was overall rare. However, our data call for critical peri-operative vigilance for bleeding events and underscore the importance of interdisciplinary emergency algorithms.

Keywords: postoperative gastrointestinal bleeding; bleeding after GI surgery; endoscopic complication management

1. Introduction

Gastrointestinal bleeding (GIB) is considered the most common indication for emergency endoscopy in clinical practice. According to the current literature, the incidence of GIB is 47/100,000 in the upper gastrointestinal tract (UGIT) or 33/100,000 in the lower gastrointestinal tract (LGIT) [1]. Depending on the cause of bleeding, localization and severity, GIB can lead to life-threatening situations and is associated with a mortality of 2–10% (UGIT) [2] and 2.4–3.9% (LGIT) [3], respectively. However, it must be considered that the respective patient populations studied mostly consist of gastroenterological patients. In contrast, the incidence, cause and therapy of GIB explicitly in surgical patients are not well studied in the current literature. Here, single studies are demonstrating an increased procedure-specific bleeding risk after surgery [4]. However, surgical patients are often older compared to the general population and commonly in a reduced general condition due to previous treatments (radio; chemotherapies) and surgical interventions, possibly with anastomoses in the GIT.

For the emergency management of GIB, endoscopic diagnosis and immediate therapy, if possible in one session, are the current gold standard. While numerous studies have

Citation: Wichmann, D.; Orlova, O.; Königsrainer, A.; Quante, M. Is There a High Risk for GI Bleeding Complications in Patients Undergoing Abdominal Surgery?. *J. Clin. Med.* **2023**, *12*, 1374. https://doi.org/10.3390/jcm12041374

Academic Editor: Paolo Aseni

Received: 27 December 2022
Revised: 25 January 2023
Accepted: 6 February 2023
Published: 9 February 2023

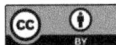

Copyright: © 2023 by the authors. Licensee MDPI, Basel, Switzerland. This article is an open access article distributed under the terms and conditions of the Creative Commons Attribution (CC BY) license (https://creativecommons.org/licenses/by/4.0/).

investigated the incidence and causes of gastrointestinal bleeding events in gastroenterological patients, data on GIB in surgical patients are scarce. Therefore, in the present study, we retrospectively analyzed our complete surgical patient population over a period of two years in regard to the incidence of GIB.

2. Materials and Methods

For the present study, all emergency endoscopies of inpatients in the Department of General, Visceral and Transplant Surgery at the University Hospital of Tübingen over a period of 2 years (1 July 2017–30 June 2019) were retrospectively analyzed. The local ethics committee approved the study (922/2018BO2), and the project was registered as a clinical trial (NCT04523753).

Inclusion criteria were inpatient care by the surgical department, indication for emergency endoscopy due to gastrointestinal bleeding and patient age > 18 years. The inclusion and exclusion criteria are listed in Table 1. For the definition of gastrointestinal bleeding, the parameters according to the DGCS "S2k-Guideline gastrointestinal bleeding" [5] were used as the basis for the analysis.

Table 1. Inclusion and exclusion criteria.

Inclusion Criteria	Exclusion Criteria
Bleeding relevant to circulation	No surgery
Hb loss greater than 2 g/dL	No emergency endoscopy
Need of transfusion	Emergency endoscopy without suspected bleeding
Need of interventions	Age < 18 years

Other aspects that were recorded and evaluated for the analysis are the clinical course, previous diseases, current medications, type of surgical intervention and the endoscopic findings as well as the success of the endoscopic therapy. The type of surgical care was described by dividing into four surgical areas (Table 2). The primary endpoint was 30-day mortality. Secondary endpoints were intensive care unit treatment duration, cause of bleeding, and therapeutic success of endoscopic intervention.

Table 2. Classification of surgical interventions into four categories.

Operating Area	Included Surgical Procedures
Upper Gastrointestinal Tract (UGIT)	Esophageal, gastric or small bowel resections, bariatric surgery
Hepatobiliary System (HPB)	Liver, pancreas, bile duct resections, liver transplantation (LTx)
Lower Gastrointestinal Tract (LGIT)	Colonic, rectal resections, hemorrhoidal procedures.
Other	Hernias, PIPAC (Pressurized Intra Peritoneal Aerosol Chemotherapy)

This study is a descriptive analysis. The statistical analysis of the data collected, as well as the graphs and tables presented in the paper, were created using Microsoft's Excel spreadsheet software. The data are presented as absolute numbers or as means with standard deviation.

3. Results

During the study period, bleeding events with indication for emergency endoscopy occurred in 2.0% (129/6455) of all surgical inhouse patients. Of these 129 patients, a total of 83.7% (*n* = 108) underwent surgery, while 21 patients (16.0%) underwent emergency endoscopy on the surgical ward without documented surgical procedures during the same inpatient stay. Patient's characteristics are shown in Table 3.

Table 3. Patient's characteristics.

Patients Groups Depended on Surgery	UGIT	HPB	LGIT	Other
Included patients (n)	26	23	51	8
Sex (m:f)	11:12	17:8	38:13	6:2
Age (years; $\bar{X}$)	65.3	59.8	70.5	56.2
Surgery for malignancy (n; %)	14 (54)	10 (43)	25 (49)	0
Surgery for mesenteric ischemia (n; %)	8 (31)	1 (4)	5 (10)	2 (25)
Anticoagulation prior to surgery (n; %)	14 (54)	15 (65)	32 (63)	2 (25)

Abbreviations: UGIT = upper gastrointestinal surgery, HPB = hepatobiliary surgery, LGIT = lower gastrointestinal surgery, n = number, $\bar{X}$ = average.

The patients without surgical procedure were excluded from further analyses. Of the analyzed 108 patients undergoing surgery and emergency endoscopy for suspected GIB events, $n = 94$ (87.01%) were examined after surgery. A total of 14 (12.96%) patients underwent endoscopy prior to surgery, where endoscopy was leading the indication for surgery in more than 50% (8/14) of the patients.

However, for the vast majority of our inhouse patients ($n = 94/108$; 87.01%), emergency endoscopy due to suspected GIB took place after surgery. In detail, fifty-one patients (47.22%) underwent surgery on the LGIT, 26 patients (24.70%) underwent surgery on the Hepato-pancreatico-biliary (HPB) system, 23 patients (21.29%) underwent surgery on the UGIT, and eight patients underwent surgery that could not be classified into the categories above. These numbers are resulting in a respective procedure-specific GIB-incidence of 1.1% for the LGIT, 7.7% for the UGIT and 8.9% for procedures in the HPB system during the study period. A diagram of the distribution of patients is shown in Figure 1.

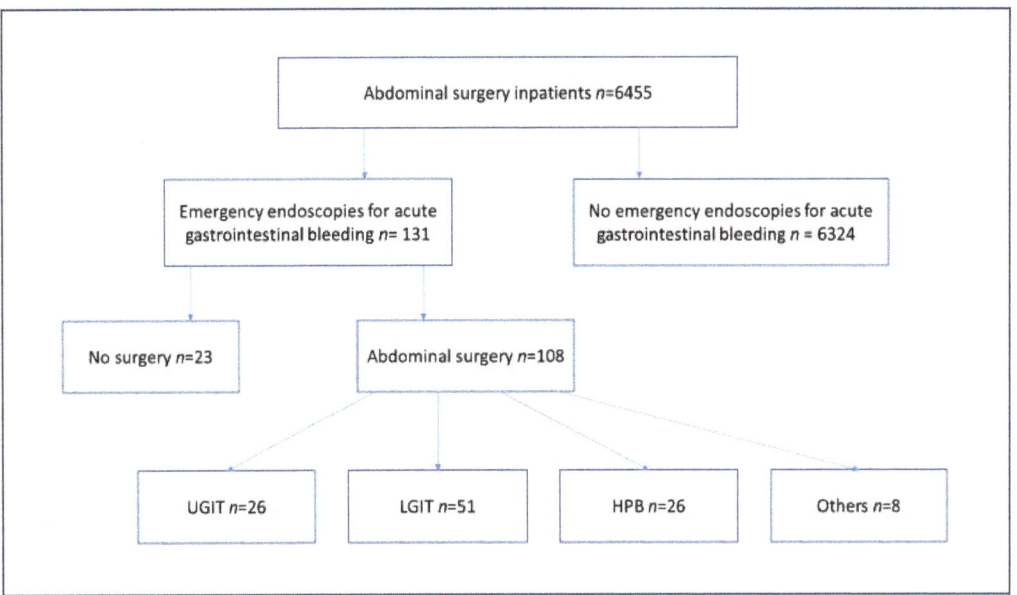

Figure 1. Patient's distribution into the four groups regarding the operation area.

The localization of bleeding detected during emergency endoscopy was found in the UGIT in $n = 46$ (52.87%), in the LGIT in $n = 18$ (20.69%), and in the HPB system in $n = 25$ (28.73%) patients. In further detail, anastomotic bleeding that led to emergency endoscopy was found in $n = 10$ (11.49%). In relation to the associated surgical site, 22.22%

of patients after UGIT procedures, 10.89% of patients after LGIT procedures, and 5.55% of patients after an HPB procedure were suffering from bleeding events in the region of their primary anastomosis. In all other patients, the bleeding event was not located in the area of the respective surgical procedures. Instead, gastroduodenal ulcerations occurred most frequently.

A detailed overview of the analyzed parameters is given in Table 4. Of the 108 patients undergoing emergency endoscopy, 80.55% ($n = 87$) had stigmata of gastrointestinal bleeding: 42 patients were found to have an active bleeding (38.89%), while 43 patients had evidence of bleeding that had occurred (39.81%). In addition, examinations of 21 further patients revealed no signs for a gastrointestinal bleeding event.

Table 4. Analyzed parameters of abdominal surgical patients with emergency endoscopies for bleeding.

Patients Groups Depended on Surgery	UGIT $n = 23$	HPB $n = 26$	LGIT $n = 51$	Others $n = 8$
Number of endoscopies per patient ($\bar{X}$) (range)	2.62 (1–7)	2.40 (1–7)	1.64 (1–5)	1.38 (1–7)
Active bleeding (n) (%)	11 (48)	15 (58)	13 (26)	1 (13)
Signs of previous bleeding (n) (%)	4 (17)	4 (15)	16 (31)	2 (26)
Endoscopic no signs of bleeding (n) (%)	8 (35)	7 (27)	22 (43)	5 (65)
Anastomotic bleeding (n) (%)	4 (17)	1 (4)	5 (10)	0
Gastroduodenal ulceration (n) (%)	13 (57)	13 (50)	19 (37)	0
Ischemic ulceration (n) (%)	1 (4)	0	12 (24)	1 (13)
Hemorrhage after endoscopic sphincterotomy (n) (%)	1 (4)	1 (4)	3 (6)	0
Bleeding esophagitis (n) (%)	0	1 (4)	3 (6)	2 (25)
Variceal bleeding (n) (%)	1 (4)	0	0	0
Bleeding gastric adenoma (n) (%)	0	0	1 (2)	0
Success of endoscopic intervention (%)	67	84	90	94
Hemostatic procedure while urgent bleeding endoscopy				
(a) injection therapy	0	3	7	0
(b) clipping solely	3	3	4	0
(c) injection + clipping	10	7	6	1
(d) hemostatic powder	2	0	3	0
(e) stent	1	1	3	0
(f) variceal banding	1	0	0	0
(g) none	4	6	26	2
Endoscopy prior surgery (n) (%)	6 (20)	0	6 (12)	2 (25)
Length of hospital stay ($\bar{X}$, days)	31.00	39.16	31.25	4.31
30-day mortality (n) (%)	6 (26)	0	2 (4)	0

Abbreviations: UGIT = upper gastrointestinal surgery, HPB = hepatobiliary surgery, LGIT = lower gastrointestinal surgery, n = number, $\bar{X}$ = average.

Anticoagulative therapy was documented in $n = 63$ patients (58.33%). Sources of GIB were gastroduodenal ulcerations ($n = 45$), bleeding esophagitis ($n = 6$), ischemic ulcerations ($n = 13$), hemorrhage after endoscopic sphincterotomy ($n = 6$), one case of variceal bleeding and one case with a bleeding gastric adenoma. Anastomotic bleeding was found in 9.26% of all analyzed patients.

Emergency endoscopic therapy was successful in 83.8% of the cases. The most common endoscopic therapy in the patients studied was fibrin glue/suprarenin injection in combination with metal clips ($n = 24$; 44.44%). Injection monotherapy or clip monotherapy was performed in $n = 10$ patients (18.52%) each. The mean length of hospital stay for the total of 14 patients who underwent endoscopy before surgical intervention was 34.9 days. For the 94 other patients who underwent endoscopy subsequent to a surgical procedure, the mean length of hospital stay was 30.9 days. An endoscopically untreatable active bleeding situation at the time of emergency endoscopy existed in $n = 5$ of the patients who died in the further course. In cases of endoscopic untreatable bleeding situation, an angiographic intervention was performed in $n = 4$, or/and an additionally or secondary surgical procedure in $n = 4$ patients.

The 30-day mortality was 9.26% ($n = 10/108$). All of these 10 patients were operated: $n = 5$ on UGIT, $n = 2$ on LGIT, and $n = 1$ on the HBP system. Two of the deceased patients could not be classified into the three respective surgical areas. The leading indication for surgery was mesenteric ischemia in $n = 19$. Of these patients, a number of $n = 5$ deceased in the clinical course.

4. Discussion

The most common location of GIB events is the UGIT according to the literature. Here, performing emergency esophago-gastro-duodenoscopy (OGD) is recommended as the gold standard. According to Oakland et al., UGIB are more common than LGIB (33/100.00) in surgical patients with an incidence of 47/10,000 [1]. According to the study by Hebert et al., 2.3% of a total of 314 patients who underwent surgical procedures in the LGIT had postoperative bleeding events in the anastomotic area [6]. In contrast, our data shed new light on the incidence and location of GIB events in a surgical patient cohort. Since one would hypothesize to find the bleeding location in the surgical area of those patients, the majority of analyzed cases provided a different picture. Here, bleeding location outside the operated organ area was found in the majority of cases, while a classical anastomotic hemorrhage could only be detected in less than 10% of the cases (17% in the UGIT, 4% in HPB and 10% in the LGIT), which is the first critical finding of our study. In more detail, there was no marked difference between stapler anastomoses (UGIT and LGIT) and manual anastomoses (HPB), which is another interesting aspect of our findings.

The average age of surgical patients at the onset of GIB is reported to be around 67 years [7,8]. However, the cited patient cohorts were reported separately according to the procedures, for example, divided into patients with resections in the right or left colon or with bariatric upper abdominal procedures. Here, the latter ones are usually representing a younger patient population in contrast to cancer patients undergoing colonic resections. As a critical amendment to the cited literature, our retrospective analysis also included surgical patients who had undergone emergency endoscopy due to GIB already before surgery. Considering only patients who underwent endoscopy for GIB after surgery, the mean age in this subgroup was 63.9 years. Of note, when considering only patients who underwent emergency endoscopy and finally died during the clinical course, the mean age was 71 years. These results demonstrate the critical impact of age, thus providing another crucial aspect being helpful for the individual perioperative risk assessment of each individual patient.

The dichotomic classification of a surgical patient population into a pre- and a postoperative group was missing in the current literature yet. Here, most retrospective analyses of surgical patients were reporting the postoperative phase only [9,10]. In our study, however, patients with bleeding events prior to surgery were also included in the analysis in order to be able to indicate the number of bleeding-related surgical procedures despite primary endoscopic therapy. In this regard, more than half of the patients with bleeding-related endoscopy prior to surgery had to undergo surgery with the indication given by endoscopy. In contrast, in patients with postoperative bleeding-related emergency endoscopy, only one-third of the patients were suffering from acute GIB while one-third of patients displayed signs of past bleeding and the remaining patients had no bleeding stigmata. Of further clinical relevance, one-third of our surgical patients underwent an invasive procedure that finally provided no benefit to them, thus calling for critical clinical evaluation and indications for emergency endoscopy.

Regarding the overall therapeutic success of endoscopic bleeding treatment, the current literature reports success rates in patient cohorts from internal medicine of approximately 80% or even higher. For example, the study by Jung et al. showed a success rate of acute endoscopic therapy of 88% [11]. Significantly lower success rates were reported by Pescatore et al. with 78.5% and 75.7%, respectively, when fibrin glue and epinephrine or epinephrine alone were used. [12]. In our study, endoscopic hemostasis could be achieved in 83.8% of cases, which is clearly within the range of the cited success rates for gastroenterological non-surgical patients. Of note, some GIB causes are not endoscopically reversible, for example in patients suffering from vascular ischemia representing a patient subgroup at highest risk with 50% mortality in our analysis. Nevertheless, these cases also represent "real-life" situations requiring first-line emergency endoscopy in surgical patients according to current emergency algorithms.

The 30-day mortality rate in the analyzed patient cohort is high and thus calling for sub-analysis to identify patients at highest risk. Here, half of the deceased patients were suffering from a mesenteric ischemia. The previously reported mortality rates in these patients is ranging from 60% up to 90% [13,14]. This high mortality rate shows the critical importance of established emergency algorithms including urgent endoscopic examinations also for surgical inpatients. In more detail, the high number of re-endoscopies is caused by relapse of bleeding, second-look endoscopies and unclear primary endoscopic results.

In summary, only a small number of surgical inhouse patients experienced a relevant GIB event. However, the associated 30-day mortality of GIB in the analyzed abdominal surgical patient population is increased at 7.75% when compared to the literature of gastroenterological patient cohorts [2,3]. Although GIB events in mostly heterogenous, postoperative patient cohorts have been poorly studied so far, the few data available report on a 30-day mortality are ranging between 0 and 13.3% for elective colonic/rectal resections [13,15]. Of note, classical anastomotic hemorrhage could only be detected in less than 10% of the cases irrespective of stapler or manual anastomosis, while for the majority of patients, the bleeding location was found to be outside the operated organ area. While our overall endoscopic therapy success rate was high and comparable to those achieved in non-surgical patients [11,12], especially vascular ischemia was not endoscopically reversible and linked to 50% specific mortality in our analysis [14,16].

The three key limitations of the present study are the retrospective and monocentric study design and the small number of cases, which are limiting the validity and generalizability of our results. Nevertheless, our results demonstrate that GIB events in surgical patients call for critical vigilance and require established, interdisciplinary emergency algorithms for rapid endoscopic diagnosis and therapy. Finally, a prospective, multicenter trial with a defined action plan in visceral surgery patients would be highly desirable.

5. Conclusions

Taken together, our study is the first to report the overall incidence of relevant gastrointestinal bleeding events in visceral surgical inpatients. Although the absolute number was rare, our analysis demonstrated several critical implications associated with the primary surgical area of the respective patients. Therefore, our data call for critical perioperative vigilance for bleeding events and underscore the importance of interdisciplinary emergency algorithms.

Author Contributions: Conceptualization, D.W. and A.K.; methodology, D.W. and O.O.; validation, D.W., O.O. and M.Q.; formal analysis, M.Q.; investigation, O.O.; data curation, D.W. and O.O.; writing—original draft preparation, D.W. and M.Q.; writing—review and editing, D.W., M.Q. and O.O.; supervision, A.K.; project administration, A.K. All authors have read and agreed to the published version of the manuscript.

Funding: This research received no external funding.

Institutional Review Board Statement: The study was conducted in accordance with the Declaration of Helsinki and approved by the Ethics Committee of the University Hospital of Tübingen (922/2018BO2; date of approval 1 October 2019), and the project was registered as a clinical trial (NCT04523753).

Informed Consent Statement: Informed consent was obtained from all subjects involved in the study.

Acknowledgments: We acknowledge support by Open Access Publishing Fund of University of Tübingen.

Conflicts of Interest: The authors declare no conflict of interest.

References

1. Oakland, K. Changing epidemiology and etiology of upper and lower gastrointestinal bleeding. *Best Pract. Res. Clin. Gastroenterol.* **2019**, *42*, 101610. [CrossRef]
2. Stanley, A.J.; Laine, L. Management of acute upper gastrointestinal bleeding. *BMJ* **2019**, *364*, l536. [CrossRef]
3. Speir, E.J.; Ermentrout, R.M.; Martin, J.G. Management of acute lower gastrointestinal bleeding. *Tech. Vasc. Interv. Radiol.* **2017**, *20*, 258–262. [CrossRef]
4. Stier, C.; May, J. Procedure-specific postoperative gastrointestinal hemorrhage. *Chirurg* **2019**, *90*, 631–639. [CrossRef] [PubMed]
5. Gotz, M.; Anders, M.; Biecker, E.; Bojarski, C.; Braun, G.; Brechmann, T.; Dechene, A.; Dollinger, M.; Gawaz, M.; Kiesslich, R.; et al. s2k guideline gastrointestinal bleeding—Guideline of the german society of gastroenterology dgvs. *Z. Gastroenterol.* **2017**, *55*, 883–936. [CrossRef] [PubMed]
6. Hebert, J.; Eltonsy, S.; Gaudet, J.; Jose, C. Incidence and risk factors for anastomotic bleeding in lower gastrointestinal surgery. *BMC Res. Notes* **2019**, *12*, 378. [CrossRef] [PubMed]
7. Amato, A.; Radaelli, F.; Correale, L.; Di Giulio, E.; Buda, A.; Cennamo, V.; Fuccio, L.; Devani, M.; Tarantino, O.; Fiori, G.; et al. Intra-procedural and delayed bleeding after resection of large colorectal lesions: The scalp study. *United Eur. Gastroenterol. J.* **2019**, *7*, 1361–1372. [CrossRef] [PubMed]
8. Susmallian, S.; Raziel, A.; Barnea, R.; Paran, H. Bariatric surgery in older adults: Should there be an age limit? *Medicine* **2019**, *98*, e13824. [CrossRef] [PubMed]
9. Jones, S.; May, A.K. Postoperative gastrointestinal hemorrhage. *Surg. Clin.* **2012**, *92*, 235–242. [CrossRef] [PubMed]
10. Fernandez de Sevilla Gomez, E.; Valls, F.V.; Basany, E.E.; Lahuerta, S.V.; Lafuente, M.P.; Medrano, A.S.; Carrasco, M.A. Postoperative small bowel and colonic anastomotic bleeding. Therapeutic management and complications. *Cirugía Española* **2014**, *92*, 463–467. [CrossRef] [PubMed]
11. Jung, J.H.; Kim, J.W.; Lee, H.W.; Park, M.Y.; Paik, W.H.; Bae, W.K.; Kim, N.H.; Kim, K.A.; Lee, J.S. Acute hemorrhagic rectal ulcer syndrome: Comparison with non-hemorrhagic rectal ulcer lower gastrointestinal bleeding. *J. Dig. Dis.* **2017**, *18*, 521–528. [CrossRef] [PubMed]
12. Pescatore, P.; Jornod, P.; Borovicka, J.; Pantoflickova, D.; Suter, W.; Meyenberger, C.; Blum, A.L.; Dorta, G. Epinephrine versus epinephrine plus fibrin glue injection in peptic ulcer bleeding: A prospective randomized trial. *Gastrointest. Endosc.* **2002**, *55*, 348–353. [CrossRef] [PubMed]
13. Du, W.; Glasgow, N.; Smith, P.; Clements, A.; Sedrakyan, A. Major inpatient surgeries and in-hospital mortality in new south wales public hospitals in australia: A state-wide retrospective cohort study. *Int. J. Surg.* **2018**, *50*, 126–132. [CrossRef] [PubMed]
14. Alhan, E.; Usta, A.; Cekic, A.; Saglam, K.; Turkyilmaz, S.; Cinel, A. A study on 107 patients with acute mesenteric ischemia over 30 years. *Int. J. Surg.* **2012**, *10*, 510–513. [CrossRef] [PubMed]
15. Mamidanna, R.; Almoudaris, A.M.; Faiz, O. Is 30-day mortality an appropriate measure of risk in elderly patients undergoing elective colorectal resection? *Color. Dis.* **2012**, *14*, 1175–1182. [CrossRef] [PubMed]
16. Tamme, K.; Blaser, A.R.; Laisaar, K.T.; Mandul, M.; Kals, J.; Forbes, A.; Kiss, O.; Acosta, S.; Bjorck, M.; Starkopf, J. Incidence and outcomes of acute mesenteric ischaemia: A systematic review and meta-analysis. *BMJ Open* **2022**, *12*, e062846. [CrossRef] [PubMed]

Disclaimer/Publisher's Note: The statements, opinions and data contained in all publications are solely those of the individual author(s) and contributor(s) and not of MDPI and/or the editor(s). MDPI and/or the editor(s) disclaim responsibility for any injury to people or property resulting from any ideas, methods, instructions or products referred to in the content.

MDPI
St. Alban-Anlage 66
4052 Basel
Switzerland
www.mdpi.com

Journal of Clinical Medicine Editorial Office
E-mail: jcm@mdpi.com
www.mdpi.com/journal/jcm

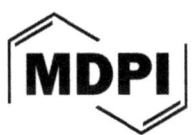

Disclaimer/Publisher's Note: The statements, opinions and data contained in all publications are solely those of the individual author(s) and contributor(s) and not of MDPI and/or the editor(s). MDPI and/or the editor(s) disclaim responsibility for any injury to people or property resulting from any ideas, methods, instructions or products referred to in the content.